THE HEALTHCARE QUALITY BOOK

Vision, Strategy, and Tools

THE HEALTHCARE QUALITY BOOK

Vision, Strategy, and Tools

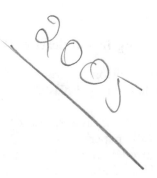

Scott B. Ransom

Maulik S. Joshi

David B. Nash

Health Administration Press, Chicago, Illinois
AUPHA Press, Washington, D.C.

AUPHA
HAP

09   08   07   06   05   5   4   3   2   1

Library of Congress Cataloging-in-Publication Data

The healthcare quality book : vision, strategy, and tools / [edited by Scott B. Ransom, Maulik Joshi, David Nash.
    p. cm.
   Includes bibliographical references and index.
   ISBN 1-56793-224-X (alk. paper)
    1. Medical care—United States—Quality control.   2. Health services administration—United States—Quality control.   3. Total quality mangement—United States.   I. Ransom, Scott B.   II. Joshi, Maulik.   III. Nash, David B.

RA399.A3H433 2004
362.11'068—dc22

2004052331

The paper used in this publication meets the minimum requirements of American National Standard for Information Sciences—Permanence of Paper for Printed Library Materials, ANSI Z39.48-1984. ♾™

Acquisitions editor: Audrey Kaufman; Project manager: Joyce Sherman; Cover designer: Megan Avery

Health Administration Press
A division of the Foundation
  of the American College of
  Healthcare Executives
One North Franklin Street
Suite 1700
Chicago, IL 60606
(312) 424-2800

Association of University Programs
  in Health Administration
2000 N. 14th Street
Suite 780
Arlington, VA 22201
(703) 894-0940

CONTENTS IN BRIEF

DETAILED CONTENTS

LIST OF FIGURES

LIST OF TABLES

ACADEMIC FOREWORD

Stephen M. Shortell

The U.S. healthcare system can be likened to a shoddily constructed building located in the pathway of an impending natural disaster. The system has been constructed by thousands of different architects, engineers, masons, and carpenters working from wildly different blueprints. For the most part, it has been built to the codes of the nineteenth century. Three major Institute of Medicine reports—the National Roundtable on Healthcare Quality's "The Urgent Need to Improve Health Care Quality," *To Err is Human*, and *Crossing the Quality Chasm*—highlighted the deficiencies in the design of the U.S. healthcare system. These reports have pointed out the inadequacies of the system for dealing with today's problems. But an even greater challenge lies in meeting the storms of the future. These include an aging population and the frequently associated increase in chronic illness; wide and growing disparities by ethnicity and income in access to care, provision of care, and outcomes of care; continued technological advances; and workforce challenges. On the chronic illness front, 125 million Americans already suffer from at least one chronic illness, and of these, approximately 50 percent suffer from two or more chronic illnesses at a cost of hundreds of billions of dollars. As our society becomes more diverse, the currently documented differences in access to care, delivery of care, and outcomes of care by ethnicity and income will grow. These disparities will further exacerbate the problems and costs associated with chronic illness. In the meantime, new diagnostic, treatment, and preventive technologies are accelerating at a pace that is overwhelming the ability of the delivery system to use them and the financing and payment systems to reimburse for them. The growth of chronic illness, existence of disparities, and advance of new technologies also have important implications for the healthcare workforce in regard to size, composition, and the nature of the work to be performed.

The major question facing us is whether the current edifice of the U.S. health system can be retrofitted and brought "up to code" through a systematic program of quality improvement reengineering and value enhancement or whether it needs to be destroyed altogether and built again from the ground up. It is the hope of most and the thesis of this book that the former is possible, namely, that the system can be retrofitted to meet the twenty-first century forces that are emerging.

Successfully meeting these challenges will require a new generation of healthcare leaders: people with the vision, strategies, and tools to make the continuous improvement of patient care quality the number one and ongoing commitment of the organizations that they lead. This must involve a marked change in the education of health professionals in which technical knowledge is married to improvement knowledge and change management knowledge centered on improving patient and community experience with the system. *The Healthcare Quality Book* by Ransom, Joshi, and Nash is an exemplary step in that direction. The book is appropriate as a graduate text for all of the health professions and focuses on improved quality for patients within the context of microsystems of care, the larger organization, and the external environment. The book provides an excellent balance of content between techniques and tools for quality improvement on the one hand and the leadership and change-management skills needed for implementation on the other hand. It also discusses the importance of environmental factors, including regulatory and accreditation processes, legal issues, and payment. The editors have done a superb job of assembling authors who have conceptual command of their subject combined with practical experience. A broad range of examples and illustrations of quality improvement applications are provided, ranging from the intensive care unit to the physician's office to the patient's home. All of the relevant topics are covered. The book will yield its greatest value when used in its entirety, but the individual chapters are strong enough to stand alone for selective use. It is hoped that future editions will incorporate the progress made by current readers in their efforts to use the knowledge and insights of this book to bring the U.S. healthcare system up to code.

Stephen M. Shortell, Ph.D.,
Blue Cross of California
Distinguished Professor of
Health Policy and Management and
Dean of the School of Public Health at the
University of California, Berkeley

EXECUTIVE FOREWORD

Gail L. Warden

The second and final report of the Institute of Medicine's (IOM) Committee on Health Care Quality in America, entitled *Crossing the Quality Chasm: A New Health System for the 21st Century*, published in 2001, calls for fundamental change in the healthcare system. Simply put, it says, "The current system cannot do the job, trying harder will not work, changing systems will." The report challenges the nation to undertake a major redesign of the delivery system and the policy environment that shapes it. Meeting those challenges requires the introduction of radical new ways of healthcare delivery, more sophisticated assessments of quality, and a commitment to continually improve it.

In the last decade the introduction of a quality philosophy in healthcare similar to other industries has stimulated extensive discussion about quality and how to improve it. However, the work of IOM, Rand Health, the Institute for Healthcare Improvement, the National Quality Forum, and the Agency for Healthcare Research and Quality has now clearly established the magnitude of the nation's problems in healthcare quality and what needs to be done about it.

Leaders in today's healthcare organizations are beginning to be very thoughtful about strategies to improve quality. They have learned that every organization must have a vision on what quality should be, a willingness to reject the status quo, and a will to improve quality that pervades the organization. They also understand that change does not happen without good leadership, transparency, and the ability to execute changes in the organization.

The editors of *The Healthcare Quality Book: Vision, Strategy, and Tools* provides a guide for quality improvement and a facilitator for dialog about quality. The chapters define quality in depth and put it into context for healthcare organizations and professionals desiring to "cross the quality chasm." They recognize the importance of quality measurement as well as reporting and analysis in relationship to clinical and operational effectiveness. Their emphasis on quality leadership will provide guidance to organizations as they take steps to bring their internal and external constituencies to an active involvement in quality improvement.

The editors acknowledge that all health constituencies, including policymakers, public and private purchasers, consumer advocates, health professionals, provider organizations, and health plans, influence both the practice and quality outcomes. A thoughtful set of study questions is provided in the book that will facilitate the right dialog in both the academic and practice settings.

The Healthcare Quality Book: Vision, Strategy, and Tools is an important contribution that will benefit all constituencies and take quality to another level. This was the aim of not only IOM but the editors as well.

Gail L. Warden
President Emeritus
Henry Ford Health System
Detroit, Michigan

PREFACE

Why do we need a textbook on healthcare quality? The question is ironic indeed. Healthcare, one of the largest industries in the United States, representing nearly 14 percent of the gross domestic product, ought to serve as a model for a consumer- or patient-focused market. Instead, as the reader will soon learn, we are faced with the realities of fragmentation, waste, deadly mistakes, and a prevailing sense of dread that little can be done to fix this mess. Virtually every adult American can retell a personal story detailing aspects of the lack of patient centeredness in our current healthcare system.

This textbook, then, seeks to provide a framework, context, and strategies and tactics enabling us to understand the complexities in the healthcare system. Most important, this book will provide an opportunity for all healthcare stakeholders to take charge and lead the way in improving health and healthcare, with a special focus on patient centeredness.

It is the editors' responsibility to articulate the purpose, audience, and scope of any assembled work. No doubt, the chapters could have been arranged differently. Some opinions are unorthodox, perhaps even irreverent. Readers will be challenged to rethink their assumptions individually and collectively. The editors have assembled a nationally prominent group of contributors to provide the best available current thinking in each of their respective disciplines. How did we organize such a broad field, and what was the overarching conceptual framework used?

Building on recent work from the Institute of Medicine (IOM), the editors chose to put the patient at the center of a discussion on improving healthcare quality. Chapter 1 (by Donald Berwick and Maulik Joshi) provides the foundation for understanding the patient with respect to the healthcare system. Chapters 2 through 4 provide an overview of the science and knowledge base of quality by discussing global topics of key quality theories and concepts (Chapter 2, by Leon Wysziewianski), the critical topic of variation in medical practice (Chapter 3, by David J. Ballard, Robert S. Hopkins III, and David Nicewander), and methods and tools for quality improvement (Chapter 4, by Mike Stoecklein).

Chapters 1 through 4 represent the core fund of knowledge for a further exploration of the complexities of healthcare quality measurement and improvement. Chapters 5 through 16 build on the theme of patient centeredness. Again, using the typology made popular by IOM, these chapters add to the understanding of quality at the organizational and so-called microsystem levels. Chapter 5 (by Robert C. Lloyd) provides the initial discussion of measurement as a building block in quality assessment and improvement. John J. Byrnes in Chapter 6 focuses on data collection and the various sources that feed into quality measurement, and Kwan Y. Lee, Linda S. Hanold, Rick G. Koss, and Jerod M. Loeb in Chapter 7 begin to discuss the analytic opportunities in quality data. David B. Nash and Adam Evans in Chapter 8 detail one specific and important measurement-profiling system in healthcare—that of physicians. Susan Edgman-Levitan in Chapter 9 tackles another often discussed, yet less well understood, area of patient satisfaction—experiences with and perspectives of care. Michael D. Pugh in Chapter 10 aggregates these multiple data points into a management tool called balanced scorecards or dashboards. Frances A. Griffin and Carol Haraden in Chapter 11 and Richard E. Ward in Chapter 12 delve deeper into two subjects—patient safety and information technology, respectively, because they are essential to furthering organizational improvements in performance.

Chapters 13 through 15 provide the triad of keys for organizations that seek to be high performers: leadership, infrastructure, and strategy for quality improvement. Chapter 16 (by Valerie Weber and John Bulger) is a compilation of the strategies and tactics necessary to change behavior, which is the basis of many of the chapter topics at the organizational and microsystem levels.

The concluding chapters, 17 through 19, provide a detailed discussion of the effect of the environment on the organizations delivering care. Specifically, Troyen A. Brennan, Ann Louise Puopolo, John L. McCarthy, Robert Hanscom, and Luke Sato in Chapter 17 examine the medicolegal implications of quality. Greg Pawlson and Paul Schyve (Chapter 18) collaborate to summarize the work of the two major accrediting bodies within healthcare quality, namely, the National Committee for Quality Assurance and the Joint Commission on Accreditation of Healthcare Organizations. Fittingly, the book concludes with an important contribution by Francois de Brantes (Chapter 19) on the power of the purchaser to select and pay for quality services.

In summary, then, the book has three major parts. Part I covers the patient and the scientific basis necessary for an understanding of the measurement and improvement of quality. Part II represents a detailed review of the systems involved in quality measurement and improvement at both the macro- and microsystem levels. Part III summarizes the environment in which the organizations that deliver care find themselves.

As evidenced by Figure 1 and the descriptions above, this textbook seeks to provide a framework, context, strategies, tactics, examples, lessons learned, and, most important, opportunity for all healthcare stakeholders to take charge and lead the way in improving health and healthcare.

The technical approaches and innovative strategies advocated in the chapters of this book all serve to address the very real inadequacies in care that occur every day, one patient at a time. The key to effective improvement is centering all of our efforts on the needs and care of our patients, every patient, every time.

Several of these chapters could, no doubt, stand alone as thorough discussions of their respective subjects. Each represents an important contribution to our understanding of the level of patient centeredness, type of organization, and environment in which we find the delivery of healthcare services. The scientific and knowledge base on which quality measurement is founded is rapidly changing. This book provides the most timely analysis of the extant tools and techniques.

Who should read this book? Of course, the editors believe that all current stakeholders would benefit from reading this text. The primary audience for the book is graduate students in healthcare and business administration, public health programs, allied health programs, and, of course, programs in medicine. Regrettably, not everyone in these fields currently shares an equal interest in furthering their understanding of the issues crucial to improving healthcare quality. It is our fervent hope that this book will go a long way toward breaking down the educational silos that currently prevent all stakeholders from sharing equally in their understanding of the patient centeredness, organizational systems, and environment of healthcare quality.

Lastly, the editors assume all responsibility for any errors of commission or omission that may have occurred in the editing of this text. We are also very interested in your feedback. What pedagogic tools would strengthen the presentation and enable the reader to more effectively grasp the complex concepts? You may communicate with all of the editors via the e-mail addresses noted below.

Scott B. Ransom   sransom@med.umich.edu

Maulik S. Joshi   joshim@dfmc.org

David B. Nash   David.Nash@jefferson.edu

FIGURE 1

The Healthcare
Quality Book
Overview

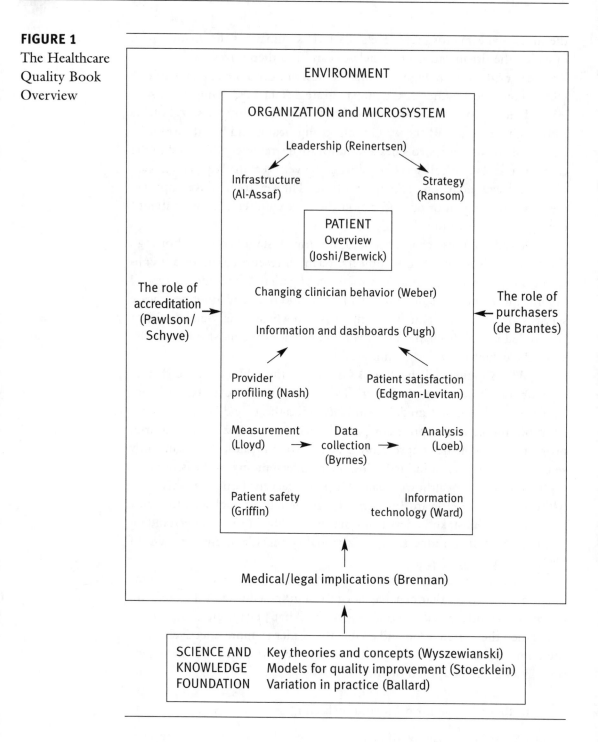

ACKNOWLEDGMENTS

To our talented collaborators, who made this book a reality.

To our mentors, colleagues, and students, from whom we continue to learn.

To our spouses, who have supported us with patience and understanding—Elizabeth, Emilie, and Esther.

To our children, who continue to provide joy and inspiration—Kelly, Christopher, Sarah, Ella, Lucas, Leah, Rachel, and Jacob.

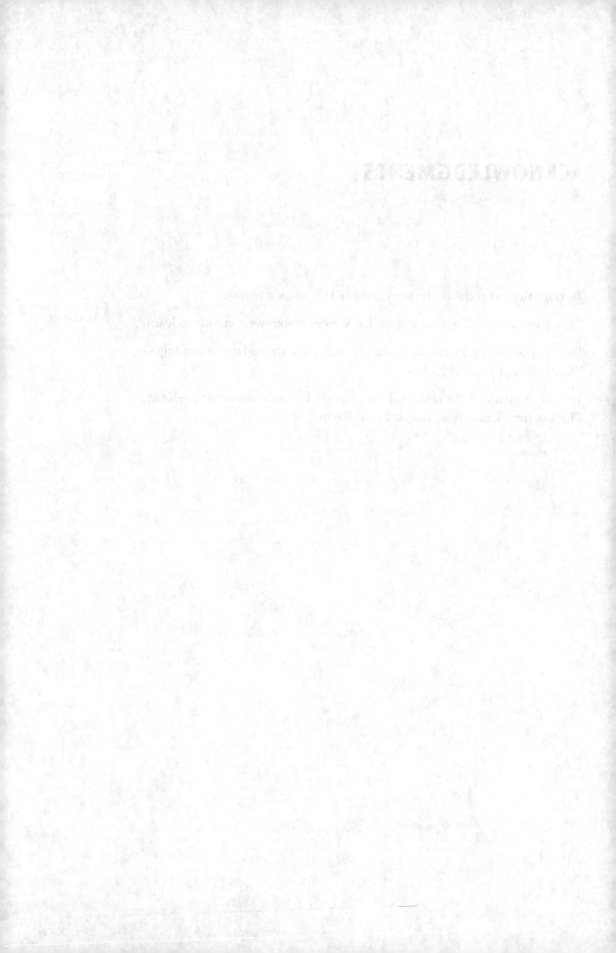

SCIENCE AND KNOWLEDGE FOUNDATION

2005

HEALTHCARE QUALITY AND THE PATIENT

Donald Berwick and Maulik S. Joshi

Quality in the U.S. healthcare system is not what it should be. We have known this to be true for years based on personal stories and anecdotes. However, beyond the single cases and story telling of terrible experiences, the evidence of this deficiency in quality came to light in three major reports:

- The Institute of Medicine's (IOM) National Roundtable on Health Care Quality report, "The Urgent Need to Improve Health Care Quality" (Chassin and Galvin 1998);
- IOM's *To Err Is Human* report (Kohn, Corrigan, and Donaldson 1999); and
- IOM's *Crossing the Quality Chasm* report (IOM 2001).

These three reports make a tremendous statement and call to action on the state of, gaps in, and opportunity to significantly improve healthcare quality in the United States to unprecedented levels.

Before we launch into the findings from these reports, let us first begin with the definition—better yet, the evolving definitions—of quality.

No text on healthcare quality can begin without a definition of quality and its implications for our work as healthcare professionals. Avedis Donabedian, one of the pioneers in understanding approaches to quality, discusses in great detail quality's various definitions, dependent on the perspective. Among his conceptual constructs of quality, one view of Donabedian's rings particularly true: "The balance of health benefits and harm is the essential core of a definition of quality" (1990). The question of balance between benefit and harm is an empirical question, and this points to medicine's essential chimerism (Mullan 2001): one part science and one part art.

An often-cited definition of quality was developed by the IOM Committee to Design a Strategy for Quality Review and Assurance in Medicare (Lohr 1990):

> Quality of care is the degree to which health services for individuals and populations increase the likelihood of desired health outcomes and are consistent with current professional knowledge. . . .

How care is provided should reflect appropriate use of the most current knowledge about scientific, clinical, technical, interpersonal, manual, cognitive, and organization and management elements of health care.

Most recently in 2001, *Crossing the Quality Chasm* states powerfully and simply that healthcare should be safe, effective, efficient, timely, patient centered, and equitable. This six-dimensional aim, which will be discussed later in this chapter, today provides the best known and most goal oriented definition, or at least conceptualization, of the components of quality.

Important Reports

The *Journal of the American Medical Association* published the National Roundtable report with two notable contributions to the industry. The first is its assessment of the state of quality: "Serious and widespread quality problems exist throughout American medicine. These problems . . . occur in small and large communities alike, in all parts of the country, and with approximately equal frequency in managed care and fee-for-service systems of care. Very large numbers of Americans are harmed." The second contribution to the knowledge base of quality was a categorization of quality defects into three broad categories: "overuse," "misuse," and "underuse." Underuse is evidenced by the fact that many scientifically sound practices are not employed as often as they should be. For example, biannual mammography screening in women aged 50 to 70 is proven to be beneficial and yet is performed less than 80 percent of the time. Overuse can be seen in areas such as imaging studies for diagnosis in acute asymptomatic low back pain or prescribing antibiotics when not indicated for infections, such as viral upper respiratory infections. Misuse is the term applied when the proper clinical care process is not executed appropriately, such as the wrong drug going to the patient or the correct drug being administered incorrectly. The classification scheme of underuse, overuse, and misuse has become a common nosology for quality defects.

Over the last several years, research findings indicating the gap between current practice and optimal practice have proliferated (McGlynn et al. 2003). The many studies range from evidence of specific processes falling short of the standard (e.g., children not getting all their immunizations by the age of two) to overall performance gaps (e.g., risk-adjusted mortality rates in hospitals varying fivefold). Although the healthcare community has known of many of these quality-related challenges for years, it was the 1998 IOM publication *To Err Is Human* that brought to light the severity of the problems in a way that captured the attention of all key stakeholders for the first time.

The Executive Summary of *To Err Is Human* begins with these headlines:

- Betsy Lehman, a health reporter for the Boston Globe, died from an overdose during chemotherapy
- Ben Kolb, an eight-year-old receiving minor surgery, died due to a drug mix-up
- As many as 98,000 people die every year in hospitals as a result of injuries from their care
- Total national costs of preventable adverse events are estimated between $17 billion and $29 billion, of which health care costs are over one-half

These data points helped focused attention on patient safety and medical errors as perhaps the most urgent of the forms of quality defect. Although many have spoken about improving healthcare, this report spoke about the negative—it framed the problem in a way that everyone could understand and demonstrated that the situation was unacceptable. One of the basic foundations for this report was a Harvard Medical Practice study done more than ten years earlier. For the first time, patient safety (i.e., ensuring safe care and not having mistakes) had arrived as a solidifying force for policymakers, regulators, providers, and consumers.

In March 2001, 18 months after publishing *To Err Is Human*, the IOM released *Crossing the Quality Chasm*, a more comprehensive report offering a potential new framework for a redesigned U.S. healthcare system.

Crossing the Quality Chasm has provided a blueprint for the future and has expanded the taxonomy and unifying framework in scoping the six aims for improvement, chain of effect, and simple rules for redesign of healthcare.

The six aims for improvement, viewed also as six dimensions of quality, are as follows (Berwick 2002):

1. *Safe:* Care should be as safe for patients in healthcare facilities as in their homes.
2. *Effective:* The science and evidence behind healthcare should be applied and serve as the standard in the delivery of care.
3. *Efficient:* Care and service should be cost effective, and waste should be removed from the system.
4. *Timely:* Patients should experience no waits or delays in receiving care and service.
5. *Patient centered:* The system of care should revolve around the patient, respect patient preferences, and put the patient in control.
6. *Equitable:* Unequal treatment should be a fact of the past; disparities in care should be eradicated.

The underlying framework for achieving these aims for improvement depicts the healthcare system in four levels, all of which require changes. *Level A* is what happens with the patient. *Level B* reflects the microsystem where care is delivered by small provider teams. *Level C* is the organizational level—the macrosystem or aggregation of the microsystems and supporting functions. *Level D* is the external environment where payment mechanisms, policy, and regulatory factors reside. Figure 1.1 provides a picture of these four cascading levels. The environment affects how organizations operate, which affects the microsystems housed in organizations, which in turn affect the patient. "True north" in the model lies at Level A, in the experience of patients, their loved ones, and the communities in which they live (Berwick 2002).

A Focus on the Patient

All healthcare organizations exist to serve their patients; so does the work of healthcare professionals. Technically, medicine has never in its history had more potential to help than it does today. The number of efficacious therapies and life-prolonging pharmaceutical regimens has exploded. Yet, the system falls far short of its technical potential. Patients are dissatisfied and frustrated with the care they receive. Providers are overburdened and uninspired by a system that asks too much and makes their work more difficult. Society's attempts to pay for and properly regulate care add complexity and even chaos. Demands for a fundamental redesign of the U.S. healthcare system are ever increasing. The IOM proposes that at the center of efforts to improve and restructure healthcare there ought to be a laserlike focus on the patient. Patient-centered care is the proper future of medicine, and the current focus on quality and safety is a step on the path to excellence.

So how do patients perceive the quality of our healthcare system today? Not very favorably. In healthcare, *quality* is a household word that evokes great emotion. These emotions include the following:

- Frustration and despair, much of which is exhibited by patients who experience healthcare services firsthand or family members who observe the care of their loved ones;
- Anxiety over the ever-increasing costs and complexities of care;
- Tension between their need for care and the difficulty and inconvenience in obtaining care; and
- Alienation from a care system that seems to have little time for understanding, much less meeting, their needs.

FIGURE 1.1
Four Levels of
the Healthcare
System

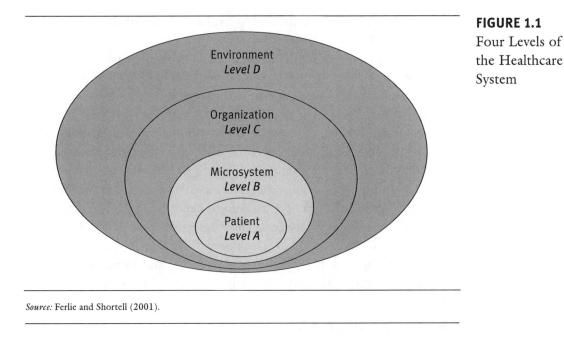

Environment
Level D

Organization
Level C

Microsystem
Level B

Patient
Level A

Source: Ferlie and Shortell (2001).

To illustrate these issues, we will explore the insights and experiences of one patient. We will examine in depth the experience of this patient who has lived with chronic back pain for almost 50 years and use this case study to understand both the inadequacies of the current delivery system and the potential for improvement. This one case study[1] is representative of the frustrations and challenges of the patients we are trying to serve and reflective of the opportunities that await us to radically improve the healthcare system. (See the section titled Case Study later in the chapter.)

Lessons Learned in Quality Improvement

We have now spent substantial time noting the gap, or chasm, in healthcare as it relates to quality. This chasm is wide, and the changes to the system are challenging. An important message is that changes are being made, patient care is getting better, and the health of communities is beginning to demonstrate marked improvement. Let us take this opportunity to highlight examples of improvement projects in various settings to provide insight into the progress.

Improvement Project: Improving ICU Care

One improvement project success story takes place in the intensive care unit (ICU) at Dominican Hospital in Santa Cruz County, California.

Dominican, a 379-bed community hospital, is part of the 41-hospital Catholic Healthcare West system.

The staff in Dominican Hospital's ICU learned an important lesson about the power of evidence over intuition. "We used to replace the ventilator circuit for intubated patients daily because we thought this helped to prevent pneumonia," explains Lee Vanderpool, vice president. "But the evidence shows that the more you interfere with that device, the more often you risk introducing infection. It turns out it is often better to leave it alone until it begins to become cloudy, or 'gunky' as the nonclinicians say."

The importance of using scientific evidence reliably in care is just the sort of lesson that people at Dominican have been learning routinely for more than a decade as they have pursued quality improvement throughout the hospital. Dominican's leaders have focused most recently on improving critical care processes, and their efforts have reduced mortality rates, average ventilator days, and other key measures (see Figure 1.2).

Ventilator Bundling and Glucose Control

After attending a conference in critical care, Dominican staff began focusing on a number of issues in the ICU. "The first thing we tackled was ventilator bundling," says Glenn Robbins, R.Ph., who is responsible for the day-to-day process and clinical support of Dominican's critical care improvement team. *Ventilator bundling* refers to a group of five procedures that, taken together, have been shown to improve outcomes for ventilator patients.[2]

"We were already doing four of the five elements," says Robbins, "but not in a formalized, documented way that we could verify." Ventilator bundling calls for ventilator patients to receive the following: the head of their bed elevated a minimum of 30 degrees; prophylactic care for peptic ulcer disease; prophylactic care for deep vein thrombosis; a "sedation vacation" (a day or two without sedatives); and a formal assessment by a respiratory therapist of readiness to be weaned from the ventilator.

The team tested ideas using Plan-Do-Study-Act (PDSA) cycles, running small tests of change, and then widening implementation of those that worked. Some fixes were complex, and some were quite simple. To ensure that nurses checked the head of the bed elevation, for example, Camille Clark, R.N., critical care manager, says, "We put a piece of red tape on the bed scales at 30 degrees as a reminder. We started with one nurse, then two, and then it spread. Now when we [perform rounds] in the ICU we always check to see that the head of the bed is right. It has become an integrated part of the routine."

Another important process change included the introduction and use of daily "therapy goal" lists as a means of identifying goals for each

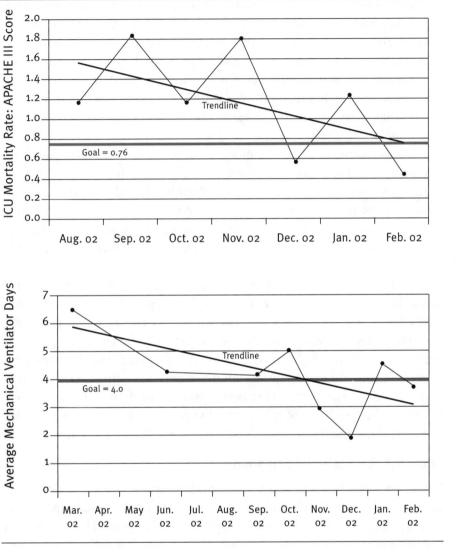

FIGURE 1.2
Improving
Critical Care
Processes:
Mortality
Rates and
Average
Ventilator
Days

Source: Dominican Hospital, Santa Cruz, CA. Used with permission.

patient and tracking progress against those goals. The form, now in use
100 percent of the time for ICU patients, went through more than 20
PDSA cycles and 25 different versions before it was final. "We got some
pushback from the nurses because it felt to them like double-charting,"
says Clark. "So we kept working on it, and incorporating their suggestions,
until it became something that was useful to them rather than simply more
paperwork." Getting physicians on board regarding the daily goal list and
other aspects of improvement was also a key factor in their success.

Next, the team turned its attention to the intravenous (IV) insulin
infusion protocol used in the ICU and intensified efforts to better control

patients' blood sugar. "The literature strongly suggests that controlling hyperglycemia helps reduce mortality in the ICU," says Aaron Morse, M.D., critical care medical director. "We initially trialed a more aggressive protocol on about 30 patients, and we've gone through seven or eight PDSA cycles on it. It is now standard protocol, and from the data we have so far it has been extremely successful. We attribute our very low rate of ventilator-associated pneumonia to changes like the ventilator bundle and glucose control."

Part of introducing the new protocol, or any new idea, involves education. "We worked to educate the staff on the importance of tight glucose control in ICU patients," says Robbins. Equally important is listening to the frontline staff who must implement the new procedures. "The nursing staff provides lots of feedback, which helps us refine our processes. We have vigorous dialogues with both nurses and physicians when we try things."

At Dominican, the culture of improvement has been pervasive for more than a decade, so everyone knows that helping to improve things is part of their job. "We are in our twelfth formal year of continuous performance improvement, and most of the people here have been a part of that from the inception," says Vanderpool. As a result of the organization's long-term commitment to quality improvement, Vanderpool says progress is steady on many fronts. "Things that were once barriers to change are not today. People know they have the ability to make changes at the work level and show the trends associated with them. People feel empowered."

"How Did You Get That to Happen?"

Vanderpool says he often gets the same question from other hospital leaders who are trying to achieve similar improvements as Dominican in their own quality journeys: "How did you get that to happen?" He underscores the value of creating a culture of improvement, which must start at the top of the organization. He demonstrates his commitment to quality by joining clinical staff on rounds in the ICU on a frequent, yet purposefully irregular, basis. "Some organizations overlook the importance of the culture change in performance improvement work," says Sister Julie Hyer, O.P., president of Dominican Hospital. "It is fundamental to create a culture that supports and respects improvement efforts."

Robbins cites physician buy-in as another key to successful improvement strategies. "We are lucky to have some very good physician champions here," he says. "They are active, creative, and knowledgeable, and their support makes a huge difference."

Vanderpool, Hyer, and Robbins all acknowledge the value of the collaborative relationships they have formed through the IMPACT network sponsored by the Institute for Healthcare Improvement (IHI). "We are not working just within our institution, but with 40 others," says Robbins. "In between learning sessions, we e-mail each other, talk on the phone, have site visits . . . we have adopted approaches others have used, and others have learned from us."

Vanderpool says that working with outside experts over the past five years has breathed new life into the hospital's well-established improvement culture. "After the first four or five years of working doggedly and diligently on our own 'home-grown' improvement projects, we found it got harder to be prophets in our own land. Bringing in expertise from the outside has strengthened our approach and our commitment."

Improvement Project: Redesigning the Clinical Office

The above improvement project case exemplifies impressive gains in quality in one specific area, the ICU. The project in this section provides evidence of the power of complete redesign of healthcare by addressing multiple parts of the healthcare system and using the six IOM dimensions of quality as a measuring stick.

CareSouth, which serves 20,000 South Carolina patients in six locations, is a heavy hitter when it comes to improvement work, determined to make significant improvements in office practice in all six categories of aim identified by IOM, plus an additional category of equal importance to the organization.

"This work is really a marriage between what we have learned about chronic care management and advanced practice concepts like advanced access," says Ann Lewis, executive director. As one of the first participants in the Health Disparities Collaborative, run jointly by IHI and the federal Bureau of Primary Health Care, which provides significant funding for CareSouth and other similar clinics throughout the nation, CareSouth focused on improving access to quality care for patients with diabetes, asthma, and depression. The results inspired Lewis to lead her organization into further improvement efforts.

"When we started the diabetes collaborative, the average HbA1c of the patients we were tracking was over 13," Lewis recalls. "I didn't even know what that meant. But I learned that every percentage drop in HbA1c represents a 13 percent drop in mortality, and that got my attention. And I would go to group visits where patients with diabetes were practically in tears with gratitude about how much our new approach to care was helping them." Lewis realized that "it's not about the business or economics of healthcare, it's about the outcomes."

The ambitious nature of CareSouth's goals is testimony to Lewis's success as a missionary in her own land. For example, the clinic aims for a

7.0 average HbA1c for patients with diabetes; to meet 80 percent of patients' self-management goals; to have 80 percent of each patient's total visit time spent face to face with a provider of care; and to have the third next available appointment (a standard measure of access) be in zero days. "To be truly patient centered," says Lewis, "it's not enough to help patients set goals. It's meeting the goals that puts the rubber to the road. We want the healthiest patients in America," she says. "Why not? The knowledge is there—we know how to make people healthy and how to make care accessible. Let's just do it."

Improvement at CareSouth Through IOM's Areas of Focus

CareSouth's work in each of the seven areas of focus reflects creativity, doggedness, and steadfast attention to the voice of the customer, its patients. "We ask the patients all the time what they want, what they think," says Lewis. "They always tell us. But you have to ask."

CareSouth is working diligently to improve in each of the IOM aim categories. Staff chose to add one more category, vitality, a measure of staff morale. While progress so far toward achieving these ambitious goals is varied, the organization's determination has been unflagging.

Effectiveness

Goal: Asthma patients will have an average of 10 or more symptom-free days out of 14. Diabetes patients will have an average HbA1c of 7.0 or less. Figure 1.3 shows CareSouth's results to date on these measures.

Action: The experience that CareSouth staff had already gained in chronic care management through the Health Disparities Collaborative gave them the tools they needed to improve effectiveness of care. "Once you know the model—self-management support, decision support, design of delivery system, clinical information system, community support—you can transfer it from one condition to another pretty smoothly," Lewis says, referring to the Chronic Care Model developed by Ed Wagner, M.D., and his colleagues, which is widely regarded as the standard for chronic care management. Wagner, a general internist/epidemiologist, is the director of Improving Chronic Illness Care and of the Seattle-based MacColl Institute for Healthcare Innovation at the Center for Health Studies, Group Health Cooperative of Puget Sound.

Patient Safety

Goal: 100 percent of all medication lists will be updated at every visit (see Figure 1.4).
Action: "Patients have a hard time remembering what medications they are taking, especially when they take several," says Lewis. "It's best if they bring

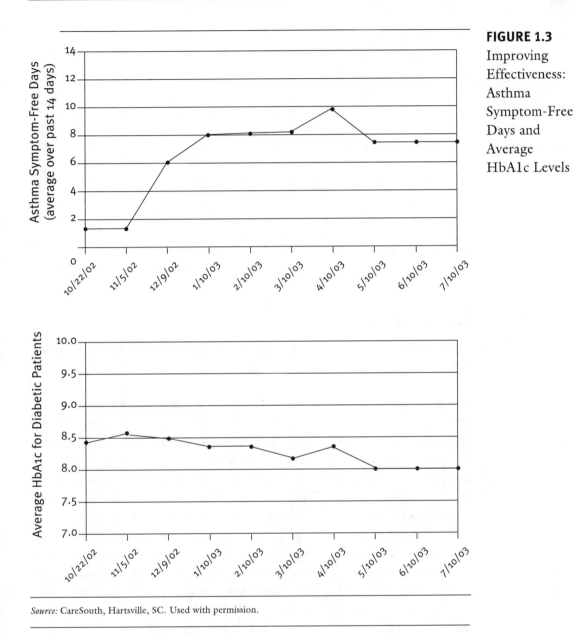

FIGURE 1.3

Improving
Effectiveness:
Asthma
Symptom-Free
Days and
Average
HbA1c Levels

Source: CareSouth, Hartsville, SC. Used with permission.

their medications to each appointment. Patients told us that it would help if they had something to bring them in. So we had very nice cloth medication bags made for everyone on three meds or more. They have our logo on them, and a reminder to bring their medications to each visit. It's a low-tech solution, but it has made a huge difference. We've had some early success in the work, as well as some recent setbacks, but I'm sure we're on the right track."

FIGURE 1.4

Improving
Patient Safety:
Percent of
Medication
Lists on All
Charts

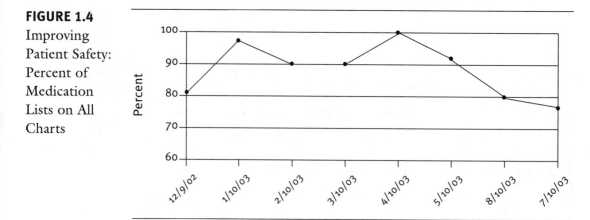

Source: CareSouth, Hartsville, SC. Used with permission.

Patient Centeredness

Goal: 80 percent of self-management goals set by patients will be met (see Figure 1.5).

Action: "One of the biggest challenges the healthcare system faces is to help patients meet their own goals," says Lewis. "We ask our patients in three ways how they want us to help them with self-management: through surveys, in one-on-one patient interviews, and in small focus groups." Through these means, CareSouth staff members are learning how to help patients tailor achievable goals. "Don't tell me to lose 40 pounds," Lewis says, explaining what patients often say. "Tell me how to do it in small steps."

CareSouth has also learned that listening to its patients is their best source of guidance regarding what system changes to make. Some of the feedback they get is surprising, according to Lewis. "Some of our elderly patients say they like it better when they can spend more time here, not less," she says. "And we've learned that centralized appointment scheduling and medical records is not what our patients want. They want to talk with the same person each time they call, someone in their own doctor's practice." Little changes also mean a lot to patients, she says. "They told us to stop weighing them in the hallway where everyone can watch."

Efficiency

Goal: The average amount of time spent with the clinician in an office visit will be 12 minutes or more (see Figure 1.6).

Action: Working to increase patient time with clinicians and decrease non-value-added time has been challenging for the CareSouth staff, but they

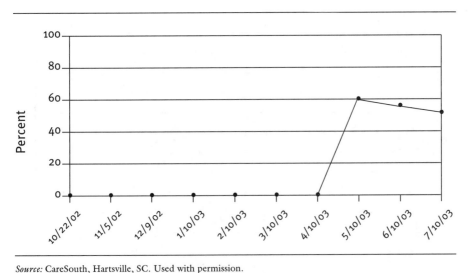

FIGURE 1.5

Improving
Patient
Centeredness:
Percent of
Patients' Self-
Management
Goals Met

Source: CareSouth, Hartsville, SC. Used with permission.

are making headway. Again, the patients told the organization what they wanted. "They didn't care about the cycle time; they wanted a rich visit, more comprehensive, where they could get more done," says Lewis. Patients like group visits, time with the nurse as well as the doctor, and opportunities for health education, so the CareSouth staff is working to organize the delivery system accordingly. The average time patients spend with their doctors is also increasing.

Timeliness

Goal: The third next available appointment shall be in zero days (see Figure 1.7).

Action: Staff began by combing the schedule for opportunities for more efficient care management of patients, in particular looking for ways to reduce unnecessary follow-up visits, substituting telephone follow-up when appropriate. "Implementing care management and deleting all those short-term return visits from the schedule gave us a big drop in appointment waiting time," says Lewis. Decentralizing appointment tracking is another means of improving timeliness because each microteam is more aware of patients' needs and able to structure providers' schedules in ways that reduce backlog (Murray and Tantau 2000).

Equity

Goal: There shall be zero disparity by race for each key effectiveness measure (see Figure 1.8). (Variation from zero equals disparity.)

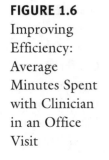

FIGURE 1.6

Improving Efficiency: Average Minutes Spent with Clinician in an Office Visit

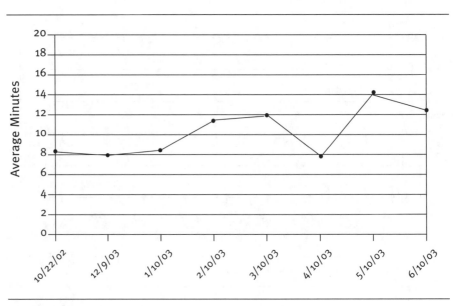

Source: CareSouth, Hartsville, SC. Used with permission.

FIGURE 1.7

Improving Timeliness: Days to Third Next Available Appointment

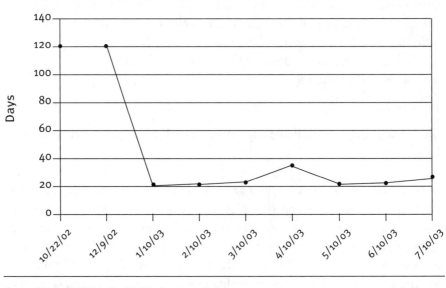

Source: CareSouth, Hartsville, SC. Used with permission.

Action: With a patient population that is 69 percent non-white, CareSouth takes equity very seriously. "This is our strong suit," says Lewis. "It is woven into our very culture." To counter the "clinic mentality" with which com-

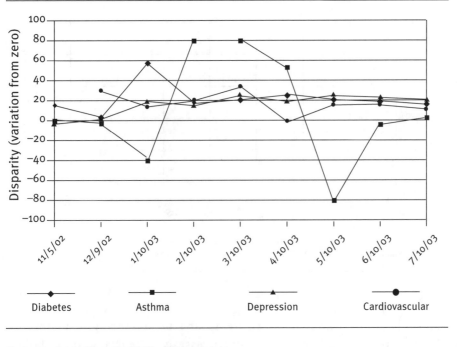

Source: CareSouth, Hartsville, SC. Used with permission.

FIGURE 1.8
Improving Equity: Disparity by Race for Key Effectiveness Measures

munity health centers are often wrongly saddled, CareSouth is conscientious not only about providing top-quality care to its patients but also about maintaining the perception of quality. "We look good," she says. "We remodeled, refurnished, repainted, and we say we offer first-class care for first-class people. Disparity is not just about outcomes, it's also about how you treat your patients."

Vitality

Goal: 0 percent of the office team shall report a somewhat or very stressful work environment (see Figure 1.9).

Actions: Organizations such as CareSouth that take on improvement work in multiple categories find that considerable overlap exists in those areas. Lewis says that all the improvements in efficiency and effectiveness are improving staff morale and "firing everyone up" about the potential for even greater changes. "We have fun here," she claims, "and we work hard. The one thing providers have told us consistently through the years is that they don't like being stuck in the office later and later each day because patients and paperwork have backed up. They want the workday to go

FIGURE 1.9
Improving
Vitality:
Percent of
Office Team
Reporting a
Somewhat
or Very
Stressful Work
Environment

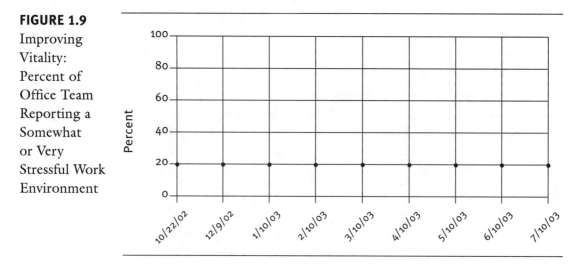

Source: CareSouth, Hartsville, SC. Used with permission.

smoothly. And all the changes we are making are addressing that. I'm sure that the stress in our workplace will decrease as these changes take hold."

Lewis is confident that all of these measures will continue to show progress as the improvement programs become fully engaged. She has seen a lot of changes in healthcare, and in her own health center, in her years as executive director. But this recent period of growth and change has been unprecedented, she says. "You go home at night dead tired," she admits, "but knowing you are doing incredible things and providing the best possible care for people who would not have access to it otherwise."

Case Study

Mr. Roberts is a 77-year-old gentleman who is retired and living in Florida with his wife. He is an accomplished and affluent person who was a child of the Depression. He worked from the time he was 13 as a longshoreman and barracks builder. He began experiencing back pain in his early 20s. At that time, he did not receive particularly good medical advice and did not pursue alternative therapies. World War II, 25 years in Asia, and life as a busy executive took priority, and the pain became a constant but secondary companion. At age 50, the pain became unbearable. He returned to New York and spent the better part of a year "on his back." In 1980, he underwent the first of four major spine surgeries. Since then, he has had multiple intervertebral discs partially or completely removed. Despite these operations, he still has pain. Over the past two to three years, his pain has been worsening, and his functional status has been decreasing.

It is hard to live in pain. Mr. Roberts is not sure he deals with it very well. He does not want to take narcotics, as they interfere with his ability to stay sharp and active, and stomach problems prohibit the use of many non-narcotic medications. Most of the time, he has only mild or temporary relief of his pain. Despite the pain, he is still active and gets out as much as he can. Although it has become more difficult, he still takes his wife dancing on Saturday nights. The pain is exhausting, limiting his ability to do what he wants. The worst part about the pain is that it is changing—getting worse—and he is uncertain of its future trajectory. As the pain becomes worse, how will he survive? What are the possibilities for remaining active and independent?

Mr. Roberts states that he has had "reasonably good" doctors. He reminds me that he is privileged because he has connections and acts as his own advocate. These assets have allowed him to expand his healthcare options and seek out the best providers and top institutions. He is also well informed and assertive and has been an active participant in his healthcare. Although his overall experience in the healthcare system has been favorable, many instances of care have been less than ideal.

Communication Deficits and Lack of a Team Approach

Mr. Roberts observed that the lack of communication between providers is a huge problem. He has multiple specialists who care for different parts of his body; however, no one person is mindful of how these systems interact to create the whole person or illness. He is never sure if one physician knows what the other is doing or how their prescriptions might interfere or interact with another's. The physicians never seem inclined to "dig deeply" or communicate as team members treating one person. On many occasions, physicians have recommended therapies that have already been tried and failed. On other occasions, they disagree on an approach to his problem and leave Mr. Roberts to decide which advice to follow. No system is in place to encourage teamwork. "Unless the physician is extremely intelligent, on the ball, or energetic, it just doesn't happen."

Record keeping and transfer of information are also faulty. Despite the fact that physicians take copious notes, the information is not put to use. Mr. Roberts might expend a great deal of time and energy ensuring that his medical records are sent to a new consultant's office. But within a few minutes of the encounter, it is apparent that the consultant has not reviewed the chart or absorbed any of the information. This realization has affected how he uses care. For instance, at one point, Mr. Roberts was experiencing worsened stomach problems. His gastroenterologist was away on vacation for four weeks and there was no covering physician. The thought of amassing his patient records for transfer to another physician (who would likely not review them and suggest the same tests and therapies) was so distasteful that he chose to go without care.

Mr. Roberts states that he spends much of his energy as a patient facilitating communication between providers and transferring information gained from one physician to another. This process is expensive, wasteful, and dangerous. If all the providers could come together and discuss the problem as a group, redundancies and mistakes could be eliminated. Instead, much time and money are wasted reproducing ineffective therapeutic plans and not treating his illness in an efficient, effective, safe, or timely manner.

In addition, effective communication between providers and patients is lacking. Despite the fact that Mr. Roberts has undergone multiple surgeries that have not resolved his pain, many new doctors he sees are quick to offer surgery as *the* solution to his problem. Seldom do physicians listen to his full story or elicit his thoughts before jumping to conclusions. This problem was painfully illustrated by the recent death of his brother, who died on the operating room table while undergoing a second spinal surgery for similar back problems. Mr. Roberts suggested that physicians carefully analyze their therapeutic personalities. They cannot assume that all patients are alike or that they will react the same to a given intervention. "Each patient needs to be treated as an individual," and service needs to be respectful of individual choice.

Taking the Question Mark Out of Patient-Provider Interactions

Mr. Roberts is particularly concerned with the inability of patients to know the true qualifications of their physicians or judge their prescriptions. At one point, he was experiencing severe arm and finger pain. Assuming these symptoms were related to his spine, he sought the advice of a highly recommended chief of neurosurgery at a premier academic center. After a brief history and examination, he was admitted to the hospital. The following day, an anesthesiologist came into the room to obtain his consent for surgery. Mr. Roberts had not been told that surgery was under consideration. He asked to speak to the neurosurgeon and insisted on some other consultations. Three days later, a hand surgeon reassured him that his problem was likely self-limiting tendonitis and prescribed conservative therapy. Within a few weeks, his pain had resolved. Mr. Roberts was grateful that he had followed his instinct but concerned for other patients who might not have asserted themselves in this manner.

Mismatch Between Supply and Demand

Mr. Roberts also stated that there is a profound disconnect between supply and demand in the healthcare system. In 1992, his pain had become particularly disabling, and his mobility was extremely restricted. His physicians suggested that he see the only neurosurgeon in the county. Despite his health emergency, he was not able to make an appointment to see this neurosurgeon for more than 10 weeks. No other solutions were offered. In pain and unable to walk because of progressively worsening foot drop and muscle weakness, he sought the help of a physician friend. This friend referred him to a "brash, iconoclastic" Harvard-trained neurologist, who, in turn, referred him to a virtuoso neurosurgeon at a county hospital 100 miles away. After only 20 minutes with this neurosurgeon, he was rushed to the operating room and underwent a nine-hour emergency procedure. Apparently, he had severe spinal cord impingement and swelling. He was later told by the neurosurgeon that he would have been a paraplegic or died if he had not received the operation that day. He subsequently underwent a series of three more spinal operations. Postoperative care was suboptimal, as he had to travel 100 miles to see the surgeon for follow-up. Eventually, this surgeon chose to travel to a more centralized location twice per month to accommodate his patients in outlying areas.

Mr. Roberts states that we need to "overcome petty bureaucracies" that do not allow matching of supply with demand. The ready availability of quality care needs to be patient driven and closely monitored by a third party that does not have a vested interest in the market.

Knowledge-Based Care

Mr. Roberts is concerned about the status of continuing medical education. He guesses that it is probably easy for physicians in large, urban teaching hospitals to keep abreast of the latest diagnostic and therapeutic advances. However, the majority of physicians may not have similar opportunities. The system does not necessarily encourage physicians to keep up to date. This lack of current, in-depth knowledge is particularly important as supply-demand issues force consumers to seek care in "instant med clinics." For example, Mr. Roberts believes emergency care to be an oxymoron. On many occasions, he has gone to the emergency room for an emergency and had to wait four to five hours before being treated. This experience is unpleasant and forces people to seek alternative sites of care that may not provide the best care for complex, chronically ill patients.

Mr. Roberts also feels that we need to learn from our errors as well as successes. We should require that groups of physicians regularly review cases and learn how to deliver care in a better way. This analysis needs to occur internally within an institution as well as externally across institutions. Ideally, the analysis would directly involve patients and families to gain their perspectives. In addition, the learning should be contextual: we should not only learn how to do better the next time but also know if what we are doing makes sense within our overall economic, epidemiological, and societal context.

Mr. Roberts believes that quality healthcare needs to be knowledge based. This knowledge comes not only from science but also from analysis of mistakes that occur in the process of delivering care. Patients need to be involved in the collection and synthesis of these data. The transfer of knowledge among patients, scientists, and practitioners needs to be emphasized and simplified.

Nonphysician/Nonhospital Care

Mr. Roberts has been very impressed with the quality of care given by people other than physicians, and he believes that the growth of alternative healthcare provider models has been a definite advance in the system. As an example, Mr. Roberts cites the effectiveness of his physical therapists as healthcare providers; they are alert, patient conscious, conscientious, and respectful. Their interventions "guide people to better life," and Mr. Roberts' functional status has improved because of their assistance. In addition, these providers are careful to maintain close communication with physicians. They function as members of a larger team.

Postoperative care has also improved. At the time of his first surgery more than two decades ago, Mr. Roberts spent two weeks in the hospital. Now, after three days, he is discharged to a rehabilitation facility that is better equipped to help him recuperate and return to full functioning.

Mr. Roberts knows how crucial his family and friends are in his medical care. Without their support, recommendations, constant questioning, and advocacy, his condition would be more precarious. The system needs to acknowledge the patient's other "carers" and involve them in shared decision making and transfer of knowledge.

Conclusion

The previous sections provide a brief insight into some successful improvement projects; it would be even easier to find examples of failures and the subsequent lessons learned. The main message is that, although the information on the gap between current practice and best practice may be daunting, improvement is occurring, albeit in pockets, and the opportunity is before us to continue to make quality a necessity, not just a nicety, in healthcare.

The aim of this textbook is to provide a comprehensive overview of the critical components of the healthcare quality landscape. You, as readers and leaders, should use this text as a resource and framework for understanding the connectivity of multiple aspects of healthcare quality from the science base, patient perspective, organizational implications, and environmental effects.

This chapter, specifically, sets the stage by highlighting

- The current state of healthcare quality;
- The importance of the patient in goals and results;
- Promising evidence of the great capacity for significant improvement in systems of care;
- Examples of breakthrough improvements happening today; and
- The call to action for all healthcare stakeholders to continue to rethink and redesign our systems for better health for all.

Building on this chapter, the book will outline healthcare quality similar to the levels of the healthcare system outlined by IOM.

Study Questions

1. Identify five ways in which you can put the patient more in control of his or her care.
2. Think of an experience you have had with healthcare or one of your family or friends. Apply IOM's six aims for improvement to the experience and identify how the experience fared according to the aims and the opportunities for improvement.
3. You are the CEO of your hospital and the local newspaper has just run a story on "how bad healthcare is." How do you respond to the reporter asking you to comment on the situation? How do you respond to your employees?

Note

1. This patient story was edited by Matthew Fitzgerald, chief scientist, Delmarva Foundation, and originally composed by Heidi Louise Behforouz, M.D., associate physician, Women's Health Division, medical director of the Prevention and Access to Care and Treatment Project; Division of Social Medicine and Health Inequalities, Brigham and Women's Hospital; and instructor, Harvard Medical School.
2. Institute for Healthcare Improvement Innovation Team.

REFERENCES

Berwick, D. M. 2002. "A User's Manual for the IOM's 'Quality Chasm' Report." *Health Affairs* May/June: 80–90.

Chassin, M. R., and R. H. Galvin. 1998. "The Urgent Need to Improve Health Care Quality. Institute of Medicine National Roundtable on Health Care Quality." *Journal of the American Medical Association* 280: 1000–05.

Donabedian, A. 1990. *The Definition of Quality and Approaches to Its Assessment, Volume I: Explorations in Quality Assessment and Monitoring.* Chicago: Health Administration Press.

Institute of Medicine. 2001. *Crossing the Quality Chasm: A New Health System for the 21st Century.* Washington, DC: National Academy Press.

Ferlie, E., and S. M. Shortell. 2001. "Improving the Quality of Healthcare in the United Kingdom and the United States: A Framework for Change." *The Milbank Quarterly* 79 (2): 281–316.

Kohn, L. T., J. M. Corrigan, and M. S. Donaldson (eds.). 1999. *To Err Is Human: Building a Safer Health System.* Washington, DC: National Academy Press.

Lohr, K. N. (ed.). 1990. *Medicare: A Strategy for Quality Assurance, Volume I.* Washington, DC: Institute of Medicine, National Academy Press.

McGlynn, E. A., S. M. Asch, J. Adams, J. Keesey, J. Hicks, A. DeCristofaro, and E. A. Kerr. 2003. "The Quality of Health Care Delivered to Adults in the United States." *New England Journal of Medicine* 348 (26): 2635–45.

Mullan, F. 2001. "A Founder of Quality Assessment Encounters a Troubled System Firsthand." *Health Affairs* Jan./Feb.: 137–41.

Murray, M., and C. Tantau. 2000. "Same-Day Appointments: Exploding the Access Paradigm." *Family Practice Management* 7 (8): 45–50.

BASIC CONCEPTS OF HEALTHCARE QUALITY*

Leon Wyszewianski

Not everyone perceives quality of healthcare services in quite the same way. Consider these two cases:

- The residents of a rural area were shocked to find out that the federal Medicare program had served notice that it would stop doing business with several of the area's physicians, alleging that the quality of care they provided was not acceptable. According to Medicare officials, the physicians had a pattern of providing unnecessary and even harmful care to Medicare patients, such as prescribing for patients with heart disease medications that were in fact likely to make the patients' condition worse. These physicians had been in the community for at least 25 years each and were known for their dedication and devotion. Their willingness to travel to remote locations without regard to time of day or weather was legendary, as was their generosity toward patients who had fallen on hard times and were unable to pay their medical bills.
- An expert panel of trauma care specialists was asked to survey and rate hospital emergency departments in a major metropolitan area. The results surprised many of the area's residents. The emergency department rated number one by the panel was known mostly for its crowded conditions, long waits, and harried and often brusque-mannered staff.

Several concepts can help make sense of these and similar apparent contradictions and inconsistencies in perceptions of quality of care. This chapter focuses on such concepts, first in relation to the definition of quality of care, and second in relation to its measurement.

* Portions of this chapter include, in modified form, material reprinted from *Clinics in Family Practice* 5 (4), Wyszewianski, L: "Defining, Measuring and Improving Quality of Care," 807–12, Copyright © 2003 Elsevier Inc. Reprinted with permission from Elsevier.

Definition-Related Concepts

The quality of healthcare services can be characterized in terms of a number of attributes. As we will see, different groups involved in healthcare—in particular physicians, patients, and health insurers—tend to attach different levels of importance to particular attributes and as a result define quality of care differently (see Table 2.1).

The Definitional Attributes

The following attributes relevant to the definition of quality of care will be discussed below:

- Technical performance;
- Management of the interpersonal relationship;
- Amenities of care;
- Responsiveness to patient preferences;
- Efficiency; and
- Cost effectiveness.

Technical Performance

Quality of technical performance refers to how well current scientific medical knowledge and technology are applied in a given situation. It is usually assessed in terms of the timeliness and accuracy of the diagnosis, appropriateness of therapy, and skill with which procedures and other medical interventions are performed (Donabedian 1980, 1988a).

Management of the Interpersonal Relationship

The quality of the interpersonal relationship is determined by how well the clinician relates to the patient on a human level. It is valued first and foremost for its own sake: by establishing a good interpersonal relationship with the patient, the clinician is able to fully address the patient's concerns, reassure the patient, and, more generally, relieve the patient's *suffering*, as distinguished from simply curing the patient's disease (Cassell 1982).

The quality of the interpersonal relationship is also important because of how it can affect technical performance (Donabedian 1988a). A clinician who relates well to a patient is better able to elicit from that patient a more complete and accurate medical history (especially with respect to potentially sensitive topics such as use of illicit drugs); that, in turn, can result in a better diagnosis. Similarly, a good relationship with the patient is often crucial in motivating the patient to follow the prescribed regimen of care, such as taking medications or making lifestyle changes, for which noncompliance rates are alarmingly high despite their obvious importance to achieving the ultimate goals of healthcare (Haynes et al. 2003).

TABLE 2.1
Stereotypical Differences in the Importance of Selected Aspects of Care to Key Participants' Definitions of Quality

Key Participant	Technical Performance	Interpersonal Relationship	Amenities and Access	Patient Preferences	Efficiency	Cost Effectiveness
Clinician	+++	+	+	+	+	—
Patient	++	++	++	+++	+	—
Payer	+	+	+	+	+++	+++

Amenities of Care

The quality of the amenities of care is determined not by what the clinician does during the encounter but by characteristics of the setting in which that encounter between patient and clinician takes place, such as comfort, convenience, and privacy (Donabedian 1980; Wyszewianski 1988). Much like the interpersonal relationship, amenities are valued both in their own right and for their potential effect on the technical and interpersonal aspects of care. Amenities such as ample and convenient parking, good directional signs, comfortable waiting rooms, and tasty hospital food are all of direct value to patients.

In addition, amenities can yield more indirect benefits. For example, in a setting that is comfortable and affords privacy and as a result puts the patient at ease, a good interpersonal relationship with the clinician is more easily established, leading to a potentially more complete patient history and therefore a faster and more accurate diagnosis. Finally, it should be noted that the notion of amenities can also be extended to include characteristics related to the accessibility of care, such as how readily the patient can see the clinician and how convenient the location of the practitioner's clinic or office is to the patient.

Responsiveness to Patient Preferences

Although taking into account the wishes and preferences of patients has long been recognized as important to achieving high quality of care, until recently this has not been singled out as a factor in its own right. In earlier formulations, responsiveness to patients' preferences was just one of the factors seen as determining the quality of the patient-clinician interpersonal relationship (Donabedian 1980). By contrast, responsiveness to patients' preferences has had a prominent role in how the physician-patient relationship was conceived in the context of economic agency theory (Arrow 1985). According to that formulation, the patient, who typically lacks the requisite medical knowledge to deal effectively with health issues, turns to the physician, who does have the requisite knowledge, to serve as the patient's agent. In that role, the physician is expected to make, on the patient's behalf, the healthcare-related choices that the patient would have made on his or her own had the patient had the necessary specialized knowledge. To be a "perfect agent," the physician must make decisions driven by the patient's goals and preferences. Although in the past the agency theory perspective had little apparent effect on how quality of healthcare was defined, the importance of responsiveness to patients' preferences to quality of care is now increasingly recognized—for example, by Donabedian (2003) under the rubric of "acceptability" and by the Institute of Medicine as "respect for patients' values, preferences and expressed needs" (IOM 2001).

Efficiency

Efficiency refers to how well resources are used in achieving a given result. Efficiency improves whenever the resources used to produce a given output are reduced. Although economists typically treat efficiency and quality as separate concepts, it has been argued that separating the two in healthcare may not be easy or meaningful. Because inefficient care uses more resources than necessary, it is wasteful care, and care that involves waste is deficient—and therefore of lower quality—no matter how good it may be in other respects: "Wasteful care is either directly harmful to health or is harmful by displacing more useful care" (Donabedian 1988a).

Cost Effectiveness

The cost effectiveness of a given healthcare intervention is determined by how much benefit, typically measured in terms of improvements in health status, the intervention yields for a particular level of expenditure (Gold et al. 1996). In general, as the amounts spent on providing services for a particular condition grow, diminishing returns set in; each unit of expenditure yields ever-smaller benefits, until a point is reached where no additional benefits accrue from adding more care (Donabedian, Wheeler, and Wyszewianski 1982). The idea that resources should be spent until no additional benefits can be obtained has been termed the "maximalist" view of quality of care. In that view, resources should be expended as long as there is a positive benefit to be obtained, no matter how small it may be. An alternative to the maximalist view of quality is the "optimalist" view, which holds that spending ought to stop earlier, at the point where the added benefits are too small to be worth the added costs (Donabedian 1988a).

The Different Definitions

Although everyone values to some extent the attributes of quality just described, different groups tend to attach different levels of importance to individual attributes, leading to differences in how clinicians, patients, payers, and society each define quality of care. Table 2.1 attempts to capture the stereotypical differences among these groups in how they value individual attributes of care when defining quality of care.

The Clinician's Definition

Clinicians, such as physicians and others who provide healthcare services, tend to perceive quality of care first and foremost in terms of technical performance. And within technical performance, clinicians' concerns focus on specific aspects that are well captured by IOM's often-quoted definition of quality of care (IOM and Lohr 1990):

> Quality is the degree to which health services for individuals and populations increase the likelihood of desired health outcomes and are consistent with current professional knowledge.

Reference to "current professional knowledge" places the assessment of quality of care in the context of the state of the art in clinical care, which constantly changes. Clinicians want it recognized that, because medical knowledge advances rapidly, it is not fair to judge care provided in 2002 in terms of what has only been known since 2004. Similarly, mention of the "likelihood of desired health outcomes" in the IOM definition is congenial to clinicians' view of quality because it signals that, with respect to outcomes, we are dealing with probabilities rather than certainties. This definition implicitly acknowledges the existence of factors that can affect outcomes of care but are beyond the clinician's control.

The Patient's Definition

Although patients, like clinicians, are deeply concerned with how good the technical aspect of care is, most patients do not possess the wherewithal to evaluate the technical elements of care. As a result, patients tend to defer to others on matters of technical quality. Many in fact take for granted that entities that ostensibly possess the requisite expertise and insight—such as accrediting bodies, state licensing agencies, and medical specialty boards—look after technical quality on the public's behalf. Patients therefore tend to form their opinions about quality of care based on their assessment of those aspects of care they are most readily able to evaluate: the interpersonal aspect of care and the amenities of care (Cleary and McNeil 1988; Donabedian 1980). In fact, because patients' reactions to the interpersonal and amenity aspects of care—rather than to the more indiscernible quality of technical aspects—largely determine their level of satisfaction with care, health maintenance organizations, hospitals, and other healthcare delivery organizations have come to view the quality of nontechnical aspects of care as crucial to attracting and retaining patients. This often dismays clinicians, to whom this focus is a slight to the centrality of technical quality in the assessment of healthcare quality.

Another aspect of care that has steadily grown in importance in how patients define quality of care is the extent to which their preferences are taken into account. Although not every patient will have definite preferences in every clinical situation, patients increasingly value being consulted about their preferences, especially in situations in which different approaches to diagnosis and treatment involve potential tradeoffs, such as between the quality and quantity of life.

The Payer's Definition

Third-party payers—health insurance companies, government programs like Medicare, and others who pay for care on behalf of the patient—tend to assess quality of care in the context of costs. From their perspective, care that is inefficient is poor-quality care. Additionally, because payers typically manage a finite pool of resources, they often have to consider whether a potential outcome justifies the associated costs. Payers are therefore more likely to embrace an optimalist definition of care, which can put them at odds with individual physicians, who generally take the maximalist view of quality. Most physicians consider cost-effectiveness calculations as antithetical to providing high-quality care, believing instead that they are duty-bound to do everything possible to help their patients, including advocating for high-cost interventions even when such measures have a small, but positive, probability of benefiting the patient (Donabedian 1988b).

By contrast, third-party payers—especially governmental units that must make multiple tradeoffs when allocating resources—are more apt to take the view that spending large sums in instances where the odds of a positive result are small does not represent high quality of care, but rather a misuse of finite resources. This perspective is reinforced, in the view of third-party payers at least, by evidence of the public's growing unwillingness to pay the higher premiums or taxes it would take to provide every patient with all the care that is technically feasible and could benefit that individual.

Society's Definition

At the broader societal level the definition of quality of care reflects concerns with cost effectiveness similar to governmental third-party payers', and much for the same reasons. In addition, however, society at large is often expected to focus on technical aspects of quality, which it is seen as better placed to safeguard than individuals are. Similarly, access to care figures prominently in societal-level conceptions of quality inasmuch as society is seen as responsible for ensuring access to care, especially to disenfranchised groups.

Are the Four Definitions Irreconcilable?

Different though they may seem, the four definitions—the clinician's, the patient's, the payer's, and society's—have a great deal in common. Although each definition clearly emphasizes different aspects of care, it is not to the complete exclusion of the other aspects (see Table 2.1). Only with respect to the cost-effectiveness aspect can it be said that the definitions directly conflict: cost effectiveness is often central to how payers and society define quality of care, whereas physicians and patients typically do not recognize cost effectiveness as a legitimate consideration in the definition of quality. But on all the other aspects of care no such clash is present; rather, the differences relate to how much weight each definition places on a particular aspect of care.

That is not to say, however, that strong disagreements do not arise among the four parties' definitions, even outside the realm of cost effectiveness. Conflicts typically arise when one party holds that a particular practitioner or clinic is a high-quality provider by virtue of having high ratings on a single aspect of care, such as the interpersonal. Those who object to such a conclusion point out that just because care rates highly on interpersonal quality does not necessarily mean that it rates equally highly on the technical, amenity, and efficiency aspects (Wyszewianski 1988). Physicians who relate especially well to their patients, and thus score high on the interpersonal aspect, still may have failed to keep up with medical advances and as a result provide care that is seriously deficient in technical terms. This is apparently what happened in the rural physicians' case mentioned at the start of the chapter.

Conversely, practitioners who are highly skilled in trauma and other emergency care but who also have a cold, even brusque, manner and who additionally work in crowded conditions may earn a facility low ratings on the interpersonal and amenity aspects of care even though, as in the second case described at the start of the chapter, the facility gets top marks from a team of expert clinicians that is presumably focusing primarily on the quality of technical performance.

In thinking about definitions of quality of healthcare, therefore, it is helpful to keep in mind that when clinicians, patients, payers, society at large, and any other involved parties refer to quality of care, they each tend to focus on the quality of specific aspects of care, sometimes to the apparent exclusion of other aspects important to the other parties. One must recognize, however, that the aspects overlooked by a given party are seldom in direct conflict with that party's own overall concept of quality (see Table 2.1).

Measurement-Related Concepts

Just as the concepts discussed above are useful in advancing our understanding of the definition of quality of care, another set of concepts can help us better understand the *measurement* of quality of care, particularly with respect to technical care. Consider the cases that follow:

- At the urging of the nurses' association, state legislators passed a law that specifies minimum nurse staffing levels for hospitals in the state.

The state nurses' association had argued that nurse staffing cutbacks around the state had affected quality of care to the point of endangering the safety of hospital patients. However, critics of the law charge that the law was passed without anyone having proven that the staffing levels stipulated in the law are "safe." In the critics' view, the law has more to do with the state's nurses fearing for their jobs than with documented quality-of-care problems.

- Several health plans are competing to be among those offered to the employees of one of the area's newest and largest employers. One of the plans, HealthBest, claims that it provides higher quality of care than any of its competitors. Among the data HealthBest cites to back its claim are statistics showing that, compared to the other plans, HealthBest has 10 percent to 20 percent higher rates of mammogram screening for breast cancer among its female population aged 52 to 69. One of the other plans, PrimeHealth, disputes that particular inference, arguing that the percentage of women screened through mammography is not a good indicator of quality of care compared to a plan's success in actually detecting breast cancers at an early stage; on that measure, PrimeHealth claims to do better than HealthBest or any of the other plans.

The following section introduces several concepts that can help make better sense of the above cases, and of similar situations involving the measurement of quality of care.

Structure, Process, and Outcomes

As Donabedian first noted in 1966, all evaluations of quality of care can be classified in terms of which of three aspects of caregiving they measure: structure, process, or outcome.

Structure

When quality is measured in terms of structure, the focus is on the relatively static characteristics of the individuals who provide care and of the settings where the care is delivered. These characteristics include the education, training, and certification of those who provide care and the adequacy of the facility's staffing, equipment, and overall organization.

Evaluations of quality that rely on such structural elements implicitly assume that well-qualified people working in well-appointed and well-organized settings will provide high-quality care. It must be remembered, however, that although good structure makes good quality more likely to ensue, it does not guarantee it (Donabedian 2003). Structure-focused assessments are therefore most revealing when deficiencies are found: good quality is unlikely, if not impossible, if those who provide care are unqualified or if necessary equipment is missing or in disrepair. Licensing and accrediting bodies have relied heavily on structural measures of quality not only because the measures are relatively stable and thus easier to capture but also because they reliably identify those who demonstrably lack the means to provide high-quality care.

Process

Care can also be evaluated in terms of the process of care, which refers to what takes place during the delivery of care. Within this process, it is useful to distinguish two further aspects on which quality can vary: *appropriateness*, which refers to whether the right actions were taken, and *skill*, that is, how well actions were carried out. Knowing that the correct diagnostic procedure was ordered for a patient tells us that the procedure was appropriate. But that is only half the story about how good the process of care was in that instance. The other half is in how well (i.e., skillfully) the procedure was carried out. Knowing that a surgical operation was successfully completed and the patient had a good recovery from it is not enough to conclude that the process of care in that case was good. It only tells us, at best, that the procedure was skillfully accomplished. For the entire process of care to be judged to have been good, we must additionally ascertain that the operation was indicated (i.e., appropriate) for that patient in the first place. Finally, similar to structural measures, use of process measures for assessing quality of care rests on a key assumption: in this case, that if the right things are done and are done right, good results for the patient (i.e., good outcomes of care) are more likely to ensue.

Outcomes

Another way quality of care can be assessed is in terms of outcome measures, which seek to capture whether the goals of care were achieved. Since the goals of care can be defined quite broadly, outcome measures have come to include the costs of care as well as patients' satisfaction with care (Iezzoni 2003). In formulations that stress the technical aspects of care, however, outcomes typically refer to health status–related indicators such as whether the patient's pain subsided, the condition cleared up, or full function was regained (Donabedian 1980; Wyszewianski 1988). Clinicians tend to be leery of such outcome measures of quality. As mentioned earlier in relation to how different parties define quality, clinicians are very aware that many factors that determine clinical outcomes—including genetic and environmental factors—are not under the clinician's control: although good process increases the likelihood of good outcomes, it does not guarantee those outcomes. Some patients do not get better in spite of the best that medicine can offer, whereas other patients regain full health even though they received inappropriate and potentially harmful care. Nevertheless, the relation between process and outcomes is not random or wholly unpredictable. We know, in particular, that the likelihood that a specific set of clinical activities—a given process—will result in desirable outcomes depends crucially on how *efficacious* that process has been shown to be.

Efficacy

A clinical intervention is said to be efficacious if it has been shown to reliably produce a given outcome when other, potentially confounding, factors are held constant. The efficacy of a clinical intervention is typically established through formal clinical trials or similarly systematic, controlled studies. Knowledge about efficacy is crucial to making valid judgments about quality of care based on either process or outcome measures. If we know that a given clinical intervention was undertaken in circumstances that match those under which the intervention has been shown to be efficacious, we can be confident that the care was appropriate and, to that extent, of good quality. Conversely, if we know that the outcome of a particular episode of care was poor, we can determine whether that result was due to an inappropriate clinical intervention by examining whether the interventions used were in conformance to what is known about those interventions' efficacy.

Which Is Best?

A frequently asked question is whether structure, process, or outcome is the best measure of quality of care. The answer—that none of them is inherently better and that all depends on the circumstances (Donabedian 1988a, 2003)—often does not satisfy those who are inclined to believe that outcome measures are the superior measure. After all, they reason, outcomes address the ultimate purpose, the "bottom line," of all caregiving: was the condition cured, did the patient get better? As previously mentioned, however, good outcomes can result even when the care (i.e., process) was clearly deficient. The reverse is also possible: although the care was excellent, the outcome was not a good one. Besides the care provided, a number of other factors—most of them, like how frail the patient is, not within the control of clinicians—can affect outcomes and must be accounted for through risk-adjustment calculations that are seldom straightforward (Iezzoni 2003).

Ultimately what a particular outcome tells us about quality of care depends crucially on whether the outcome can be *attributed* to the care provided. In other words, we have to examine the link between the outcome and the antecedent process and determine whether the care provided was *appropriate*—a determination that is made based on what we know about efficacy—and whether it was provided *skillfully*. Outcomes are therefore very useful in identifying possible problems of quality ("fingering the suspects"), but not in ascertaining whether poor quality was actually provided ("determining guilt"). The latter determination requires delving into the antecedent process of care to establish whether the care provided is actually the likely cause of the observed outcome.

Criteria and Standards

In practice, to assess quality using structure, process, or outcome measures we need to know what constitutes good structure, good process, or good outcomes. In other words, we need *criteria* and *standards* for those aspects of care.

Definitions

Criteria refer to specific attributes that are the basis for assessing quality. *Standards* express quantitatively what level the attributes must reach to satisfy preexisting expectations about quality. An example unrelated to healthcare may help clarify the difference between criteria and standards. Graduate programs at most universities evaluate applicants for admission based on, among other things, the applicants' scores on standardized tests. The scores are thus one of the criteria by which programs judge the quality of their applicants. However, although two programs may use the same criterion—standardized scores—to evaluate applicants, the programs may differ markedly on their standards: one program may consider applicants acceptable if they have scores above the 50th percentile, whereas scores above the 90th percentile may be the standard of acceptability at the other. Table 2.2 provides illustrative healthcare examples of criteria and standards for structure, process, and outcome measures.

Sources

A shift in the way criteria and standards are derived has been occurring in the healthcare field. Prior to the 1970s, formally derived criteria and standards for quality-of-care evaluations for the most part relied on consensus opinions of groups of clinicians selected for their clinical knowledge and experience and for the respect they commanded among their colleagues (Donabedian 1982). This approach to formulating criteria took for granted that in their deliberations the experts would incorporate the latest scientific knowledge relevant to the topic under consideration, but formal requirements that they do so seldom existed.

It was not until the mid-1970s that the importance of the scientific literature in relation to criteria and standards was highlighted, notably by

Type of Measure	Focus of Assessment	Criterion	Standard
Structure	Primary care group practice	Percent of board-certified physicians in internal or family medicine	100% of physicians in the practice must be board certified in internal or family medicine
Process	Treatment of patients hospitalized for heart attack	Percent of post–heart attack patients prescribed beta-blockers on discharge	At least 96% of heart attack patients receive a beta-blocker prescription on discharge
Outcome	Blood pressure of patients with diabetes	Percent of patients with diabetes whose blood pressure is at or below 130/85	At least 50% of patients with diabetes have blood pressure at or below 130/85

TABLE 2.2
Illustrative Examples of Criteria and Standards

Williamson's (1977) work. At about the same time, Brook and his colleagues at RAND were the first to use systematic reviews and evaluations of the scientific literature as the starting point for the deliberations of panels charged with defining criteria and standards for studies of quality (Brook et al. 1977). This focus on the literature—and especially on the validity of the studies within that literature—was reinforced in the 1990s by the evidence-based medicine movement, which seeks to put into practice what the best evidence has to say about what is and is not efficacious under a given set of clinical circumstances (Evidence-Based Medicine Working Group 1992; Sackett et al. 2000). Thus, criteria and standards have come to revolve increasingly around the strength and validity of the scientific evidence and less on the unaided consensus opinions of experts (Eddy 1996).

It must be noted, however, that although estimates vary, efficacy has not been definitely established for at least half of what physicians do in their daily practice (Eddy 1993; Sackett et al. 2000). Definitive, efficacy-based assessments of quality are therefore impossible to make about much care clinicians provide. On the other hand, even when we do not know what is the right thing to do, we often know what is *not* the right thing to do (e.g., prescribing antibiotics for viral infections), and that knowledge can certainly be translated into useful and meaningful criteria and standards.

Levels

When formulating standards, a critical decision that must be made is the level at which the standards should be set: minimal, optimal, achievable, or something in between (Muir Gray 2001). *Minimal* standards specify what level must be met for quality to be considered acceptable. The implication is that if care does not meet a minimal standard, remedial action is called for. *Optimal* standards denote the level of quality that can be reached under the best conditions, typically conditions similar to those under which efficacy is determined. Optimal standards are probably most useful as a reference point for setting *achievable* standards—the level of performance that should be reached by everyone to whom the standards are being applied. One way to define achievable standards is in relation to the level of performance of the top quartile of providers of care. The reasoning is that if the top quartile can perform at that level, the other three quartiles should be able to reach it as well (Muir Gray 2001). Since there is no a priori level at which a particular standard ought to be set, a sensible and frequently adopted approach is to choose the level based on why the underlying evaluation is being conducted in the first place.

Using Measurement-Related Concepts

How does understanding structure, process, and outcomes; efficacy; and criteria and standards give us insight into quality-of-care measurement issues? The two cases cited at the beginning of this section provide some illustrations.

In the first case, minimum standards of quality were specified in terms of nurse staffing levels, a structural measure of quality. The critics are not questioning the choice of measure, nor should they, since structural measures are well suited to detecting lack of capacity to deliver care of acceptable quality. In this case, hospitals that do not meet minimum staffing levels by definition cannot deliver care of acceptable quality ("safe care").

Put another way, the critics do not challenge nurse staffing levels as a *criterion* for assessing quality of care. However, they do contend, in effect, that the law's *standards* specifying minimum staffing levels are not evidence based but were set instead at levels intended to minimize job losses among members of the state nurses' association. To effectively rebut the critics' charge, evidence supporting the staffing standards in the law is needed. The evidence would have to come from properly controlled studies showing that quality of care falls below what can be considered safe levels when nurse staffing ratios are reduced, holding all else constant. In other words, silencing the critics requires evidence from the kind of studies on which efficacy determinations are based.

In the second case, both measures under discussion are process measures. However, mammograms belong to a subset of process measures that represent a kind of resting point along the continuum of the activities that make up the process of care. These kinds of resting points share with most outcomes the characteristic of being discrete events that are relatively easily counted; hence, the label *procedural endpoints* has been applied to them (Donabedian 1980).

PrimeHealth's challenge may be interpreted as meant to underline that mammograms are *not* an outcome (i.e., they are not an end in themselves, but rather the means for the early detection of breast cancer). Because performing mammograms is certainly the right thing to do for the target population, *appropriateness* is not in question. But PrimeHealth's challenge implicitly reminds us that the *skill* with which the mammograms are done matters just as much. If mammograms are not done right—if, because of deficiencies in skill, mammograms are performed incorrectly, resulting in incorrect interpretations, or if they are done correctly but read incorrectly— the mammograms will fail as a means for early detection of breast cancer. Early detection of breast cancer can therefore be claimed to be the better alternative measure of quality: it reflects not just whether mammograms were performed when indicated (appropriateness), but also how well they were done and interpreted (skill).

Conclusion

The main insight that can be drawn from a deeper understanding of the concepts related to the measurement of healthcare quality is that it matters less what type of measure is used—structure, process, or outcome— than what we know about that measure's link to the others. Structural measures are only as good and useful as the strength of their relation to desired processes and outcomes. So, too, process and outcome measures must relate to each other in measurable and reproducible ways—as demonstrated by efficacy studies—to be truly valid measures of quality.

Additionally, structure, process, and outcome measures are the building blocks for the criteria on which all evaluations of healthcare quality rest. But whereas the decision on which measures ought to become criteria ideally is evidence based—and thus driven by considerations of efficacy, along with the recognition of the distinction between appropriateness and skill—the setting of standards that correspond to the criteria is not based

on the scientific literature. Instead, the decision to set standards at a minimal, ideal, or reachable level should properly be driven by the goals behind
the specific quality-of-care evaluation in which the standards are to be used.

Study Questions

1. An article in *Consumer Reports on Health* offered the following
    advice on how to find a new personal physician (Lipman 1997):

    > There's no sure way to find a new personal physician who
    > will meet all your needs. . . . Many people simply ask a satis-
    > fied friend or relative. A better approach . . . is to ask a
    > healthcare professional—a physician, nurse, therapist, techni-
    > cian, or social worker—who has seen many doctors in action.
    > Almost anyone who works in a hospital can tell you which
    > doctors are regarded highly by their patients and colleagues.

    In terms of the attributes of care that typically enter into the
    definition of quality, what does it mean to say that it would be
    preferable to rely on a healthcare professional's opinion—rather
    than that of a friend or relative who is *not* a healthcare profes-
    sional—when choosing a personal physician?
2. Describe an instance in which outcomes would not be a good meas-
    ure of healthcare quality. Please spell out why outcomes would not
    be a good indicator of quality in that instance.
3. Some third-party payers have been criticized for making judgments
    about quality of healthcare based almost exclusively on whether a
    given service should or should not have been provided. In terms of
    concepts relevant to the definition and measurement of quality of
    care, what else might these third-party payers take into considera-
    tion when making judgments about quality of care?

REFERENCES

Arrow, K. 1985. "The Economics of Agency." In *Principals and Agents: The
    Structure of Business*, edited by J. D. Pratt and R. J. Zechauser. Boston:
    Harvard Business School.
Brook, R. H., A. Davies-Avery, S. Greenfield, L. J. Harris, T. Lelah, N. E.
    Solomon, and J. E. Ware, Jr. 1977. "Assessing the Quality of Medical
    Care Using Outcome Measures: An Overview of the Method." *Medical
    Care* 15 (9 Suppl.): 1–165.
Cassell, E. J. 1982. "The Nature of Suffering and the Goals of Medicine." *New
    England Journal of Medicine* 306 (11): 639–45.

Cleary, P. D., and B. J. McNeil. 1988. "Patient Satisfaction as an Indicator of Quality Care." *Inquiry* 25 (1): 25–36.

Donabedian, A. 1966. "Evaluating the Quality of Medical Care." *The Milbank Quarterly* 44: 166–203.

———. 1980. *Explorations in Quality Assessment and Monitoring. Vol. I: The Definition of Quality and Approaches to Its Assessment.* Chicago: Health Administration Press.

———. 1982. *Explorations in Quality Assessment and Monitoring. Vol. II: The Criteria and Standards of Quality.* Chicago: Health Administration Press.

———. 1988a. "The Quality of Care: How Can It Be Assessed? *Journal of the American Medical Association* 260 (12): 1743–48.

———. 1988b. "Quality and Cost: Choices and Responsibilities." *Inquiry* 25 (1): 90–99.

———. 2003. *An Introduction to Quality Assurance in Health Care.* New York: Oxford University Press.

Donabedian, A., J. R. C. Wheeler, and L. Wyszewianski. 1982. "Quality, Cost, and Health: An Integrative Model." *Medical Care* 20 (10): 975–92.

Eddy, D. M. 1993. "Three Battles to Watch in the 1990s." *Journal of the American Medical Association* 270: 520–26.

———. 1996. *Clinical Decision Making: From Theory to Practice.* Sudbury, MA: Jones and Bartlett.

Evidence-based Medicine Working Group. 1992. "Evidence-Based Medicine. A New Approach to Teaching the Practice of Medicine." *Journal of the American Medical Association* 268: 2420–25.

Gold, M. R., J. E. Siegel, L. B. Russell, and M. C. Weinstein (eds.). 1996. *Cost-Effectiveness in Health and Medicine.* New York: Oxford University Press.

Haynes, R. B., H. McDonald, A. X. Garg, and P. Montague. 2003. *Interventions for Helping Patients to Follow Prescriptions for Medications (Cochrane Review). The Cochrane Library (Issue 2).* Oxford: Update Software.

Iezzoni, L. I. (ed.) 2003. *Risk Adjustment for Measuring Healthcare Outcomes,* 3rd ed. Chicago: Health Administration Press.

Institute of Medicine. 2001. *Crossing the Quality Chasm: A New Health System for the 21st Century.* Washington, DC: National Academy Press.

Institute of Medicine, and K. N. Lohr (ed.). 1990. *Medicare: A Strategy for Quality Assurance.* Washington, DC: National Academy Press.

Lipman, M. M. 1997. "When to Fire Your Doctor—and How to Find Another." *Consumer Reports on Health* 9 (3): 35.

Muir Gray, J. A. 2001. *Evidence-Based Healthcare,* 2nd ed. Edinburgh: Churchill Livingstone.

Sackett, D. L., S. E. Straus, W. S. Richardson, W. Rosenberg, and R. B. Haynes. 2000. *Evidence-Based Medicine,* 2nd ed. Edinburgh: Churchill Livingstone.

Williamson, J. W. 1977. *Improving Medical Practice and Health Care: A Bibliographic Guide to Information Management in Quality Assurance and Continuing Education.* Cambridge, MA: Ballinger Publishing.

Wyszewianski, L. 1988. "Quality of Care: Past Achievements and Future Challenges." *Inquiry* 25 (1): 13–22.

VARIATION IN MEDICAL PRACTICE AND IMPLICATIONS FOR QUALITY

David J. Ballard, Robert S. Hopkins III, and David Nicewander

Despite the growing interest in and use of evidence-based medicine, the art of medical practice remains largely empirical and is subject to considerable differences in process and outcome, even among the finest medical centers (Reinertsen 2003). Indeed, in examining the 50 best hospitals noted for their "compassionate geriatric and palliative care," the *Dartmouth Atlas of Health Care* project found that the percentage of patients admitted one or more times to an intensive care unit during the last six months of life differed widely by region, from 23 percent to 45 percent (*Dartmouth Atlas of Health Care* 2003; Wennberg 2002) (see Figure 3.1). It might be tempting to suggest that this variation is important and has profound consequences on quality of care. Such an assertion, however, presumes that variation really exists in the observed data and that variation is inherently understood as undesirable. As we shall see, several distinct types of variation can be applied to studies of medical processes and outcomes. In addition, variation can be just as illuminating for what it offers in terms of innovation and improvement as it is instructive for what it can reveal in terms of irregularity and incompatibility (Wheeler 2000).

Background and Terminology

Statisticians, medical researchers and practitioners, and hospital administrators use and understand variation in ways that are sometimes compatible and sometimes mutually exclusive. Each definition is valuable in its particular application, so no one definition should be inferred as absolutely "correct" at the expense of another. For purposes of the present discussion, *variation* is the difference between an observed event and a standard or norm. Without this standard, or best practice, measurement of variation offers little beyond a description of the observations, with minimal, if any, understanding of what they mean (Gelbach 1993; Katz 2003; Wheeler 2000). Consequently, any measurement of variation in healthcare and its application to quality improvement must begin with the identification and

FIGURE 3.1
Percent of Medicare Enrollees Admitted to Intensive Care During the Last Six Months of Life, by Hospital Referral Regions (1995–96)

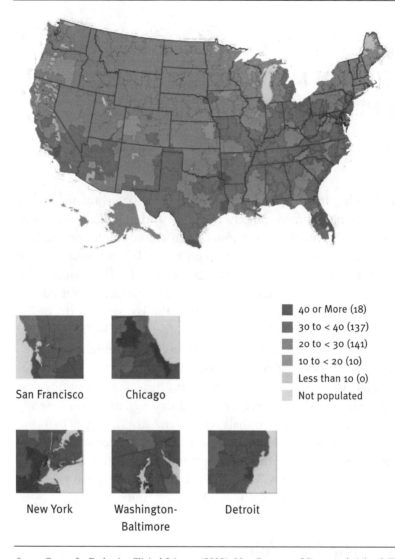

San Francisco

Chicago

New York

Washington-Baltimore

Detroit

■ 40 or More (18)
■ 30 to < 40 (137)
■ 20 to < 30 (141)
■ 10 to < 20 (10)
Less than 10 (0)
Not populated

Source: Center for Evaluative Clinical Sciences (2000). Map Courtesy of *Dartmouth Atlas.* © Trustees of Dartmouth College.

articulation of what is to be measured and the gold standard against which it is to be compared, a process based on extensive research, trial and error, and collaborative discussion.

Random Versus Assignable Variation

Variation can be either random or assignable (Wheeler 2000). *Random variation* is a physical attribute of the event or process, adheres to the laws of probability, and cannot be traced to a root cause. This is what one traditionally thinks of as "background noise" or "expected variation," and it is usually not worth studying in any great detail. *Assignable variation* arises from a single or small set of causes that are not part of the event or process and can therefore be traced, identified, and implemented or eliminated. In general, researchers are interested in assignable variation because they can link—or assign—variation to a single specific cause and act accordingly. This type of variation is generally easy to measure given the widespread training of healthcare quality researchers in statistical methods, breadth of tests and criteria for determining whether variation is assignable or random, and increasing sensitivity and power of numerical analysis. Measurement of assignable variation, however, is subject to potential misunderstanding because of complexity of design and interpretation, particularly in understanding true variation versus artifact or statistical error (Powell, Davies, and Thomson 2003; Samsa et al. 2002).

Process Variation

Our discussion uses three different categories of variation of quality in medical practice. The first of these is *process variation*, which is the difference in procedure throughout an organization. In this case, for example, one might measure the degree to which physicians use various screening methods for colorectal cancer. Some might prefer fecal occult blood testing, others might elect to use sigmoidoscopy or colonoscopy, and yet others might prescribe a combination of these tests. It is essential to distinguish between process and technique, however, the latter being the multitude of ways in which any given procedure can be performed within the realm of acceptable medical practice (Mottur-Pilson, Snow, and Bartlett 2001).

Outcome Variation

Another category is *outcome variation*, which is the difference in the results of any single process. This is ultimately what most healthcare quality researchers and medical practitioners want to know: which process yields the optimum results (Samsa et al. 2002). In some cases, this is easily determined, as the results of a particular process can be observed in relatively short order or procedural changes can be undertaken in a timely fashion. Unfortunately, genuine outcome variation requires study over an extended period, often years or decades, and many studies labeled as "outcome research" are largely "process research."

Performance Variation

The third category, and arguably the most important, is *performance variation*, which is the difference between any given result and the optimal or ideal result (Ballard 2003). This threshold, or best practice, is the standard against which all other measurements of variation are compared, although some key analytical tools, such as statistical process control, do not directly address performance relative to a gold standard. "From the perspective of the quality of care," argues one physician, "the variation that is the greatest cause for concern is that between actual practice and evidence-based 'best practice,'" and ultimately this is what performance variation measures (Steinberg 2003). Without knowing what is optimal, assignable variation is merely descriptive and of little value. Without some concept of a best practice, process variation offers little beyond an enumeration of methods to fulfill some task. Without a threshold value, outcome variation reveals only what happened over time, not the desirability of a particular outcome. Performance variation tells us where we are and how far we are from where want to be, as well as suggests ways to achieve the desired goal.

Variation in Medical Practice

The language of quality improvement in medical practice suggests a subjective and occasionally pejorative view of variation. Standard procedures, operating protocols, flowcharts, prescriptive guidelines, handbooks, and checklists are all intended to reduce or eliminate variation and hence the potential for error or excessive costs (Mottur-Pilson, Snow, and Bartlett 2001). There is also a widespread tendency to assume that variation implies ranking, that "measures reflect quality and that variations in the measures reflect variations in quality" (Powell, Davies, and Thomson 2003). This interpretation results from the attribution of causality between the processes of care provided and the observed quality measures—high measured performance reflects good actual performance, and low measured performance reflects poor actual performance. In many cases, this link between variation and quality is valid, but far too many times the link is tenuous at best, subjective, and not always supportable by research focused on the relation between process and outcome of care.

Variation, however, can be a profoundly desirable goal, as a successful procedure that differs from other, less successful procedures is by definition a variation. The objective, then, for quality improvement researchers is not simply to identify variation but to determine its *value*. If variation reveals a suboptimal process, the task at hand is to identify how the variation can be reduced or eliminated in ways that focus on the variation rather than the people involved. If the variation is good or desirable, it is essential to understand how can it be applied across an organization in an effort to improve quality more broadly. Put plainly, understanding the implications for quality of variation in medical practice is not simply learning how to eliminate variation per se but learning how to improve performance by identifying and accommodating good or suboptimal variation from a predefined best practice.

Scope and Use of Variation in Healthcare

The origins of quality assessment in healthcare in the United States can be traced to the pioneering work of Ernest A. Codman and the Mayo brothers during the early twentieth century (Codman 1984, 1996; Mallon 2000). By 1990, the National Academy of Sciences' Institute of Medicine (IOM) defined quality of care as the "degree to which health services for individuals and populations increase the likelihood of desired health outcomes and are consistent with current professional knowledge." A decade later, IOM further articulated the healthcare quality improvement challenge for the United States in three seminal reports (IOM 2000, 2001a, 2001b). Over the next ten years, the Joint Commission on Accreditation of Healthcare Organizations (Joint Commission 2003), U.S. Preventive Services Task Force (2003), National Quality Forum (2002), and Centers for Medicare & Medicaid Services (CMS 2003a) produced explicit indicators for quality measures.

Quality researchers use a variety of categories to measure improvements and detect variation in quality of care, including fiscal, service, and clinical indicators. Hospital-based clinical indicators, for example, incorporate those derived from the CMS Seventh Scope of Work measures and other advisory directives and include indicators pertaining to acute myocardial infarction (AMI), community-acquired pneumonia, and congestive heart failure (CMS 2003a). For each case, organizations may define a threshold, or green light, level, which indicates satisfactory compliance with acceptable standards of care (Ballard 2003). One example of a process-of-care measure for AMI is the administration of beta-blockers within 24 hours of admission: the threshold level is 90 percent; that is, based on the total number of AMI admissions at any one hospital or clinic or across any healthcare delivery system, at least 90 percent of admitted patients are afforded the preferred process of care.

Quality in healthcare is also measured by its ability to satisfy qualitative standards as well as quantitative thresholds. As mentioned throughout the book, IOM has established six aims for healthcare improvement to ensure that medical care is safe, timely, effective, efficient, equitable, and patient centered (Ballard 2003; IOM 2001a). As such, clinical indicators that address timeliness of care, for example, from several clinical domains—AMI, surgical infection prevention, community-acquired pneumonia—are aggregated to assess the appropriate level of time-dependent quality of care at a medical facility.

Variability plays an obvious role in identifying, measuring, and reporting these quality indicators and process-of-care improvements (Goldberg et al. 1994). For example, patient mix may make it difficult to compare process-of-care measures across multiple hospitals in the same system, creating the appearance of variation among facilities in providing these services. Consequently, some healthcare services administrators are reluctant to utilize quality improvement measures and indicators because they are perceived to be biased toward academic medical research centers or large healthcare organizations, which are not believed to experience broad variation (Miller et al. 2001). This is an unfortunate and false assumption, as quality improvement efforts can be and have been successfully applied to small organizations and practices, including single-physician practices (Geyman 1998; Miller et al. 2001).

Clinical and Operational Issues

Implementing best practices, establishing clinical indicators, and measuring and interpreting variation all involve considerable effort to create and sustain an environment conducive to sustaining these quality improvement efforts. An organization's size and complexity create functional, geographical, and other systemic constraints to success. The ability to collect appropriate and accurate data that can be rigorously analyzed requires assiduous planning (Ballard 2003). Patient demographics and physician case mix affect the data to be studied and can arbitrarily skew the conclusions.

Organizational Size

The size of an organization also affects the ability to disseminate best practices. One group of physicians in a large healthcare delivery system might have developed an effective method to achieve high levels of colorectal cancer screening (Stroud, Felton, and Spreadbury 2003), but the opportunity to describe, champion, and implement such process redesign across dozens of other groups within the system is much more challenging and typically will require incremental resource commitment. Large organizations tend to have rigid frameworks or bureaucracies; change is slow and requires perseverance and the ability to make clear to skeptics and enthusiasts alike the value of the new procedure in their group and across the system. Small practices may be equally difficult, especially if only one or two physicians or decision makers are involved and they are unwilling or uninterested in pursuing quality improvements. Irrespective of organizational size, there is often a complex matrix of demands for quality improvement and change agents, so simply changing one process in one location will not necessarily result in quality improvement, especially throughout an organization.

Large organizations also create the potential for multiple layers of quality assessment. The Baylor Health Care System (BHCS), located in the Dallas–Fort Worth area, includes 11 hospitals with 83,000 admissions per year and 47 primary care and senior centers with more than 500,000 visits annually. Consequently, BHCS evaluates its quality improvement efforts at both the hospital level and an outpatient level. Obviously, inpatient and outpatient processes of care differ; quality improvement efforts may be widely applicable for inpatient services at all 11 hospitals, but such process redesigns might not necessarily be applicable to the 47 outpatient clinics and senior centers.

Organizational Commitment

An organization's commitment to paying for quality improvement studies and implementation is equally affected by its size and infrastructure. Value-based purchasing is increasing, whereby consumers and insurers utilize those healthcare facilities that embrace quality improvement efforts and hence provide better processes of care and, arguably, outcomes. The Joint Commission, CMS, and Medicare have established minimum standard levels of quality and linked reimbursement schemes to achieving these goals. Although all healthcare organizations are obligated to meet these standards, a number of hospitals and delivery systems chose to use these standards before they were mandatory or have set higher threshold levels because of the compelling business case to do so. Increasing numbers of healthcare organizations fund these efforts internally, both for inpatients and outpatients, because it makes sense to do so in terms of outcomes, patient satisfaction, and long-term financial picture (happy patients return for additional care or recommend that friends and relatives use the same services) (Ballard 2003; Leatherman et al. 2003; Stroud, Felton, and Spreadbury 2003).

Planning the collection and analysis of suitable data for quality measures requires significant forethought, particularly when considering strategies to assess true variation and minimize false variation, and includes using appropriate measures, controlling case mix and other variables, minimizing chance variability, and using high-quality data (Powell, Davies, and Thomson 2003).

The initial results of a study that compared generalists to endocrinologists in providing care to patients with diabetes showed what most people might expect, that specialists provided better care. Adjusting for patient case-mix bias and clustering (physician-level variation) substantially altered the results: there was no difference between generalists and endocrinologists in providing care to diabetes patients. Studies must be designed with sufficient power and sophistication to account for a variety of confounding factors and require sufficient numbers of physicians and patients per physician to avoid distorting differences in quality of care between physician groups (Greenfield et al. 2002). Another study evaluated the relationship of complication rates of carotid endarectomy to processes of care and reported findings similar to the original diabetes survey. Initial analysis showed that facilities with high complication rates likely had substandard processes of care. By repeating the study at the same location but at a different time, researchers found substantially different complication rates and concluded that the "inability, in practice, to estimate complication rates at a high degree of precision is a fundamental difficulty for clinical policy making" (Samsa et al. 2002).

Strength of Data

Moreover, the data must also pass muster. Physicians and administrators alike may challenge results they do not like on the grounds that they consider the data "suspect" because of collection errors or other inaccuracies. For example, despite the impartiality of external records abstractors in gathering data from patient medical charts, critics might claim that these independent abstractors lack an insider's understanding or select data to fit an agenda, capriciously affecting the results. Patient socioeconomic status, age, gender, and ethnicity also influence physician profiles in medical practice variation and analysis efforts (Franks and Fiscella 2002).

Keys to Successful Implementation and Lessons Learned from Failures

Despite the inherent appeal in improving quality, considerable limits and barriers to the successful implementation of quality improvement projects exist. These barriers are subject to or the result of variation in culture, infrastructure, and economic influences across an organization, and overcoming them requires a stable infrastructure, sustained funding, and the testing of sequential hypotheses as to how to improve care.

Administrative and Physician Views

Issues that must be addressed to implement quality improvements include organizational mind-set, administrative and physician worldviews, and patient knowledge and expectations. The pace of quality improvement efforts is subject to considerable variability given an organization's propensity to change. In one example in a primary care setting, screening for colorectal cancer improved steadily from 47 percent to 86 percent over a two-year period (Stroud, Felton, and Spreadbury 2003). This evolutionary change minimized the barriers of revolutionary change, especially physician and administrator push-back, as well as other personal issues that are difficult to identify and alter (Eisenberg 2002). Success in adjusting culture to embrace quality improvement requires a long view that is sympathetic to converting daily practice into an environment that adapts accordingly. Many decision makers expect immediate and significant results and are sensitive to short-term variation in results that might suggest the improvements are inappropriate or not cost effective. A monthly drop in screening rates, for example, could be viewed as an indication that the screening protocol is not working and should be modified or abandoned altogether to conserve scarce resources. Then again, the observed decrease could be random variation and no cause for alarm or change (Wheeler 2000). Cultural tolerance to variation and change is a critical issue when considering successful factors to implementing quality improvement efforts, and it can be addressed by systemic adjustments and educational and motivational interventions (Donabedian and Bashur 2003; Palmer, Donabedian, and Povar 1991).

Physicians often think in terms of treating disease as it presents within each unique patient rather than in terms of population-based preventive care. As such, physician buy-in is critical to reducing undesired variation or creating new and successful clinical preventive services systems of care (Stroud, Felton, and Spreadbury 2003). The process includes training physician champions and investing in them to serve as models, mentors, and motivators, and it reduces the risk of alienating the key participants in quality improvement efforts. Physicians' failure—or refusal—to follow best practices is often linked inextricably to the presence—or absence—of adequate physician champions who have both the subject matter expertise and professional respect of their peers (Mottur-Pilson, Snow, and Bartlett 2001).

Patient Knowledge

Patient education is equally subject to variation in quality of care. Increasingly patients are aware of the status of their healthcare providers in terms of national rankings, public revelations of quality successes (and failures), and participation in reimbursement schemes (e.g., insurance, Medicare) that favor healthcare delivery systems that embrace quality improvement efforts. Participation in public awareness efforts such as the CMS Public Domain program, which makes variation and processes of care measures available to the public (both consumers and researchers), is another opportunity to educate patients about a healthcare organization and its commitment to quality (CMS 2003b; Hibbard, Stockard, and Tisler 2003; Lamb et al. 2003; Shaller et al. 2003).

Organizational Mind-set

Organizational infrastructure is an essential component in minimizing variation, disseminating best practices, and supporting a research agenda associated with quality improvements. Electronic medical records (EMRs), computerized physician order entry systems, and clinical decision support tools may reduce errors, allow sharing of specific best practices across large organizations, and enable the widespread automated collection of data to support quality improvement research (Bates and Gawande 2003; Bero et al. 1998; Casalino et al. 2003; Hunt et al. 1998). Healthcare organizations therefore are addressing the challenge to articulate and implement a long-term strategy to employ EMR resources. Unfortunately, the economic implications of both short- and long-term infrastructure investments undermine these efforts. Working in an environment that embraces short-term financial gain (in the form of either the quarterly report to stockholders or the report to the chairman of the board), physicians and hospital administrators "often face an outright disincentive to invest in an infrastructure that will improve compliance with best practices" (Leatherman et al. 2003).

Those same economic incentives may be effective in addressing variation in healthcare by awarding financial bonuses to physicians and administrators who meet quality targets or withholding bonuses from those who do not. This economic wake-up call makes it clear that future success within an organization is dependent on participating in quality improvement efforts, reducing undesirable variation in processes of care, and encouraging an environment conducive to quality research and improvement. In one such model being developed by the Health Texas Provider Network (the medical group practice component of BHCS), 5 percent of a physician's salary is withheld for quality targets based on preventive health services (70 percent) and patient satisfaction (30 percent). The threshold for quality parameters is to meet or exceed 25 percent of the overall group performance from the previous year. Quality performance money is awarded at the group level, with 10 percent of the total performance fund pool awarded to the group staff (Ballard 2003). The goal of such incentives is to help people understand that their organization is serious about implementing quality changes and minimizing unwanted variation to ensure alignment with national standards and directions in quality of care, and to encourage them to avail themselves of an organization's resources to help achieve these goals (Casalino et al. 2003).

Case Study

For the period of care from September 1999 to September 2002, BHCS measured its pneumococcal vaccine screening and administration performance for patients hospitalized with community-acquired pneumonia. At the Baylor-Irving Hospital, only 2 of 51 patients (4 percent) had medical record documentation that they received these processes of care, substantially below the goal of 90 percent specified by the BHCS Best Care

Committee (Ballard 2003). Initial assessments of this suboptimal performance showed superficial or incomplete medical history, lack of commitment to the screening process, and difficulty in obtaining accurate information from the admission source (e.g., nursing home) or patients, who often confused pneumococcal vaccination with a "flu shot" and therefore reported false prior vaccination.

Irving began a number of process improvement efforts designed to increase screening and vaccination rates, including improved physician and nurse education, improved history and immunization record assessment, and improved liaison with nursing homes. Screening levels improved substantially, but the immunization rate did not. The hospital staff next identified a physician champion and began developing a protocol and physician order set (a group of orders that relate to a specific health condition) that specifically included the pneumococcal vaccine. This proved time intensive, taking some ten months to approve and implement, and the delay hindered the rollout sufficiently to undermine its overall success. Physicians and nurses also disliked the presence of an additional step in the order process. Consequently, immunization rates improved somewhat but then dropped because of physician and nurse resistance to use of the order set. Additional physician-related interventions included multiple chart-based reminders and computer-generated forms that ordered vaccination prior to discharge. Despite these efforts, vaccination rates improved little, as the vaccination order was often overlooked or the patient was unwilling to delay hospital departure to await the vaccine.

Ultimately, Irving decided to implement automatic insertion by a case manager of a preprinted order in the chart for all patients older than 65 years of age who reported no prior pneumococcal vaccination; mandatory vaccination would be required within 72 hours of admission unless the patient's physician specifically canceled the order within 24 hours and included a compelling reason for cancellation (unjustified cases were referred to the Internal Medicine Peer Review Committee). Although there has been some fluctuation, this action led to the sustained improvement of vaccination rates at Irving.

The screening and vaccination rate at Irving rose from 4 percent in January 2000 to 91 percent in June 2003. The XmR chart in Figure 3.2 depicts the average moving range (hence its name) of the screening and vaccination results by month as compared to the weighted average, bounded by an upper process limit and a lower process limit. Although gaps in the data during 1999, 2000, and 2001 exist, a large jump in screening and vaccination percentages occurred, from single digits to figures ranging from 70 percent to 100 percent. Applying a run chart for the period from June 2001 to June 2003 shows fewer than seven data points on one side of the weighted average, so Figure 3.2 shows that the change in screening rates at Irving was the result of assignable variation (Hart and Hart 2002).

This assignable variation tells us that the screening and vaccination protocols Irving implemented resulted in real improvements at one hospital. We can compare Irving's results with other BHCS hospitals to see if other facilities improved independently during the same time frame. Figure 3.3 compares Irving's average screening and vaccination rate of 84 percent to the 53 percent average at five other BHCS hospitals. Moreover, Irving's rate exceeded the Joint Commission–accredited hospitals' national median rate of 29 percent and was substantially above the 64 percent rate achieved nationwide by 90 percent of Joint Commission–accredited hospitals. The difference in the rates at Irving and at other BHCS hospitals suggests that Irving is doing something different from the remaining BHCS hospitals, although this conclusion is largely intuitive and does not necessarily exclude random variation in accounting for this difference.

The process control chart (or "p chart") in Figure 3.4 shows that Irving's performance in screening and vaccination rates is indeed statistically different from that of the other BHCS hospitals. The screening rate (expressed here as a proportion) of 0.84 falls outside the upper confidence limit (which measures the same thing as an upper process limit) and is therefore by definition the result of assignable variation (Hart and Hart 2002). Not only does this process control chart demonstrate that Irving's standing order protocol is *different* from those of other BHCS hospitals, but it also shows that Irving's results are significantly *better* than those of other BHCS hospitals. Based on this clearly identified and positive variation, BHCS leaders and medical staff can evaluate changes to existing protocols at other BHCS hospitals to take advantage of Irving's successful experience and implement changes systemwide. Indeed, in September 2003 both Baylor-Garland and Baylor University Medical Center implemented Irving's standing order protocol. Over time, these improvements can be measured to determine their broader success.

Conclusion

Contemporary industrial and commercial methods to improve quality, such as Six Sigma and ISO 9000, emphasize the need to minimize variation, if not eliminate it altogether. While certainly appropriate in a setting that requires the repetitive manufacturing of mass quantities of identical products, these tools may unnecessarily mask variation in the healthcare environment and consequently obscure opportunities to change or improve essential processes of care. The keys to successful management—rather than elimination—of variation in pursuit of quality healthcare are to be able to

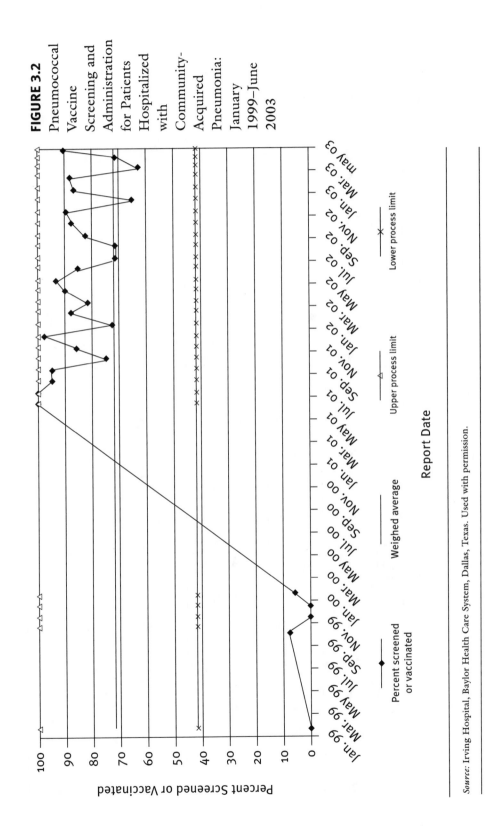

FIGURE 3.2

Pneumococcal Vaccine Screening and Administration for Patients Hospitalized with Community-Acquired Pneumonia: January 1999–June 2003

Source: Irving Hospital, Baylor Health Care System, Dallas, Texas. Used with permission.

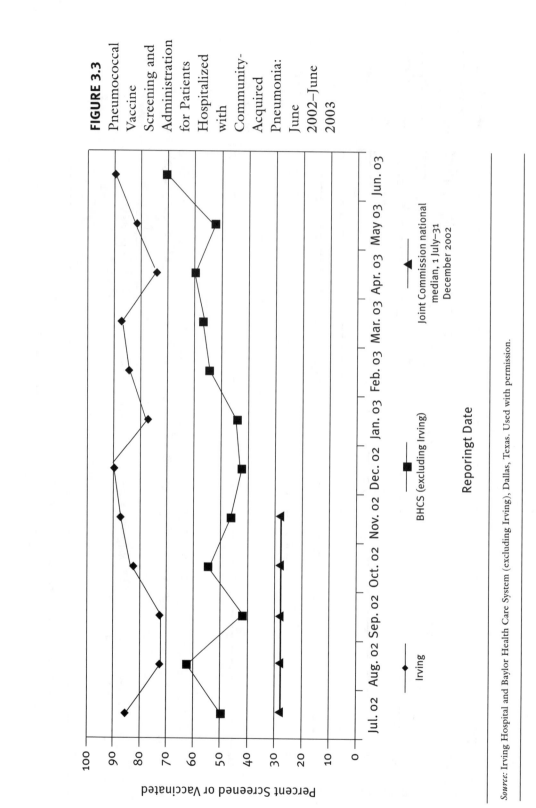

FIGURE 3.3

Pneumococcal Vaccine Screening and Administration for Patients Hospitalized with Community-Acquired Pneumonia: June 2002–June 2003

Source: Irving Hospital and Baylor Health Care System (excluding Irving), Dallas, Texas. Used with permission.

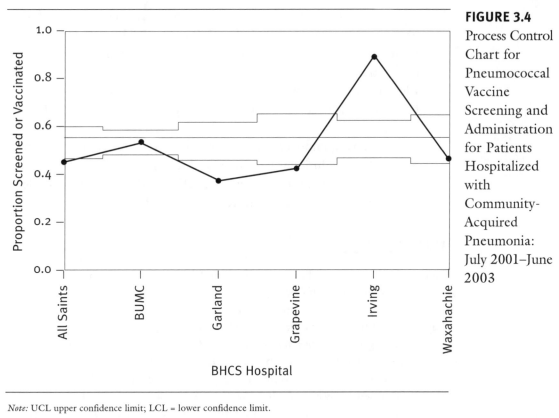

FIGURE 3.4
Process Control Chart for Pneumococcal Vaccine Screening and Administration for Patients Hospitalized with Community-Acquired Pneumonia: July 2001–June 2003

Note: UCL upper confidence limit; LCL = lower confidence limit.

Source: Baylor Health Care System, Dallas, Texas. Used with permission.

identify variation; distinguish between random and assignable variation; determine the meaning, importance, or value of the observed variation relative to some standard; and then implement methods that will take advantage of or rectify what the variation reveals. Ultimately, variation tells us what is working and what is not and how far from optimal our healthcare processes really are. Rather than avoiding variation in pursuit of quality healthcare, we are better off embracing it as an essential method of assessing our progress toward success.

Study Questions

1. While exploring opportunities to improve processes of care for a group practice, you find no variability across physicians over time for colorectal cancer screening based on the recommendation of the U.S. Preventive Services Task Force. Is this optimal? Why or why not?

2. Discuss the role of financial compensation strategies as part of the process to reduce variation in medical practice. How effective are these financial incentives, especially in terms of timing or use with other strategies?
3. Identify different ways to distinguish between random and assignable variation. Be sure to assess the strengths and weaknesses of each method.
4. In many cases, improvements in healthcare quality are small "incremental," or evolutionary, changes and not necessarily "breakthrough," or revolutionary, changes. Discuss the value of multiple small variations to effect long-term, sustained improvement.

REFERENCES

Ballard, D. J. 2003. "Indicators to Improve Clinical Quality Across an Integrated Health Care System." *International Journal of Quality in Health Care* 15 (6 Suppl.): 1–11.

Bates, D. W., and A. A. Gawande. 2003. "Improving Safety with Information Technology." *New England Journal of Medicine* 348: 2526–34.

Bero, L. A., R. Grilli, J. M. Grimshaw, E. Harvey, A. D. Oxman, and M. A. Thomson. 1998. "Closing the Gap Between Research and Practice: An Overview of Systematic Reviews of Interventions to Promote the Implementation of Research Findings." *British Medical Journal* 317: 465–68.

Casalino, L., R. R. Gillies, S. M. Shortell, J. A. Schmittdiel, T. Bodenheimer, J. C. Robinson, T. Rundall, N. Oswald, H. Schauffler, and M. C. Wang. 2003. "External Incentives, Information Technology, and Organized Processes to Improve Health Care Quality for Patients with Chronic Diseases." *Journal of the American Medical Association* 289 (4): 434–41.

Center for Evaluative Clinical Sciences. 2000. *Dartmouth Atlas*. Hanover, NH: Dartmouth College.

Centers for Medicare & Medicaid Services. 2003a. "Quality Improvement Organizations (QIOs) Statement of Work." [Online information; retrieved 9/22/03.] http://cms.hhs.gov/qio/2.asp.

———. 2003b. "Overview of Hospital CAHPS." [Online information; retrieved 9/22/03.] www.cms.hhs.gov/quality/hospital/HCAHPSqanda3.pdf.

Codman, E. A. 1934, Reprinted 1984. *The Shoulder: Rupture of the Supraspinatus Tendon and Other Lesions in or About the Subacromial Bursa*. Malabar, FL: Krieger Publishing.

———. 1917, Reprinted 1996. *A Study in Hospital Efficiency as Demonstrated by the Case Report of the First Five Years of a Private Hospital*. Oakbrook Terrace, IL: Joint Commission on Accreditation of Healthcare Organizations.

Dartmouth Atlas of Health Care. 2003. [Online information; retrieved
    9/22/03.] www.dartmouthatlas.org/99US/chap_6_sec_3.php.

Donabedian, A., and R. Bashur (eds.). 2003. *An Introduction to Quality
    Assurance in Health Care.* New York: Oxford University Press.

Eisenberg, J. M. 2002. "Measuring Quality: Are We Ready to Compare the
    Quality of Care Among Physician Groups?" *Annals of Internal Medicine*
    136: 153–54.

Franks, P., and K. Fiscella. 2002. "Effect of Patient Socioeconomic Status on
    Physician Profiles for Prevention, Disease Management, and Diagnostic
    Testing Costs." *Medical Care* 40 (8): 717–24.

Gelbach, S. H. 1993. "Study Design: The Experimental Approach." In
    Interpreting the Medical Literature, 3rd ed., pp 78–108. New York:
    McGraw-Hill.

Geyman, J. P. 1998. "Evidence-Based Medicine in Primary Care: An Overview."
    Journal of the American Board of Family Practice 11 (1): 46–56.

Goldberg, H. I., M. A. Cummings, E. P. Steinberg, E. M. Ricci, T. Shannon, S.
    B. Soumerai, B. S. Mittman, J. Eisenberg, D. A. Heck, S. Kaplan, et al.
    1994. "Deliberations on the Dissemination of PORT Products:
    Translating Research Findings into Improved Patient Outcomes."
    Medical Care 32 (7 Suppl.): JS90–110.

Greenfield, S., S. H. Kaplan, R. Kahn, J. Ninomiya, and J. L. Griffith. 2002.
    "Profiling Care Provided by Different Groups of Physicians: Effects of
    Patient Case-Mix (Bias) and Physician-Level Clustering on Quality
    Assessment Results." *Annals of Internal Medicine* 136: 111–21.

Hart, M. K., and R. F. Hart. 2002. *Statistical Process Control for Health Care.*
    Pacific Grove, CA: Duxbury.

Hibbard, J. H., J. Stockard, and M. Tisler. 2003. "Does Publicizing Hospital
    Performance Stimulate Quality Improvement Efforts?" *Health Affairs* 22
    (2): 84–94.

Hunt, D. L., R. B. Haynes, S. E. Hanna, and K. Smith. 1998. "Effects of
    Computer-Based Clinical Decision Support Systems on Physician
    Performance and Patient Outcomes: A Systematic Review." *Journal of the
    American Medical Association* 280: 1339–46.

Institute of Medicine. 1990. *Medicare: A Strategy for Quality Assurance. Vol. 1,*
    p. 4. Washington, DC: National Academy Press.

———. 2000. *To Err Is Human: Building a Safer Health System.* Washington,
    DC: National Academy Press.

———. 2001a. *Crossing the Quality Chasm: A New Health System for the 21st
    Century.* Washington, DC: National Academy Press.

———. 2001b. *Envisioning the National Health Care Quality Report.*
    Washington, DC: National Academy Press.

Joint Commission on Accreditation of Healthcare Organizations. 2003. "A
    Comprehensive Review of Development and Testing for National
    Implementation of Hospital Core Measures." [Online information;

retrieved 9/10/03.] www.jcaho.org/pms/core+measures/cr_hos_
cm.htm.

Katz, M. H. 2003. "Multivariable Analysis: A Primer for Readers of Medical
Research." *Annals of Internal Medicine* 138: 644–50.

Lamb, R. M., D. M. Studdert, R. M. J. Bohmer, D. M. Berwick, and T. A.
Brennan. 2003. "Hospital Disclosure Practices: Results of a National
Survey." *Health Affairs* 22 (2): 73–83.

Leatherman, S., D. Berwick, D. Iles, L. S. Lewin, F. Davidoff, T. Nolan, and M.
Bisognano. 2003. "The Business Case for Quality: Case Studies and an
Analysis." *Health Affairs (Millwood)* 22 (2): 17–30.

Mallon, W. J. 2000. *Ernest Amory Codman: The End Result of a Life in
Medicine.* Philadelphia: W.B. Saunders.

Miller, W. L., R. R. McDaniel, B. F. Crabtree, and K. C. Stange. 2001.
"Practice Jazz: Understanding Variation in Family Practices Using
Complexity Science." *Journal of Family Practice* 50 (10): 872–78.

Mottur-Pilson, C., V. Snow, and K. Bartlett. 2001. "Physician Explanations for
Failing to Comply with 'Best Practices.'" *Effective Clinical Practice* 4:
207–13.

National Quality Forum. 2002. "National Consensus Standards Endorsed for
Monitoring the Quality of Care for Diabetes [Press Release]." [Online
information; retrieved 9/22/03.] www.qualityforum.org/prdiabetes10-
01-02FINAL.pdf.

Palmer, R. H., A. Donabedian, and G. J. Povar. 1991. *Striving for Quality in
Health Care: An Inquiry into Practice and Policy.* Chicago: Health
Administration Press.

Powell, A. E., H. T. O. Davies, and R. G. Thomson. 2003. "Using Routine
Comparative Data to Assess the Quality of Health Care: Understanding
and Avoiding Common Pitfalls." *Quality and Safety in Health Care* 12:
122–28.

Reinertsen, J. L. 2003. "Zen and the Art of Physician Autonomy Maintenance."
Annals of Internal Medicine 138: 992–95.

Samsa, G., E. Z. Oddone, R. Horner, J. Daley, W. Henderson, and D. B.
Matchar. 2002. "To What Extent Should Quality of Care Decisions Be
Based on Health Outcomes? Application to Carotid Endarectomy."
Stroke 33: 2944–49.

Shaller, D., S. Sofaer, S. D. Findlay, J. H. Hibbard, D. Lansky, and S. Delbanco.
2003. "Consumers and Quality-Driven Health Care: A Call to Action."
Health Affairs 22 (2): 95–101.

Steinberg, E. P. 2003. "Improving the Quality of Care—Can We Practice What
We Preach?" *New England Journal of Medicine* 348: 2681–83.

Stroud, J., C. Felton, and B. Spreadbury. 2003. "Collaborative Colorectal
Cancer Screening: A Successful Quality Improvement Initiative." *BUMC
Proceedings* 16: 341–44.

U.S. Preventive Services Task Force. 2003. "Guide to Clinical Preventive Services, 3rd ed., 2000–2002." [Online information; retrieved 9/22/03.] www.ahrq.gov/clinic/cps3dix.htm.

Wennberg, J. E. 2002. "Unwarranted Variations in Healthcare Delivery: Implications for Academic Medical Centres." *British Medical Journal* 325 (26 Oct.): 961–64.

Wheeler, D. J. 2000. *Understanding Variation: The Key to Managing Chaos,* 2nd ed. Knoxville, TN: SPC Press.

QUALITY IMPROVEMENT SYSTEMS, THEORIES, AND TOOLS

Mike Stoecklein

This chapter describes some of the tools and methods that can be used to improve the quality of healthcare. Included are a number of different tool-kits and approaches to quality improvement. Although they may have different names and categories, you will recognize core commonalities in methods across these approaches. As a starting point, Figure 4.1, an adaptation of the work of Barbara Lawton (1996), is a framework for understanding the tools and methods—the "tip of the iceberg"—and the ideas and theories behind the tools—the "base of the iceberg."

Theories, Paradigms, and Assumptions: Foundation of the Iceberg Model

The following section describes some of the theories that form the foundation of the quality improvement iceberg, and ultimately the tools and methods used for improvement. The contributions of some of the primary quality improvement thought leaders are summarized.

Walter Shewhart

As part of his work at Western Electric Co., Walter Shewhart had the task of ensuring the reliability of the national system of telephone exchanges and the production of telephones. Although his Ph.D. was in physics, Shewhart used his understanding of statistics to design a tool to help guide the appropriate action to take in response to variation. In 1924, Shewhart explained how a control chart can differentiate random variation (common cause) from assignable (special) causes. Prior to this, workers reacted to each new data point in an effort to improve the future output. The result of this tampering actually made matters worse. Shewhart felt that his most important contribution was not the control chart, but rather his work on "operational definitions," ensuring that people used common operations to define what they measured (Kilian 1988).

FIGURE 4.1
Framework for
Viewing
Quality-
Improvement
Tools and
Methods

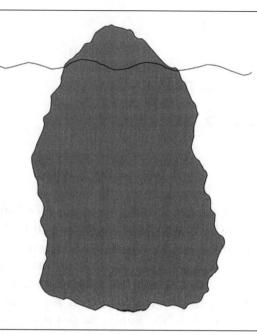

Tools, methods, and procedures
(what we can see and do)

Systems and processes
(under the surface—unseen;
shaped by our theories)

Theories, paradigms, and
assumptions
(deep under the surface,
we are largely unaware of
them; shape the systems
and processes we design)

W. Edwards Deming

Deming combined what he learned from Shewhart and others and, over the course of several decades, developed a theory of improvement. In the 1970s, Deming provided his "14 Points for Western Management" in response requests from U.S. managers for the secret to the radical improvement that Japanese companies were achieving in a number of industries. Deming was one of several statisticians and advisors who provided guidance at the request of Japanese industry leaders in the 1950s. Deming's 14 points represented a unified body of knowledge that ran counter to the conventional wisdom of most U.S. managers. Deming's 14 points for management are as follows (Neave 1990):

1. Create constancy of purpose for continual improvement of products and service to society.
2. Adopt the new philosophy. We are in a new economic age created in Japan.
3. Eliminate the need for mass inspection as a way of life to achieve quality.
4. End the practice of awarding business solely on the basis of price tag.
5. Improve constantly and forever every process for planning, production, and service.

6. Institute modern methods of training on the job for all, including management.
7. Adopt and institute leadership aimed at helping people to do a better job.
8. Encourage effective two-way communication and other means to drive out fear throughout the organization.
9. Break down barriers between departments and staff areas.
10. Eliminate the use of slogans, posters, and exhortations for the workforce that do not provide methods.
11. Eliminate work standards that prescribe quotas for the workforce and numerical goals for people in management.
12. Remove the barriers that rob hourly workers, and people in management, of their right to pride of workmanship.
13. Institute a vigorous program of education and encourage self-improvement for everyone.
14. Clearly define top management's permanent commitment to ever-improving quality and productivity and their obligation to implement all of these principles.

Over time, Deming spoke less about the 14 points and more about their source—"a system of profound knowledge." Deming described this system as an understanding of four components: (1) variation (Shewhart's influence); (2) theory of knowledge; (3) appreciation for a system; and (4) psychology and the interactions between the components (Neave 1990).

Deming described the Plan-Do-Study-Act (PDSA) cycle, which can be traced to Shewhart. Deming referred to PDSA as a cycle for learning and a cycle for improvement. Some have changed the "S" to "C" (PDCA cycle), but Deming preferred the use of *study* rather than *check* (Neave 1990, 139).

Joseph M. Juran

Juran, specializing in managing for quality, is the coauthor of *Juran's Quality Control Handbook* (Juran and Gryna 1951) and also consulted with Japanese companies in the 1950s. Juran defined quality as consisting of two different but related concepts. The first form of quality is income oriented and consists of those features of the product that meet customer needs and thereby produce income. In this sense, higher quality costs more. The second form of quality is cost oriented and consists of freedom from failures and deficiencies. In this sense, higher quality usually costs less (American Society for Quality 2000). "The Juran Trilogy" describes three interrelated processes: quality planning, quality control, and quality improvement (Juran 1989).

Taiichi Ohno

Ohno is generally credited with developing the Toyota Production System (or lean thinking). He described *muda* (a Japanese word that means "waste") and identified seven categories of muda (Heim 1999):

1. Overproduction
2. Inventory
3. Repairs/rejects
4. Motion
5. Processing
6. Waiting
7. Transport

The seven types of waste all represent activities that do not add value to the process.

Philip B. Crosby

Crosby introduced the idea of zero defects in 1961 and defined quality as "conformance to requirements," with quality measured as the "cost of non-conformance." Crosby equated quality management with prevention, believing that inspecting, checking, and other nonpreventive techniques have no place in quality management. Crosby also felt that statistical levels of compliance tend to program people for failure and that there is absolutely no reason for having errors or defects in any product or service. He felt that companies should adopt a quality "vaccine" to prevent nonconformance, with the three ingredients being determination, education, and implementation (American Society for Quality 2000).

Armand V. Feigenbaum

Feigenbaum originated the concept of total quality control (TQC) in his 1951 book. Feigenbaum approached quality as a strategic business tool that requires awareness by everyone in the company, in the same manner that most companies view cost and revenue. He felt that quality reaches far beyond managing defects in production and should be a philosophy and a commitment to excellence. Feigenbaum defined TQC as excellence driven rather than defect driven. His approach to quality is outlined in "Three Steps to Quality: Quality Leadership, Modern Quality Technology, and Organizational Commitment" (American Society for Quality 2000).

Kaoru Ishikawa

Ishikawa was a student of Deming and a member of the Union of Japanese Scientists and Engineers. Ishikawa edited the *Guide to Quality Control* and is also known for developing the cause-and-effect diagram. Ishikawa described TQC as follows (American Society for Quality 2000):

- The responsibility of all workers and all divisions.
- A group activity that calls for teamwork that cannot be done by individuals.
- An activity that will not fail if everyone (from the president to the line workers) cooperates.
- TQC will likely generate discussion and criticism about middle management.
- Quality control circles are a part of TQC.
- Objectives should not be confused with the means to attain them.
- TQC will not work miracles.

Systems and Processes: Middle of the Iceberg Model

We now turn our attention to the middle level of the iceberg model to describe some of the systems and processes that guide quality improvement efforts. To reiterate, these are logical consequences derived from some of the ideas and theories developed by thought leaders, some of whom were described in the previous section. A number of the more formally recognized systems and models are listed below (in alphabetical order).

API Improvement Model

Tom Nolan and Lloyd Provost, cofounders of Associates for Process Improvement (API), developed a simple model for improvement based on Deming's PDSA cycle. The model (see Figure 4.2) contains three fundamental questions that form the basis of improvement: What are we trying to accomplish? How will we know that a change is an improvement? What changes can we make that will result in improvement? Focus on the three questions and the PDSA cycle allows for the application of the model to be as simple or sophisticated as necessary (Langley et al. 1996).

Baldrige Criteria and Related Systems

The Malcolm Baldrige National Quality Award—named for Malcolm Baldrige, who served as Secretary of Commerce from 1981 until his death in 1987—was created by Public Law 100-107, signed in 1987. This law led to the creation of a new public-private partnership to improve the United States's competitiveness.

The Baldrige criteria were originally developed and applied to businesses; however, in 1997, healthcare-specific criteria were created to help healthcare organizations address challenges such as focusing on core competencies, introducing new technologies, reducing costs, communicating

FIGURE 4.2
API
Improvement
Model

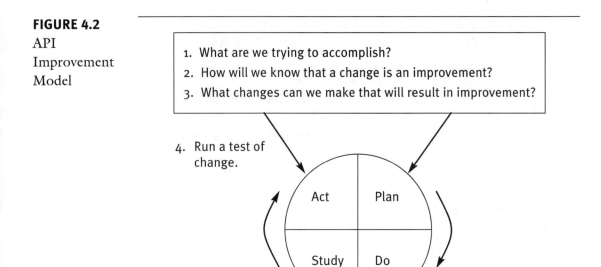

1. What are we trying to accomplish?
2. How will we know that a change is an improvement?
3. What changes can we make that will result in improvement?

4. Run a test of change.

Act | Plan
Study | Do

Source: Langley et al. (1996).

and sharing information electronically, establishing new alliances with healthcare providers, or just maintaining market advantage. The criteria can be used to assess performance on a wide range of key indicators: healthcare outcomes; patient satisfaction; and operational, staff, and financial indicators. The criteria can also help organizations to align resources and initiatives such as ISO 9000, PDSA cycles, and Six Sigma; improve communication, productivity, and effectiveness; and achieve strategic goals.

The Baldrige healthcare criteria are built on the following set of interrelated core values and concepts:

- Visionary leadership
- Patient-focused excellence
- Organizational and personal learning
- Valuing staff and partners
- Agility
- Focus on the future
- Managing for innovation
- Management by fact
- Social responsibility and community health
- Focus on results and creating value
- Systems perspective

The criteria are organized into seven interdependent categories (National Institute of Standards and Technology 2003):

1. Leadership
2. Strategic planning
3. Focus on patients, other customers, and markets
4. Measurement, analysis, and knowledge management
5. Staff focus
6. Process management
7. Organizational performance results

Similar models are in place in Europe and in individual U.S. states.

FOCUS-PDCA

In the 1980s, Dr. Paul Batalden formed the Quality Resource Group, part of the Hospital Corporation of America, as an internal consulting division in the application of continual improvement. The Quality Resource Group designed the FOCUS-PDCA model to help guide a team's improvement efforts (Strickland 2003): FOCUS-PDCA is an acronym for the following:

- Find an opportunity for improvement.
- Organize an effort (includes assigning a team).
- Clarify current understanding of how the process works.
- Understand the process variation and capability.
- Select a strategy for improvement.
- The PDCA cycle tests the strategy to determine if it results in improvement.

IHI Breakthrough Series Model

The Institute for Healthcare Improvement (IHI) has designed a model to support its breakthrough collaborative series. A collaborative consists of 20 to 40 healthcare organizations working together for six to eight months on improving a specific clinical or operational area. Under the guidance of an IHI panel of national experts, team members study, test, and implement the latest knowledge available to produce rapid improvements in their organizations. A collaborative represents an intensive effort of healthcare professionals making significant changes that improve clinical outcomes and reduce costs (IHI 2003). An adaptation of the Breakthrough Series model is shown in Figure 4.3.

ISO 9000

The International Organization for Standardization (ISO) is a non-governmental entity founded in 1947 by 25 countries to develop volun-

FIGURE 4.3

IHI
Breakthrough
Series Model

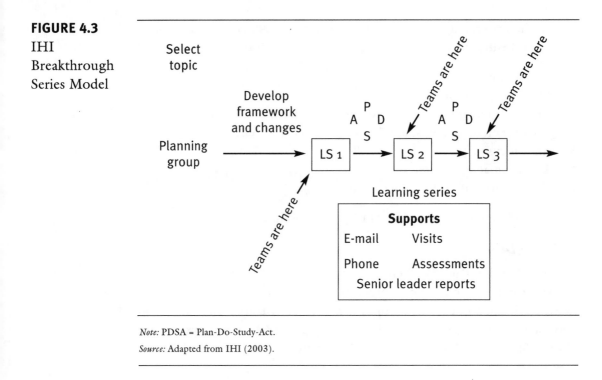

Note: PDSA = Plan-Do-Study-Act.

Source: Adapted from IHI (2003).

tary technical standards for international businesses. Its intent was to provide consensus for an approved methodology that would ensure consistency in manufacturing through standardization of processes and services to conform with and fulfill world-market customer requirements.

The ISO 9000 Quality Management System was created in 1987 to provide a nonprescriptive management system quality standard for non-technical business functions. It was further improved in 1994 and released as three distinct standards (ISO 9001, 9002, and 9003). The most recent version of ISO 9000 is ISO 9001:2000 (Dillon 2002). ISO 9000 has been more widely accepted and applied in countries other than the United States but appears to be the focus of increased interest as a model for organizing quality improvement activities (Tsiakals, Ciavrani, and West 2002).

Kaizen

Kaizen is a Japanese word for "improvement." The term indicates ongoing improvement involving everyone, including both managers and workers. The kaizen philosophy assumes that our way of life (work, social, home) deserves to be constantly improved. The kaizen concept includes a number of improvement practices (Imai 1986), including the following:

- Customer orientation
- TQC
- Robotics
- Quality control circles
- Suggestion system
- Automation
- Discipline in the organization
- Total productive maintenance
- Kamban
- Quality improvement
- Just-in-time
- Zero defects
- Small-group activities
- Cooperative labor-management relations
- Productivity improvement
- New-product development

Lean Thinking

Lean thinking, sometimes called lean manufacturing or the Toyota Production System, focuses on the removal of waste, which is defined as anything not necessary to produce the product or service. One common measure is touch time—the amount of time the product is actually being worked on, or touched, by the worker. Frequently, the focus of lean thinking is manifested in an emphasis on flow (Nave 2002). Its starting point is value, and the ultimate customer defines what value is; anything in excess of this value is waste.

Lean thinking consists of five steps:

1. Identify which features create value.
2. Identify the sequence of activities, called the value stream.
3. Make the activities flow.
4. Let the customer pull the product or service through the process.
5. Perfect the process.

While lean thinking focuses on removing waste and improving flow, it also has some secondary effects. Quality is improved. The product spends less time in process, reducing the chances of damage or obsolescence. Simplification of processes results in less variation, more uniform output, and less inventory (Heim 1999). As the company looks at all the activities in the value stream, the system constraint is removed and performance is improved.

The lean methodology also makes the following assumptions:

1. People value the visual effect of flow.
2. Waste is the main restriction to profitability.

3. Many small improvements in rapid succession are more beneficial than analytical study.

4. Process interaction effects will be resolved through value stream refinement.

5. People in operations appreciate this approach.

6. Lean involves many people in the value stream. Transitioning to flow thinking causes vast changes in how people perceive their roles in the organization and their relationships to the product.

Six Sigma

Six Sigma is a system for improvement that was developed over time by Hewlett-Packard, Motorola, General Electric, and others in the 1980s and 1990s (Pande, Neuman, and Cavanagh 2000). The tools used in Six Sigma are not new. The thinking behind this system came from the foundations of quality improvement from the 1930s through 1950s. What makes Six Sigma appear new is the rigor of tying improvement projects to key business processes and clear roles and responsibilities for executives, champions, master black belts, black belts, and green belts.

The aim of Six Sigma is to reduce variation (eliminate defects) in key business processes. By using a set of statistical tools to understand the fluctuation of a process, management can begin to predict the expected outcome of that process. If the outcome is not satisfactory, associated tools can be used to further understand the elements influencing that process. Six Sigma includes five steps—define, measure, analyze, improve, and control—commonly known as DMAIC:

- *Define:* Practitioners begin by defining the process. They ask who the customers are and what their problems are. They identify the key characteristics important to the customer along with the processes that support those key characteristics. They then identify existing output conditions along with the process elements.
- *Measure:* Next, the focus is on measuring the process. Key characteristics are categorized, measurement systems are verified, and data are collected.
- *Analyze:* Once data are collected, they are analyzed. The intent is to convert the raw data into information that provides insights into the process. These insights include identifying the fundamental and most important causes of the defects or problems.
- *Improve:* The fourth step is to improve the process. Solutions to the problem are developed, and changes are made to the process. Results of process changes are seen in the measurements. In this step, the company can judge whether the changes are beneficial or if another set of changes is necessary.

- *Control:* If the process is performing at a desired and predictable level, it is put under control. This last step is the sustaining portion of the Six Sigma methodology. The process is monitored to ensure that no unexpected changes occur.

For Six Sigma, the primary theory is, "If we focus on reducing variation, we will have more uniform process output." Secondary effects include less waste, less throughput time, and less inventory (Heim 1999).

Theory of Constraints

Theory of constraints (TOC) is a thinking process that focuses on system improvement to maximize customer value while minimizing expense. An analogy for a system is the chain—a group of interdependent links working together toward the overall goal. The constraint is a weak link; the performance of the entire chain is limited by the strength of the weakest link. TOC concentrates on the process that slows the speed of product through the system (Nave 2002).

TOC consists of the following five steps:

1. *Identify the constraint.* The constraint is identified through various methods. The amount of work in queue ahead of a process operation is a classic indicator; another example is where products are processed in batches.
2. *Exploit the constraint.* Once the constraint is identified, the process is improved or otherwise supported to achieve its utmost capacity without major expensive upgrades or changes.
3. *Subordinate other processes to the constraint.* When the constraining process is working at maximum capacity, the speeds of other subordinate processes are paced to the speed or capacity of the constraint. Some processes will sacrifice individual productivity for the benefit of the entire system. Subordinate processes are usually found ahead of the constraint in the value stream. Processes after the constraint are not a major concern—they are probably already producing under capacity because they have to wait for the constraining process.
4. *Elevate the constraint.* If the output of the overall system is not satisfactory, further improvement is required. The company may now contemplate major changes to the constraint. Changes can involve capital improvement, reorganization, or other major expenditures of time or money. Elevating the constraint involves taking whatever action is necessary to eliminate it.
5. *Repeat the cycle.* Once the first constraint is broken, another part of the system or process chain becomes the new constraint. Now is the time to repeat the cycle of improvement. The performance of the

entire system is reevaluated by searching for the new constraint process, exploiting the process, subordinating, and elevating.

By focusing on constraints, this methodology produces positive effects on the flow time of the product or service through the system. Reduction of waste in the constraint increases throughput and improves throughput time. When the constraint is improved, variation is reduced and quality is improved. Constraint focus does not require intimate knowledge of data analysis or that a large number of people understand the elements of the system. The understanding of a few people with the power to change things is all that is necessary; the effort can be localized with minimum involvement of the workforce.

TOC methodology operates on the following assumptions:

1. As in the case of lean thinking, the organization places a value on the speed at which its product or service travels through the system. Speed and volume are the main determinants of success.
2. Current processes are essential to produce the desired output.
3. The product or service design is stable.
4. Value-added workers do not need to have an in-depth understanding of this improvement methodology. Suggestions by the workforce are not considered vital for successful implementation of TOC.

For TOC, the primary theory is, "If we focus on constraints, throughput volume will improve." Secondary effects include less inventory and a different accounting system. TOC uses five tools (current reality tree, conflict resolution diagram, future reality tree, prerequisite tree, and transition tree) in its ongoing improvement process (Heim 1999).

Total Quality Management

Total quality management (TQM) has been defined as a holistic approach to running an organization such that every facet earns the description *quality* (Grandzol 1997). TQM systems range from the all inclusive (Pegels 1995) to the common sense and concise (Cohen and Brand 1993). Some are based on various dimensions of quality (Garvin 1987), whereas others stress management commitment, structure/strategy, training, problem identification, measurement, and culture (Talley 1991). Some emphasize TQM as a philosophy (Drummond 1992), whereas others proclaim that it represents a social revolution in the workplace (Hutchins 1992). Some have incorrectly attributed the term TQM to W. Edwards Deming, who abhorred it. Any attendee who used the term during the question-answer period of Deming's four-day seminar learned that lesson quickly and publicly.

Tools, Methods, and Procedures:
Tip of the Iceberg Model

As with icebergs, where only a small portion is actually visible above the surface, what we see in an organization (behaviors, methods, practices) is only the tip of the iceberg. The visible part of the iceberg is supported by a large, unseen structure.

Tools, methods, and procedures are analogous to the tip of the iceberg. We can observe people using tools and methods for improvement. We can see them making a flowchart, plotting a control chart, or using a checklist. These tools and procedures are the logical results of systems and models that people put in place (knowingly and unknowingly). People may use several tools and procedures to make improvements, and these tools might form one part of an improvement system. Although we can observe people using the tools of the system, the system itself is invisible and cannot be observed. These systems come from theories that might be shared among many people who work together to improve quality, or they may come from ideas held by individuals. People do not often consider why they do what they do. Several probing questions may be necessary to bring to the surface the underlying assumptions behind the systems in place.

One of the difficult things about quality is explaining how a *tool* is different from a *process* or *system*. For example, the previous section described ISO 9000 and the Baldrige criteria. ISO 9000 is a quality management system, and the Baldrige criteria represent a framework to assess an organization's performance management system to achieve excellence. Neither are tools, but rather models that describe how tools can be used. Another example is the current emphasis on lean production and Six Sigma in U.S. industry. Neither is actually a tool; both are systems that provide an effective integration of many different tools. Much of Six Sigma's success can be attributed to the fact that its DMAIC methodology is a logical and proven way to apply nearly all the quality tools to their correct purposes. But had Six Sigma been introduced earlier in the quality revolution, it likely would not have been successful. Because many organizations have developed greater levels of quality maturity over the past two decades they can now better understand Six Sigma.

This section is not intended to be an all-inclusive reference for quality tools, but rather a summary of more than two dozen of the most widely used tools that have been organized into six categories: (1) basic; (2) management; (3) creativity; (4) statistical; (5) design; and (6) measurement.

Basic Tools

Basic tools are used to define and analyze discrete processes that usually produce quantitative data. The first four are used primarily to help understand the process, identify potential causes for process performance problems, and collect and display data indicating which causes are most prevalent. The last five tools are used for more precise data analysis; they can help identify trends, distribution, and relationships.

Flowchart

The flowchart is a map of each step of a process, in the correct sequence, showing the logical sequence for completing an operation. The flowchart is a good staring point for a team seeking to improve an existing process or attempting to plan a new process or system.

Cause-and-Effect Diagram

Cause-and-effect analysis is sometimes referred to as the Ishikawa, or fishbone, diagram. In a cause-and-effect diagram, the problem (effect) is stated in a box on the right side of the chart, and likely causes are listed around major headings (bones) that lead to the effect. Cause-and-effect diagrams can assist in organizing the contributing causes to a complex problem (American Society for Quality 2000).

Pareto Chart

Vilfredo Pareto, an Italian economist in the 1880s, observed that 80 percent of the wealth in Italy was held by 20 percent of the population. Juran later applied this "Pareto principle" to other applications and found that 80 percent of the variation of any characteristic is caused by only 20 percent of the possible variables. A Pareto chart is a display of the frequency of occurrences that helps to show the "vital few" contributors to a problem so that management can concentrate resources on correcting these major contributors (American Society for Quality 2000).

Check Sheet

Check (or tally) sheets are simple tools used to measure the frequency of events or defects over short intervals. This tool initiates the process of information gathering, is easy to use, can be applied almost anywhere, is easily taught to most people, and immediately provides data to help to understand and improve a process.

Run Chart

Run charts are plots of data, arranged chronologically, that can be used to determine the presence of some types of signals of special cause variation in processes. A center line (usually the median) is plotted along with the data to test for shifts in the process being studied.

Control Chart

A control chart consists of chronological data along with upper and lower control limits that define the limits of common cause variation. A control chart is used to monitor and analyze variation from a process to determine if that process is stable and predictable (comes from common cause variation) or unstable and not predictable (shows signals of special cause variation).

Histogram

A histogram is a graphical display of the frequency distribution of the quality characteristic of interest. A histogram makes variation in a group of data readily apparent and assists in an analysis of how data are distributed around an average or median value.

Scatter Diagram

Scatter diagrams (or plots) show the relationship between two variables. The scatter diagram can help to establish the presence or absence of correlation between variables, but it does not indicate a cause-and-effect relationship.

Management Tools

These tools are used to analyze conceptual and qualitatively oriented information that may be prevalent when planning organizational change or project management.

Affinity Diagram

The affinity diagram can encourage people to develop creative solutions to problems. A list of ideas is created, then individual ideas are written on small note cards. Team members study the cards and group the ideas into common categories. The affinity diagram is a way to help achieve order out of a brainstorming session (American Society for Quality 2002).

Current Reality Tree

The current reality tree is commonly part of the TOC toolkit and employs cause-and-effect logic to determine what to change by identifying the root causes or core problems. Another purpose of the current reality tree, whether developed by an individual or a team, is to create a consensus among those involved with a problem (Heim 1999).

Interrelationship Diagraph

While the affinity diagram can help organize and make visible the initial relationships in a large project, the interrelationship diagraph (or relationship diagram) helps to identify patterns of cause and effect between ideas. The interrelationship diagraph can help management recognize the patterns, symptoms, and causes of systems of resistance that can emerge through the development of plans and actions. It can help to pinpoint the cause(s) of problems that appear to be connected symptoms (American Society for Quality 2000).

Matrix Diagram

The matrix diagram helps to answer two important questions when sets of data are compared: Are the data related? and, How strong is the relationship? The quality function deployment (QFD) House of Quality is an example of a matrix diagram. It lists customer needs on one axis and the in-house standards on the second axis. A second matrix diagram is added to show the in-house requirements on one axis and the responsible departments on the other. The matrix diagram is helpful to identify patterns in relationships and serves as a useful checklist for ensuring that tasks are being completed (American Society for Quality 2000).

Priorities Matrix

The priorities matrix uses a series of planning tools built around the matrix chart. This matrix helps when there are more tasks than available resources and management needs to prioritize based on data rather than emotion. A priorities matrix allows a group to systematically discuss, identify, and prioritize the criteria that have the most influence on the decision and study the possibilities (American Society for Quality 2000).

Tree Diagram

A tree diagram helps to identify the tasks and methods needed to solve a problem and reach a goal. It creates a detailed and orderly view of the complete range of tasks that need to be accomplished to achieve a goal. The tree diagram can be used once an affinity diagram or interrelationship diagraph has identified the primary causes and relationships (American Society for Quality 2000).

Process Decision Program Chart

The process decision program chart is a type of contingency plan that guides the efforts of a team when things do not turn out as expected. The actions to be completed are listed, then possible scenarios about problems that could occur are developed. Management decides in advance which measures will be taken to solve those problems should they occur. This chart can be helpful when a procedure is new and little or no experience is available to predict what might go wrong (American Society for Quality 2000).

Failure Mode and Effects Analysis

Failure mode and effects analysis (FMEA) is a method for looking at potential problems and their causes as well as predicting undesired results. FMEA was developed in the aerospace and defense industries and has been widely applied in many others. FMEA is normally used to predict product failure from past part failure, but it can also be used to analyze future system failures. This method of failure analysis is generally performed for design and process. By basing their activities on FMEA, people are more able to focus energy and resources on prevention, monitoring, and response plans where they are most likely to pay off.

Poka-Yoke

Poka-yoke (*POH-kuh yoh-KAY*), the Japanese name for "mistake proofing," means paying careful attention to every activity in a process to place checks and problem prevention measures at each step. Mistake proofing can be thought of as an extension of FMEA. Whereas FMEA helps in the prediction and prevention of problems, mistake proofing emphasizes the detection and correction of mistakes before they become defects delivered to customers. Poka-yoke puts special attention on human error.

Creativity Tools

Although this group is not known as a fixed list of specific tools—that would be incongruent with the concept of creativity—it typically includes brainstorming, mind maps, Edward deBono's (1999) six thinking hats, and the use of analogies. These tools help one look at processes in new ways and identify unique solutions.

Statistical Tools

Statistical tools are used for more sophisticated process data analysis. They help understand the sources of variation, the relative contribution of each variable, and the interrelationships between variables. Statistical process control is a graphic means used to monitor and respond to special causes of variation. "Design of experiments," a wide range of statistical techniques that can be applied to both parametric and nonparametric data, allows the analysis of the statistical significance of more complex interrelationships.

Design Tools

Design tools, such as QFD and FMEA, are used during the design and development of new products and processes. They can help to better align customer needs, product characteristics, and process controls.

Measurement Tools

Measurement is a core need for effective process management. Tools such as cost of quality, benchmarking, auditing, and surveys enable the collection and analysis of different types of data that can then be used to guide and evaluate the effectiveness of improvement efforts.

Application of Quality Improvement Science in Healthcare

While quality improvement theory and methodology have been available since the early 1900s, widespread acceptance and application by the healthcare industry have not occurred. Reemerging concerns about double-digit healthcare cost inflation are placing the healthcare industry under increased scrutiny.

Two landmark reports from the Institute of Medicine (IOM) document the alarming state of U.S. healthcare relative to safety and quality (IOM 2000, 2001). As it turns out, the same system accomplishing technical miracles is responsible for an estimated 44,000 to 98,000 preventable annual deaths caused by medical errors. A report from the Midwest Business Group on Health (2001) estimates that about one-third of the $390 billion spent on healthcare produces nothing (is waste) and that the annual cost of poor quality per covered employee is as high as $2,000 per year.

The factors that have allowed healthcare's isolation from mainstream industries relative to quality science can be understood through study of the two historical traditions that influence the theories and assumptions of today's healthcare managers (the foundation of the current healthcare system iceberg). These two traditions are shown in Figure 4.4.

Column 1 represents regulatory and punitive practices that can be traced to the Code of Hammurabi from approximately 2100 B.C. (The penalty for surgical malpractice was to amputate the hands of the surgeon!) The historical influences of column 1 focused on "bad care" and evolved into minimum standards, which, while serving some useful purpose, cannot result in the achievement of excellence (Merry and Crago 2001).

Column 1, regulation, has dominated the learning tradition from column 2, which dates to Hippocrates (third century B.C.), and both columns have remained largely impenetrable to the quality science available from column 3. In 1987, a few healthcare organizations worked with quality experts from manufacturing and service industries to launch the

Column 1: Regulation	Column 2: Learning Science	Column 3: Management Science
Hammurabi	Hippocrates	Industrial revolution
⇩	⇩	⇩
Legal system	F. Nightingale	Taylor: "scientific management"
⇩	⇩	
State boards	A. Flexner, E. A. Codman, American College of Surgeons/Hospital Standardization Program	⇩
⇩ ⇨		W. Shewhart
Joint Commission "inspection"		⇩
		⇩
⇩	⇐ ⇩	W. E. Deming, J. M. Juran, total quality
⇩	M&M conferences	
⇩	⇩	⇩
	A. Donabedian, structure, process, outcome	⇐ ⇩
PRO/NCQA		Six Sigma, human ⇐⇐⇐factors
⇩	⇩	
Report cards, HEDIS, ORYX	Outcomes, disease management ⇨	

FIGURE 4.4
Three
Histories

introduction of column 3 management practices. The experiment proved to be successful, demonstrating that quality science techniques could achieve in healthcare what they had accomplished in all other industries (Berwick, Godfrey, and Roessner 1991; Merry and Crago 2001).

Bolstered by the evidence that quality improvement can simultaneously improve quality and lower cost, healthcare organizations spent millions in the 1980s and 1990s on improving processes, realizing some impressive results and some failures. Eventually, the wave passed by and quality science methods failed to take hold in a critical mass of healthcare organizations. Most managers who experimented with column 3 reverted to columns 1 and 2, and the assumptions behind these columns are the implicit paradigms (the foundation of the iceberg) in most healthcare organizations today (Merry and Crago 2001).

Healthcare's crises with falling provider payment, Balanced Budget Act implications, ambulatory fixed payment systems, rising costs, and insurance premiums are forcing healthcare organizations to look again to column 3 for solutions. Only quality science knowledge can bridge the current quality chasm, and it is the only body of knowledge that leaders can use to address the economic and quality issues simultaneously.

The First and Second Curves of Healthcare Quality Improvement

Although widespread application of quality improvement principles has not occurred in the healthcare system, some organizations have used the quality methods, tools, and procedures outlined in this chapter, implementing quality systems such as ISO 9000 and Six Sigma. There is growing interest in the use of the Baldrige criteria, based in part on the recent accomplishment of SSM Health Care in St. Louis as the first recipient of the Malcolm Baldrige National Quality Award for Healthcare. A number of healthcare professionals have successfully tapped into the management science field (column 3 in Figure 4.4) to produce "second curve" results. A brief explanation of the first and second curve model is provided below.

Influenced by the work of Thomas Kuhn (1962) and Ian Morrison (1996), Dr. Martin Merry describes a model that synthesizes the influences of the three historical traditions from Figure 4.4. The model is shown in Figure 4.5.

Healthcare's first curve of quality improvement has produced advances in performance from the early 1900s to the present. However, it has achieved the maximum capability of 4 sigma, which is as much as can be expected from a craft-age culture dependent on humans inspecting each other. The performance of the system is actually worsening. It is becoming evident that modern healthcare has ignored the systems infrastructure. We are now paying a huge price for having isolated medical and nursing practice from the management of resources. New knowledge is needed to design the essential physical and information infrastructures.

As with the paradigm shifts described by Kuhn (1962) and Morrison (1996), the shift from first to second curve will be discontinuous, derived from an entirely different set of assumptions and beliefs. Nothing less than the wholesale importation of management science knowledge will suffice to achieve the performance levels needed at a cost that our economy can bear (Merry 2003).

Case Study: A Second Curve Example

Figure 4.6 describes the process for diagnosing breast cancer as it was practiced in the 1920s and continues to be practiced today within most organizations. This system is built primarily around the needs of physicians (primary care, surgeon, and radiologist). It asks an anxious woman with possible breast cancer to go from doctor to doctor, facility to facility, healthcare silo to healthcare silo before she learns whether she has cancer. The

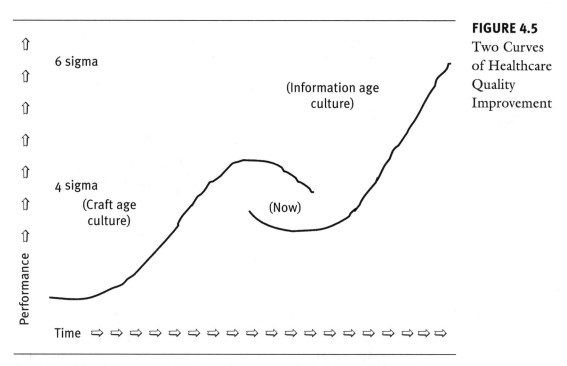

⇧ 6 sigma

⇧

⇧   (Information age
                                         culture)
⇧

⇧

⇧

⇧ 4 sigma
      (Craft age   (Now)
⇧   culture)

⇧

Performance

Time ⇨

FIGURE 4.5
Two Curves
of Healthcare
Quality
Improvement

Source: Adapted from I. Morrison, *The Second Curve: Managing the Velocity of Change*, Ballantine Books, 1996.

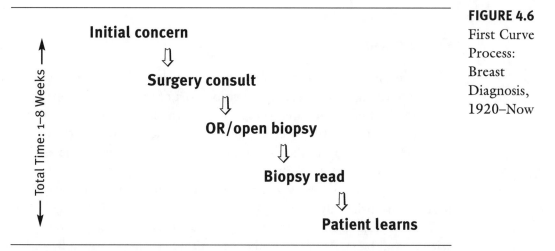

Initial concern
⇩
Surgery consult
⇩
OR/open biopsy
⇩
Biopsy read
⇩
Patient learns

◄— Total Time: 1–8 Weeks —►

FIGURE 4.6
First Curve
Process:
Breast
Diagnosis,
1920–Now

Source: Adapted from I. Morrison, *The Second Curve: Managing the Velocity of Change*, Ballantine Books, 1996.

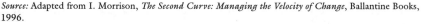

FIGURE 4.7
Second Curve
Process: Breast
Diagnosis,
Park-Nicollet,
1995–Now

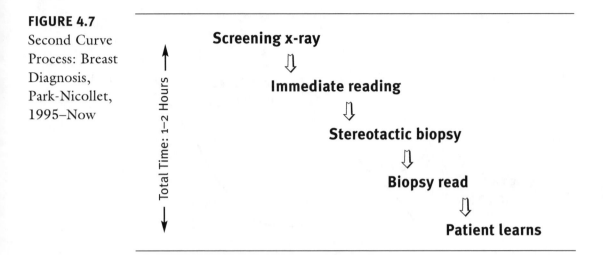

process in Figure 4.6 takes from a few days to *almost 2 months* in some locations. For the patient, this can mean up to 56 sleepless nights.

Figure 4.7 represents a radically different process, by which the Park-Nicollet Medical Center dealt with this sleepless night issue. In 1993, a thoughtfully conceived and interlinked system was designed that produced a definitive diagnosis in *2 hours*. To conceive of the new system required unlearning long-standing and strongly held beliefs and the willingness to think in a completely different way (Merry 2003).

Conclusion

The tools and methods used by an organization—what we see—can be likened to the tip of an iceberg; the visible part of the iceberg is supported by a large, unseen structure. These tools are the logical outcomes of systems and models that have been put in place. These systems are, in turn, the logical extensions of the paradigms and assumptions held by leaders in organizations, which form the base of the iceberg.

The paradigms and assumptions that currently drive the healthcare industry are primarily influenced by two historical paths: (1) regulatory and (2) learning science. A third body of knowledge (quality improvement science) will be necessary to bridge the quality chasm described by IOM. Quality improvement science is also the only source of knowledge that will adequately address the escalating cost of healthcare, which is placing a tremendous drain on limited economic resources.

Since the 1950s, quality improvement principles have helped many organizations to better meet customer needs, improve productivity, reduce costs, and stay in business to, in turn, better meet the needs of society. These principles have demonstrated success in many healthcare organizations where leadership has developed a long-term commitment; however, their application is not widely distributed.

Study Questions

1. How would one go about selecting and implementing one or more of these approaches in his or her own institution?
2. What are the quality paradigms and assumptions currently driving most healthcare organizations?
3. Considering the different tools discussed, what are some of their key common elements?
4. What is the difference between a quality improvement system and a tool? Provide examples of each.

REFERENCES

American Society for Quality, Quality Management Division. 2000. *Certified Quality Manager Handbook*. Milwaukee, WI: Quality Press.

Berwick, D., A. Godfrey, and J. Roessner. 1991. *Curing Health Care*. San Francisco: Jossey-Bass.

Cohen, S., and R. Brand. 1993. *Total Quality Management in Government*. San Francisco: Jossey-Bass.

deBono, E. 1999. *Six Thinking Hats*. New York: Little, Brown.

Dillon, R. 2002. "Health Care and ISO 9000: An Interview with Dr. Michael Crago." *Infusion* July/Aug.

Drummond, H. 1992. *The Quality Movement: What Total Quality Management Is Really About*. London: Kogan Page.

Feigenbaum, A. V. 1951. *Total Quality Control*. New York: McGraw-Hill.

Garvin, D. A. 1987. "Competing on the Eight Dimensions of Quality." *Harvard Business Review* Nov./Dec.

Grandzol, J. R. 1997. "Which TQM Practices Really Matter: An Empirical Investigation." *Quality Management Journal* 4 (4): 43–59.

Heim, K. 1999. "Creating Continuous Improvement Synergy with Lean and TOC," Presented at the ASQ Annual Quality Congress, May 1999, Anaheim, CA.

Hutchins, D. 1992. *Achieve Total Quality Management*. Cambridge, UK: Director Books.

Imai, M. 1986. *Kaizen: The Key to Japan's Competitive Success*. New York: Random House.

Institute for Healthcare Improvement. 2003. [Online information; retrieved 7/7/04.] www.ihi.org.

Institute of Medicine. 2000. *To Err Is Human: Building a Safer Health System.* Washington, DC: National Academy Press.

———. 2001. *Crossing the Quality Chasm: A New Health System for the 21st Century.* Washington, DC: National Academy Press.

Juran, J. M. 1989. *Juran on Leadership for Quality.* New York: The Free Press.

Juran, J. M., and F. M. Gryna (eds.). 1951. *Juran's Quality Control Handbook.* New York: McGraw-Hill.

Kilian, C. 1988. *The World of W. Edwards Deming.* Knoxville, TN: SPC Press.

Kuhn, T. 1962. *The Structure of Scientific Revolutions.* Chicago: University of Chicago Press.

Langley, G., K. Nolan, T. Nolan, C. Norman, and L. Provost. 1996. *The Improvement Guide: A Practical Approach to Enhancing Organizational Performance.* San Francisco: Jossey-Bass.

Lawton, B. 1996. "Transitioning to the Knowledge Age." Presented at the Ninth Annual Hunter Conference, Pre-Conference Workshop, 15 May 1996, Madison, WI.

Merry, M. 2003. "Health Care's 2nd Curve: The Future Begins!" Unpublished manuscript.

Merry, M., and M. Crago. 2001. "The Past, Present and Future of Health Care Quality." *The Physician Executive* Sept./Oct.: 30.

Midwest Business Group on Health. 2001. *Reducing the Cost of Poor Quality Through Responsible Purchasing Leadership.*

Morrison, I. 1996. *The Second Curve, Managing the Velocity of Change.* New York: Ballantine Books.

National Institute of Standards and Technology. 2003. *Baldrige National Quality Program Health Care Criteria for Performance Excellence.* Gaithersburg, MD: NIST.

———. "President and Commerce Secretary Announce Recipients of Nation's Highest Quality Award." [Online information.] www.nist.gov.

Nave, D. 2002. "How to Compare Six Sigma, Lean and Theory of Constraints." *Quality Progress* 3 (3): 73–78.

Neave, H. R. 1990. *The Deming Dimension.* Knoxville, TN: SPC Press.

Pande, P. S., R. P. Neuman, and R. R. Cavanagh. 2000. *The Six Sigma Way: How GE, Motorola, and Other Top Companies Are Honing Their Performance.* New York: McGraw-Hill.

Pegels, C. C. 1995. *Total Quality Management: A Survey of Its Important Aspects.* New York: Boyd & Fraser.

Strickland, R. 2003. Personal communication.

Talley, D. J. 1991. *Total Quality Management Performance and Cost Measures: The Strategy for Economic Survival.* Quality Press.

Tsiakals, J. J., C. A. Ciavrani, and J. E. West. 2002. *The ASQ ISO 9000:2000 Handbook.*

ORGANIZATION AND MICROSYSTEM

THE SEARCH FOR A FEW GOOD INDICATORS

Robert C. Lloyd

Increasingly, healthcare professionals are using Shewhart control charts to analyze the variation that resides within data. Yet, many still struggle with an essential aspect of quality measurement—identifying and developing appropriate indicators to be placed on control charts. Control charts based on inappropriate or poorly developed indicators are of no value; they merely provide chart junk. To obtain good data, therefore, it is necessary to approach its collection in a systematic way. This chapter provides a template and practical recommendations for selecting and developing indicators. Seven milestones in the quality measurement journey are discussed, and recommendations for avoiding pitfalls along the way are offered. This chapter also reviews the leading national indicator initiatives and the data expectations related to each initiative.

It may seem hard to believe, but there actually was a time when the only group that cared about measuring the efficiency and effectiveness of healthcare services was providers themselves. Today, it is a very different story. While providers are more focused than ever on performance measurement, they must balance their own measurement efforts against those being demanded by the following:

- Purchasers of care (individuals and companies)
- Business coalitions (representing companies within defined geographical areas)
- Insurance companies interested in structuring contractual agreements around quality outcomes
- Accrediting organizations (e.g., the Joint Commission on Accreditation of Healthcare Organizations [Joint Commission], National Committee on Quality Assurance [NCQA], and state departments of health and welfare)
- The Centers for Medicare & Medicaid Services (CMS), formerly known as the Health Care Financing Administration
- The media (especially newspapers and television)

Not only are more organizations demanding healthcare data but they are also making a strong argument for the release of these data to the public. This is a fundamental switch from how healthcare data have historically been treated. Prior to the early 1980s, the only way one could obtain data on hospitals or physicians was through the subpoena process. Today, the public release of provider data is quite common. Such data can be obtained from various Internet sites, state data commissions, CMS, *Consumer Reports*, and various proprietary vendors. The basic theory behind such releases is that they will make providers more accountable for the outcomes they produce, improve quality, and help to contain costs. Consistent support of this theory remains elusive.

National Indicator Initiatives

Along with the growing interest in reporting healthcare performance data to the public has come a related challenge. Specifically, those who endorse the public release of provider data have quickly realized that the indicators being reported must be

1. Standardized across all providers (common definitions and data collection procedures);
2. Produced within reasonable time frames (which has been a widely debated issue);
3. Developed at a reasonable cost to both providers and those assembling the data; and
4. Easy to read and interpret (especially by consumers and purchasers).

In my 20-plus years in the healthcare field, I have never seen one set of indicators satisfy all four of these criteria simultaneously.

Numerous groups and organizations have sponsored national indicator sets. Several of the more well known indicator initiatives are summarized below.

Minimum Data Set

The idea of creating a small set of indicators that captures the essential aspects of any healthcare experience is very appealing. As healthcare has become more complex, the idea of a minimum data set (MDS) has gained even more appeal than it had when it was first introduced in the late 1960s. What started as a general concept has emerged, over time, into a variety of specific data sets. MDSs have been proposed for everything from inpatient services to ambulance services. The basic idea behind an MDS is that a small core set of indicators is defined and used for mandatory collection and reporting at the state, regional, or national level. The basic problem with implementing this concept, however, is that agreement on what constitutes a "minimum" set of indicators has been elusive. The other major challenge has been determining who will be the end user of the MDS. Providers have different data needs than policymakers, and both groups have different needs than the purchasing managers of large corporations or the public.

In the long and interesting history associated with the development of MDSs, several key developments and structures deserve to be mentioned.

In 1969, the National Committee on Vital and Health Statistics developed the first formal outline for an MDS for hospital discharge data elements. This led to the creation of the Uniform Hospital Abstract Minimum Data Set in 1973.

The Uniform Hospital Discharge Data Set (UHDDS) emerged in the early 1970s as the standard MDS referent for hospital-based services. The 14 data elements contained in the original UHDDS were then used to create the first Uniform Bill (UB) for hospital services, popularly known as UB-82 (82 refers to 1982, when the structure of the UB was first accepted). In the mid 1990s, UB-82 was updated and is now referred to as UB-92. This one-page form contains 86 fields, some of which allow for multiple entries or subcategories. While UB-92 is used primarily for processing Medicare claims, the format has been adopted by other groups (e.g., most state data commissions) to collect data on other payer groups. The elements included in UB-92 were determined by the National Uniform Billing Committee (NUBC),[1] which was established in 1975. Each state has its own UBC that can recommend limited revisions to UB-92. In terms of physician billing, the CMS-1500 form (originally called HCFA-1500) is the standard reference. This form was last revised in 1992 and is accepted by nearly all insurance plans.[2]

New MDSs are being developed each year. An area that has been particularly active has been the nursing profession. The Nursing Minimum Data Set was initially proposed in the early 1970s. Today, the Nursing Management Minimum Data Set is undergoing research and development (Huber et al. 1992), with the intention of having a common set of indicators that captures the essence of the nursing component of care.

The most recent development in this area is being sponsored by the Agency for Healthcare Research and Quality (AHRQ). This agency, basically the research arm of the U.S. Department of Health and Human Services, has been charged by Congress to report annually on the status of healthcare quality in the United States. The National Healthcare Quality Report is the structure for reporting on a broad set of performance and outcome indicators believed to measure the current quality of healthcare services. Related to this initiative is AHRQ's National Quality Measures Clearinghouse, a web-based repository of tools and data evaluating quality.

Long-Term Care MDS

CMS has been involved with the development of several MDSs that are tied directly to reimbursement and used to evaluate the quality of care. One of the better known of these data sets is the Long Term Care Resident Assessment Instrument (RAI) MDS (version 2.0). The RAI has three components.

1. The *Minimum Data Set Version 2.0* is a core set of indicators capturing the clinical and functional characteristics of the long-term care facility's residents. The four-page assessment form used to capture the core set of data elements contains more than 72 fields that have to be completed on every patient four times each year. While this data set is referred to as an MDS, ironically, the completion of these forms has placed additional data collection burdens on most facilities. Yet, Chapter 1 of the RAI manual states that "The RAI should not be, nor was it ever meant to be, an additional burden for nursing facility staff."
2. *Resident Assessment Protocols* are built around the MDS data elements. These protocols are intended to assist staff in addressing the individual patient's social, medical, and psychological problems so that personalized care plans can be developed.
3. *Utilization Guidelines* basically provide direction on when and how to use the RAI.

This MDS, along with site inspection data, serves as the primary source for the public release of long-term care data, which was initiated in 2002.[3]

Home Health Care (OASIS)

The Outcome Assessment Information Set (OASIS) is a CMS-sponsored MDS designed to capture core indicators for adult home care visits. It also serves as the basic data tool for measuring what is known as outcome-based quality improvement (OBQI). OASIS was initially conceived in 1990 and sponsored jointly at that time by HCFA and the University of Colorado. In 1996, it was pilot tested with 50 home care agencies. Further refinements were achieved during a three-year demonstration project (1996–1999). Today, any home care agency wishing to participate in the Medicare program is required to participate in the OASIS initiative. The basic idea behind OASIS and OBQI is that if home care agencies understand the outcomes they produce, they will engage in "remediation" to improve the negative outcomes and "reinforcement" to maintain the positive outcomes. The OASIS system is built around 45 indicators that capture the following aspects of a home care encounter:

- Sociodemographic characteristics of the patient
- Environmental characteristics (of the patient's home setting)
- The patient's support system
- Functional status of the patient
- Utilization of health services

In 2003, CMS began using the OASIS data system to issue public reports on home health care agencies.[4]

The Joint Commission Core Measures

The Joint Commission has a long and rich history in the development of indicators. The organization started its measurement journey in 1987 with the Agenda for Change. The most recent initiatives are referred to as ORYX and Core Measures. ORYX began as a fairly flexible and open approach to meeting the Joint Commission accreditation requirements. Hospitals were allowed to select from a broad range of indicators, but the problem was maintaining consistency across myriad indicators that did not have standardized definitions. Currently, the ORYX initiative is in the process of transitioning to what are known as Core Measures. This approach offers a more specific and limited set of indicators that have standardized definitions and more clear specifications for data collection. After a pilot study on the proposed core measures, the following four clinical topics now form the basis of the Joint Commission Core Measures project:

- Hospital acute myocardial infarction (AMI): nine specific indicators
- Heart failure (HF): four specific indicators
- Community-acquired pneumonia (CAP): six specific indicators
- Pregnancy and related conditions (PR): three specific indicators

Currently, hospitals are expected to select two of these four areas and submit data to the Joint Commission. Eventually, it is anticipated that all hospitals will be expected to submit data on all four clinical topics. The Joint Commission has also suggested that additional clinical areas (e.g., critical care, diabetes, asthma) will be addressed in the near future. The ultimate goal of the Joint Commission initiatives is to be able to offer uniform aggregated results that can be compared across all hospitals. To further establish the credibility of these measures, the Joint Commission has joined into a collaborative arrangement with CMS, the American Hospital Association (AHA), and a number of state hospital associations to collect and share the Core Measures results. This is seen as a positive step, since it is an attempt to minimize the burden of data collection being placed on hospitals and work toward a common MDS that can serve numerous purposes. Since this collaboration is still new, however, the exact details of how the data sharing will work need to be finalized; the value-added contribution of the collaborative remains to be seen.[5]

NCQA HEDIS Measures

NCQA is a private, not-for-profit organization located in Washington, DC. Its primary purpose is to accredit health plans, primarily health maintenance organizations (HMOs) and preferred provider organizations (PPOs). But NCQA has also been involved with developing measures of quality and certification standards for individual physician offices, large medical groups, disease management entities, and credentialing organizations. Participation in the NCQA accreditation process is strictly voluntary. Of all HMOs in the country, about half are NCQA accredited. Far fewer PPOs have gone through the accreditation process, basically because the PPO accreditation process was initiated in 2000 and it takes several years to gear up for a successful accreditation review. The NCQA Health Plan Report Card is the primary reference for large companies and other organizations interested in evaluating which health plans to offer to their employees. The Health Plan Employer Data and Information Set (HEDIS) is the MDS that NCQA has created to evaluate the quality of care and customer service provided by each health plan. The HEDIS data elements include quality of care, access to care, and member satisfaction with the health plan and the doctors they see.[6]

The Measurement Challenge

This renewed focus on and mandate for healthcare data place healthcare providers in a very different situation than they have experienced in the past. Providers are being asked to document what they do, evaluate the outcomes of their efforts, and then be prepared to share their results with the public. Unfortunately, many providers struggle to proactively address the measurement mandate. This leads organizations to assume a defensive posture when their data are released. In such cases, the usual responses by the provider include the following:

- The data are old (one to two years, typically) and do not reflect our current performance.

- The data are not stratified and do not represent appropriate comparisons.
- Our patients are sicker than those at the other hospitals in our comparison group (i.e., no risk adjustments were made to the data).

While these responses frequently have some degree of merit, they are generally regarded, especially by those who release the data, to be feeble excuses and attempts by providers to justify their current ways of delivering care. A more proactive posture would be to develop an organizationwide approach to quality measurement that meets both internal and external demands. Such an approach is not a task to be completed once, but rather a journey that has many potential pitfalls and detours. As on any worthwhile journey, key milestones exist and can be used to mark your progress and help to chart your direction. The remainder of this chapter outlines seven major milestones that will aid in your search for a few good indicators.

Milestones Along the Quality Measurement Journey

The primary objective of this section is to provide an overview of the seven key milestones summarized in Table 5.1. Because of space limitations, all the details associated with each milestone are not provided. Some of the detail is presented in other chapters of this book, and additional detail can be found in references that address quality measurement topics (Caldwell 1995; Carey 2003; Carey and Lloyd 2001; Gaucher and Coffey 1993; Langley et al. 1996).

Milestone 1

The first step in the quality measurement journey is strategic in nature. It is achieved by engaging in a serious dialog within the organization on the role of performance measurement. Many organizations do not have a sense of *why* they are measuring. In most of these instances, the organization ends up either taking a defensive posture toward data or assumes the "Let's wait and see what we're asked to provide" position. Is measurement a part of your organization's day-to-day functioning? Or is it something that is done periodically to prepare reports for board meetings or respond to external requirements? Does everyone in the organization understand the critical role of performance measurement? Or do employees think that the development of indicators is something only management does?

The first step toward this milestone is the creation of an organizational statement on the role of measurement. Another way to view this step is to consider developing a measurement philosophy. Advocate Health Care,

TABLE 5.1	Milestone	Activities Performed
Quality Measurement Journey Milestones and Their Related Activities	1	Develop a measurement philosophy
	2	Identify the concepts to be measured (types and categories of indicators)
	3	Select specific indicators
	4	Develop operational definitions for each indicator
	5	Develop a data collection plan and gather the data (giving special consideration to stratification and sampling)
	6	Analyze the data using statistical process control (SPC) methods (especially run and control charts)
	7	Use the analytic results (data) to take action (implement cycles of change, test theories, and make improvements)

the largest integrated delivery system in the Chicago metropolitan area, was established in 1995 as a result of the merger of Lutheran General Health System and EHS Health Care. Advocate Health Care owns eight hospitals with more than 24,000 employees and 5,000 affiliated physicians. It also has the largest home health care service organization in the state of Illinois. Advocate's measurement philosophy statement indicates that organizations should sponsor their own dialogs that produce a consistent view on the role of performance measurement.

Milestone 2

The second milestone is both strategic and operational. It consists of deciding which concepts (sometimes called types or categories of indicators) the organization wishes to monitor. Donabedian (1980, 1982) provided a simple and clear approach to organizing a measurement journey. He proposed three basic categories of indicators: structures (S), processes (P), and outcomes (O). The relationship between these three categories is usually shown as follows:

$$S + P = O$$

Structures represent both the physical and organizational aspects of the organization (e.g., design of the outpatient testing area, hiring practices, tuition reimbursement policies). As Deming (1995) constantly pointed out, "Every activity, every job is part of a process." *Processes* are created by management and refined by workers. Structures combine with processes to produce *outcomes* (results).

Donabedian's model has served as a general rubric for many organizations. Frequently, however, organizations need to be a little more specific than structures, processes, and outcomes. In this case, most organizations turn to either their strategic plan or the literature. One of the more frequently referenced sources is the Institute of Medicine's (IOM 2001) report *Crossing the Quality Chasm*, which identifies the following six aims for improvement:

1. Safety
2. Effectiveness
3. Patient centeredness
4. Timeliness
5. Efficiency
6. Equity

The Joint Commission (1993) has also identified the following dimensions of clinical performance that could be used to categorize indicators:

- Appropriateness
- Availability
- Continuity
- Effectiveness
- Efficacy
- Efficiency
- Respect and caring
- Safety
- Timeliness

Irrespective of the method used, it is critical that an organization decide which concepts, types, or categories of indicators it wishes to measure. If consensus around this issue is not reached, the rest of the journey will be a mere random walk through the data.

Milestone 3

Once an organization has decided on the types of indicators it wishes to track, the next step in the journey is to identify specific indicators. Many people do not see how this step differs from milestone 2. A helpful comparison to clarify these two milestones is the analogy of finding your seat at a baseball game. Milestone 2 identifies the section in which you are to sit (e.g., Section 110). Milestone 3, on the other hand, focuses on the specific row and seat you have been assigned (e.g., Row N, Seat 21).

A healthcare example should provide further clarification. Imagine that your organization has identified patient safety as one of its strategic objectives. This seems like a perfectly good thing to monitor, but patient safety cannot be directly measured because it is a concept. Concepts by their very nature are vague. You need to specify, therefore, (1) what aspect of patient safety you intend to measure and (2) the actual indicators. Figure 5.1 shows how this cascading process works. Note that even within the broad category of patient safety, we need to identify what aspect (i.e., what section in the ballpark) will be measured. Within patient safety, for example, you could focus on medication errors, patient falls, wrong-site surgeries, missed/delayed diagnoses, or blood product errors.

This example uses medication errors as the selected aspect of patient safety. Now, we need to get very specific. Within the medication error area, many things could be measured. The decision as to which indicator is selected (from the list shown in Figure 5.1 or a new list of indicators a team might develop) depends on what questions a quality improvement team is trying to answer. If you phrase the question in terms of the absolute volume of an activity you might be interested in tracking, a simple count of the number of medication errors might be sufficient. If, on the other hand, you are interested in a relative measure, you would be better off measuring the percentage of medication errors or the indicator most frequently used, the medication error rate. Life is full of options. When it comes to indicator selection, there are more options than most people realize. The challenge is to be very specific about what section, row, and seat you have selected.

Milestone 4

The real work of indicator development begins when you hit milestone 4—developing an operational definition of the specific indicator. This activity requires inquisitive minds (left-brained people are often good at developing operational definitions) and patience.

Every day, we are challenged to think about operational definitions. They are not only essential to good measurement but also critical to successful communication between individuals. For example, a neighbor of mine just returned from vacation. I asked whether he had a good vacation. He responded, "It was better than good, it was great!" When I asked him where he went, he said that he had gone away for a week with four of his friends (all male) and played golf all day and cards all night and smoked cigars. This may not meet everyone's definition of a good vacation, but for my neighbor it met all the criteria in his operational definition.

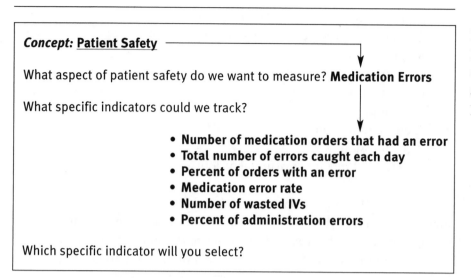

FIGURE 5.1
Relationship
Between a
Concept and
Specific
Indicators

Basically, an *operational definition* is a description, in quantifiable terms, of what to measure and the specific steps needed to measure it consistently. A good operational definition

*   Gives communicable meaning to a concept or an idea;
*   Is clear and unambiguous;
*   Specifies the measurement method, procedures, and equipment (when appropriate);
*   Provides decision-making criteria when necessary; and
*   Enables consistency in data collection.

Remember, however, that operational definitions are not universal truths. They can be debated and argued ad nauseam. A good operational definition represents, therefore, a statement of consensus by those responsible for tracking the indicator. Note also that the operational definition may need to be modified at some future point, which is not unusual. When this is done, it will be necessary to note when the definition was changed, as this could have a dramatic effect on the results.[7]

In healthcare, many terms beg for more precise operational definitions. How does your organization define the following terms?

*   A patient fall (a partial fall versus an assisted fall)
*   A complete history and physical
*   A successful physical therapy session
*   A restraint (physical versus chemical restraint)

- A prompt response to a call button
- A good employee performance review
- Surgical start time
- An accurate patient bill
- Quick turnaround time
- A clean patient room
- A quick admission
- A readmission
- A successful quality measurement journey

The problem poor operational definitions create for good measurement is obvious. If you are part of a multihospital system or plan on comparing provider outcomes, each provider *must* define the indicator in the same way. For example, CMS released data on nursing homes to the public in 2002. In 2003, CMS released home health care comparative reports. In 2004, CMS follows with data on inpatient hospitals. Lack of consistency in the operational definitions used by CMS poses the risk of not having apples and oranges when comparisons are made; fruit salad will be the result! The pieces will not be comparable, which means that ultimately the conclusions derived from the data will not be accurate or will be challenged by the providers. All good measurement begins and ends with operational definitions.

Milestone 5

Data collection is the billboard for this milestone. Unfortunately, many people begin their quality measurement journey at this marker. Faced with the challenge of presenting data, their first reaction is that they have to "go get some data." This orientation typically directs them toward convenient data that are readily available and familiar to everyone. It can also lead to collecting the wrong data in the wrong amounts (too little or too much).

The major problem with using readily available, convenient data is that the data usually do a very poor job of answering the questions being asked. For example, it is not uncommon for quality improvement teams to use average length of stay and average cost (or charges) per discharge as proxy measures for quality. Both average length of stay and average cost are gross outcome (the O part of the Donabedian model) measures. What is the team doing to measure the structures or processes of care? When asked this question, teams frequently respond, "Well, we currently don't collect anything on these components, and it's easier for us to go with what we have always used and what is available. It's good enough, isn't it?"

Ten or twenty years ago, the "good enough" approach to data collection might have been acceptable. Today, however, with the myriad growing pressures to demonstrate effectiveness of care and efficiency of health-care processes, this mind-set is not acceptable. Quality and excellence of performance do not occur because organizations do what they have always done or what is convenient. This behavior leads to the perpetuation of the status quo, what most healthcare observers feel the industry definitely does not need.

The data collection phase of the journey consists of two parts: (1) planning for data collection and (2) the actual gathering of the data. A well-thought-out data collection plan should address issues such as the following:

- What processes will be monitored?
- What specific indicators will be collected?
- What are the operational definitions of the indicators?
- Why are you collecting these data? What is the rationale for collecting these data rather than some other type of data?
- Will the data add value to your quality improvement efforts?
- Have you discussed the effect of stratification on the indicators?
- How often (frequency) and for how long (duration) will you collect the data?
- Will you employ sampling? If so, what sampling design do you propose?
- How will you collect the data? (Will you use data sheets, surveys, focus group discussions, phone interviews, or some combination of methods?)
- Will you conduct a pilot study before you collect data throughout the entire organization?
- Who will actually collect the data? (Most teams ignore this question.)
- What costs (monetary plus time costs) will be incurred by collecting these data?
- Will collecting these data have any negative effects on patients or employees?
- What is the current baseline for this indicator?
- Do you have targets and goals?
- How will the data be coded, edited, and verified?
- Will you tabulate and analyze these data by hand or by computer?
- How will these data be used to make a difference?
- What plan do you have for disseminating the results of your data collection efforts?

Once these issues have been resolved, the actual collection of the data usually goes smoothly. Unfortunately, many quality improvement teams do not spend sufficient time discussing their data collection plans; they want to move immediately to the data collection step. This is usually a sure guarantee that they will (1) collect too much (or too little) data; (2) collect the wrong data; or (3) become frustrated with the entire measurement journey. When individuals or groups become frustrated with the measurement process, they begin to lose faith in the data and results. This leads to a major detour in the quality measurement journey. As a result, if the team or management is presented with data they do not believe reflects their preconceived views of reality, they tend to (1) distort the data (which is unethical and illegal); (2) distort the process that produced the data; or (3) kill the messenger![8] A well-thought-out data collection plan will contribute significantly to a team's ability to avoid these data pitfalls.

Two key data collection skills—stratification and sampling—will enhance any data collection effort. These skills are based more on logic and clear thinking than on statistics. Yet, most healthcare professionals have received limited training in both concepts.

Stratification

Stratification is the separation and classification of data into homogeneous categories. The objective of stratification is to create strata, or categories, within the data that are mutually exclusive and allow discovery of patterns that would not be observed if the data were all aggregated together. Stratification allows understanding of differences in the data caused by

- Day of the week (are Mondays different than Wednesdays?);
- Time of day (registration is busier between 9 a.m. and 10 a.m. than between 2 p.m. and 3 p.m.);
- Time of year (do we see more of this diagnosis in February than in June?);
- Shift (does the process differ by day and night shifts?);
- Type of order (stat versus routine);
- Experience of the worker;
- Type of procedure (nuclear medicine films versus routine X-rays); and
- Machine (such as ventilators or lab equipment).

If you do not think about how these factors might influence your data *before* you collect it, you run the risk of (1) making incorrect conclusions about your data and (2) having to manually try to tease out the stratification effect after the data have been collected. Consider the following example of how stratification could be applied to the pharmacy process. A quality improvement team is interested in the following question: What percentage of medication orders are delivered to the nursing stations within one hour of receipt in the pharmacy? Before collecting data on this question, someone on the team ought to ask the following stratification question: Do we believe that this percentage might differ by floor, time of day, day of week, type of medication ordered, pharmacist on duty, or volume of orders received? If your answer to any part of this question is yes (i.e., the team believes that one or more of these factors will influence the outcome), steps should be taken to make sure that the relevant factors are collected each time an order is received in the pharmacy.

Stratification is an essential aspect of data collection. If you do not spend some time discussing the implications of stratification, you will end up thinking that your data are worse (or better) than they should be.

Sampling

Sampling is the second key skill that healthcare professionals need to develop. If a process does not generate a lot of data, you will probably analyze all the occurrences. In this case, sampling is not required. This happens most often when the indicator is a percentage or a rate. For example, computation of the percent of no-shows for magnetic resonance imaging (MRI) typically does not use a sampling plan; all the scheduled MRIs that do not show up for the procedure (the numerator) are divided by the total number of scheduled MRIs (the denominator). When a process generates considerable data, however (e.g., turnaround times for medication orders), a sampling plan is usually appropriate. Sampling is probably the single most important thing you can do to reduce the amount of time and resources spent on data collection.

Like stratification, however, many healthcare professionals receive little training in sampling procedures. As a result, they collect either too much or too little data or question the results they obtain, which is an issue with the reliability and validity of the data. Ishikawa's classic work *Guide to Quality Control* (1982) identified four conditions for developing a sampling plan: accuracy, reliability, speed, and economy. It is nearly impossible to obtain a sample that meets all four criteria simultaneously. Sampling, therefore, really consists of a series of compromises and trade-offs. The key to successful sampling lies in understanding the overall purpose of selecting a sample and the specific sampling methodologies that can be applied to the data.

The basic purpose of sampling is to be able to draw a limited number of observations and be reasonably confident that they represent the larger population from which they were drawn. What happens, though, when a sample is not representative of the population from which it was drawn? The sample presents a picture that is either more positive than it should be (a positive sampling bias) or more negative than it should be (a negative sampling bias). A well-drawn sample, therefore, should be representative of the larger population. For example, if you use a mailed survey to gather patient satisfaction feedback, you probably do not send a survey to every patient.[9] You would start by sending surveys to roughly 50 percent of the patients and see how many are returned. This allows you to determine the response rate. Assume that you get back 25 percent of the surveys. The next task is to determine how representative of the total population these respondents are. To test this question, you need to develop a profile of the total population. Typically, this profile is based on standard demographics such as gender, age, type of visit, payer class, and whether this was the patient's first visit. If the distribution of these characteristics in the sample is similar (within 5 percent) to those found in the total population, you can be comfortable that your sample is reasonably representative of the population. If the characteristics for the sample and the population show considerable variation, however, the sampling plan needs to be adjusted.

Inevitably, the number one question asked during a discussion on sampling is, "So, how much data do I need?" There is no simple answer; it depends on the size of the population, importance of the question being asked, and resources available for drawing the sample. If, for example, you are drawing a single sample at a fixed point in time (what Deming called an enumerative study), the general rule of thumb places a "reasonable" minimum sample size at between 20 and 30 observations (e.g., selecting the wait times for 20 emergency department patients on Monday of next week). On the other hand, if you are sampling for quality improvement purposes (what Deming called analytic studies), a different approach should be taken. Analytic studies are dynamic in nature and look at a process as it lays itself out over time. Sampling for analytic studies therefore requires the selection of a smaller number of observations (e.g., five to ten) drawn at multiple (as opposed to single) points in time.

There are two basic approaches to sampling, *probability* and *non-probability*. The dominant sampling techniques associated with each approach are shown in Figure 5.2 and briefly described below. A more detailed discussion on sampling can be found in any basic text on statistical methods or research design.[10]

Probability sampling is based on a simple principle, statistical probability. That is, within a known population of size n, there will be a fixed probability of selecting any single element (n_i). The selection of this element (and subsequent elements) must be determined by objective statistical means if it is to be a true random process (not by judgment, purposeful intent, or convenience).

FIGURE 5.2
Probability
and Non-
probability
Sampling
Techniques

Probability Sampling Techniques	• Systematic sampling
	• Simple random sampling
	• Stratified random sampling
	• Stratified proportional random sampling
Nonprobability Sampling Techniques	• Convenience sampling
	• Quota sampling
	• Judgment sampling

Campbell (1974) lists three characteristics of probability sampling:

1. A specific statistical design is followed.
2. The selection of items from the population is determined solely according to known probabilities by means of a random mechanism, usually using a table of random digits.
3. The sampling error (i.e., the difference between results obtained from a sample survey and those that would have been obtained from a census of the entire population conducted using the same procedures as in the sample) can be estimated, and, as a result, the precision of the sample result can be evaluated.

There are numerous ways to draw a probability sample. All are essentially variations on the simple random sample. The most frequently used probability sampling methods are listed below.

*   *Systematic sampling.* This is what most healthcare professionals think is random sampling. While systematic sampling is a form of random sampling, it is one of the weakest approaches to probability sampling. Its chief advantage is that it is easy to do and inexpensive. Systematic sampling (sometimes called mechanical sampling) is achieved by numbering or ordering each element in the population (e.g., time order, alphabetical order, medical record order) and then selecting every kth element. The key point that most people ignore when doing a systematic sample is that the starting point to pull every kth element should be selected through a random process and

equal to or less than *k* but greater than zero. The selection of a random starting point is usually achieved by using a random number table (found in the back of any good statistics book) or computer-based random number generator (found in all statistical software programs and spreadsheet packages). For example, if you wanted to select a systematic sample of 60 medical records from a total of 600, you would pull every tenth record. To determine the starting point for the sample, however, you would need to pick a random number between 1 and 10. Say that the random draw produces the number 8. To start our systematic sample, we would go to the eighth medical record on our list, pick it, and then select every tenth record after this starting point. Technically, this is known as a systematic sample with a random start (Babbie 1979). The major problem with systematic sampling is that chunks of data that could provide knowledge about the process are eliminated. If, for example, you are selecting every tenth record, you have automatically eliminated from further consideration records 1 through 9. If something occurs regularly in the data or something causes your data to be organized into bunches of, say, six or seven, these records would be automatically eliminated from consideration. The other problem with this form of sampling in healthcare settings is that the people drawing the sample do not base the start on a random process; they merely pick a convenient place to start and then apply the sampling interval they have selected. This introduces bias and greatly increases the sampling error.

- *Simple random sampling.* A random sample is one that is drawn in such a way that it gives every element in the population an equal and independent chance of being included in the sample. As mentioned in the previous section, this is usually accomplished by using a random number table or computer-based random number generator. A random sample could also be drawn by placing equally sized pieces of paper with a range of numbers on them (e.g., 1 to 100) into a bowl and merely picking out a predetermined number to be the sample. The major problem with simple random samples is that they may over- or underrepresent certain segments of the population.
- *Stratified random sampling.* Stratifying the population into relatively homogeneous strata or categories *before* the sample is drawn increases the representativeness of the sample and decreases the sampling error. Once the stratification levels have been identified, a random selection process is applied within each level of stratification. For example, you might stratify a clinic's appointments into

well-baby visits, follow-up visits, and unscheduled visits and then sample randomly within each category. This would help to ensure that one group is not overrepresented (or underrepresented) in the sampling plan. The major challenge in this form of sampling is that it requires detailed knowledge of the population and how the characteristics of interest are distributed within it.

- *Stratified proportional random sampling.* In this case, the approach outlined for stratified random sampling is used, with another twist. The proportion that each stratum represents in the population is determined, and this proportion is replicated in the sample. For example, if we knew that well-baby visits represent 50 percent of the clinic's business, follow-up visits represent 30 percent, and unscheduled visits represent 20 percent, we would draw 50 percent of the sample from well-baby visits, 30 percent from follow-up visits, and 20 percent from unscheduled visits. This would produce a sample that was not only representative but also proportionally representative of the population distribution. This would further increase the precision of the sample and further reduce the sampling error. The stratified proportional random sample is one of the more sophisticated sampling designs and requires considerable knowledge about the population being sampled. It can also be more costly in terms of both money and time.

Nonprobability sampling techniques should be used when estimating the reliability of the selected sample or generalizing the results of the sample to a larger population is not of concern. The basic objective of nonprobability sampling is to select a sample that the researchers *believe* is "typical" of the larger population. The problem is that there is no way to actually measure how typical or representative a nonprobability sample is with respect to the population it supposedly represents. In short, nonprobability samples can be considered "good enough samples" (i.e., they are good enough for the people pulling the sample). The major problem with nonprobability sampling is that people have a tendency to generalize the sample results to larger populations.

For example, a local TV news reporter conducts a "man on the street" survey by nabbing ten people as they come out of the grocery store. The reporter asks them how they feel about the proposed local tax increase to support teacher salary increases. Only eight of the ten agree to be interviewed. After assembling the footage and her notes, the reporter looks into the camera and says, "There you have it, a unanimous opinion that the tax increase is not warranted. . ." The implication is that there is public consensus against the proposal, when in fact the reporter has merely selected a limited convenience sample and jumped to a conclusion. This same situation could happen if you decide to interview ten patients in your emergency department on a given day and draw conclusions about your emergency services from these people. This is a classic example of "driving beyond your headlights." You have taken a little bit of data and made a huge jump in logic, gone beyond the limits of your vision. This is also known as the *ecological fallacy*, that is, taking a small microcosm (i.e., the sample) and generalizing to the entire ecology (i.e., the entire population).

There are three major forms of nonprobability sampling: convenience, quota, and judgment.

- *Convenience sampling.* This approach to sampling is designed to obtain a small number of observations that are readily available and easy to gather. Convenience sampling is also known as chunk sampling (Hess, Riedel, and Fitzpatrick 1975) or accidental sampling (Maddox 1981; Selltiz et al. 1959). There is essentially no science behind convenience sampling. It produces a biased sample that is basically a collection of anecdotes that cannot be generalized to larger populations. The primary question that should be asked when a convenience sample is drawn is, "How important is it to know if the sample of elements selected is representative of the larger population?" If the consequences of being wrong do not matter, the convenience sample might be good enough.
- *Quota sampling.* Quota sampling was developed in the late 1930s and used extensively by the Gallup Organization. Babbie (1979) nicely describes the steps involved in developing a quota sample.
  1. Develop a matrix describing the characteristics of the target population. This may entail knowing the proportion of male and female; various age, racial, and ethnic proportions; as well as the educational and income levels of the population.
  2. Once the matrix has been created and a relative proportion assigned to each cell in the matrix, data are collected from persons having all the characteristics of a given cell.
  3. All persons in a given cell are then assigned a weight appropriate to their proportion of the total.
  4. When all the sample elements are so weighted, the overall data should provide a reasonable representation of the total population.

Theoretically, an accurate quota sampling design should produce results that are reasonably representative of the larger population. Remember, however, that the actual selection of the elements to fill the quota is left up to the individual gathering the data, not to random chance. If the data collectors are not diligent and honest about their work, they will end up obtaining their quotas in a manner that is more like a convenience sample than a true quota sample. The final threat involves the process by which the data collectors actually gather the data. For example, if a quota sample was established to gather data in the emergency department, but only during the day shift, you would run the risk of missing key data points during the afternoon and evening shifts.

- *Judgment sampling.* In judgment sampling, the knowledge and experience of the person drawing the sample are the key driving factors. No objective mechanical means are used to select the sample. The assumption is that experience, good judgment, and appropriate strategy can select a sample that is acceptable for the objectives of the researcher. Obviously, the major challenge to this form of sampling is related to the knowledge and wisdom of the person making the judgment call. If everyone believes that this person exhibits good wisdom, they will have confidence in the sample the person selects. If, on the other hand, people doubt the person's knowledge, the sample will be discredited. Deming considered judgment sampling to be the method of choice for quality improvement research. Langley et al. (1996) maintain that "A random selection of units is rarely preferred to a selection made by a subject matter expert." In quality improvement circles, this type of sampling is also known as expert sampling, acceptance sampling, or rational sampling. It essentially consists of having those who have expert knowledge of the process decide how to arrange the data into homogeneous subgroups and pull the sample. The subgroups can be selected by either random or nonrandom procedures. The other important distinction about Deming's view of judgment sampling is that the samples should be selected at regular intervals over time, not at a single point. Most sampling designs, whether probability or nonprobability, are static in nature. The researcher decides on a time frame, then picks as much data as possible. In contrast, Deming's view of sampling was that it should be done in small doses and pulled as a continuous stream of data (Deming 1950, 1960, 1975). The primary criticism of judgment sampling is that the "expert" may not fully understand all facets of the population under investigation and may therefore select a biased sample. The counter to this criticism is that by selecting multiple samples over time, the potential bias of the expert will be mitigated by the inherent variation in the process.

Building knowledge about the various sampling techniques is one of the best ways to reduce the amount of time and effort spent on collecting data. Done correctly, sampling is also one of the best ways to ensure that the data collected are directly related to the questions at hand. Done incorrectly, sampling will inevitably lead to the proverbial debate that challenges the data, the process that produced the data, or the collector's credibility.

Milestone 6

After collecting data, many quality improvement teams think the majority of their work has been completed, when in fact it has just begun; data do not turn into information magically or because the team has good intentions. The analytical and interpretive steps that must be applied to the data are critical to the team's success. All too often, however, the lack of planning for the analytic part of the quality measurement journey causes a team to run into a dead end and either give up or die of boredom. Many teams put considerable effort into defining indicators and collecting data only to hit a major roadblock because they did not take time to figure out how they would analyze the data and who would actually churn the numbers.

A dialog about reaching this milestone must take place or all the effort put into the earlier part of the journey will leave you far short of your destination. Figure 5.3 provides a list of discussion questions that should be considered as an analysis plan is developed. Remember, however, that the time to think through the components and specific activities of an analysis plan is before the data start arriving.

If you are engaged in a quality improvement initiative, the best analytic path to follow is one guided by statistical process control (SPC) methods. This branch of statistics was developed by Dr. Walter Shewhart in the early 1920s while he worked at Western Electric Co. (Schultz 1994). Shewhart's primary analytic tool, the control chart, serves as the cornerstone for all quality improvement work. Statistical analysis conducted with control charts is very different from what some label as "traditional research" (e.g., hypothesis testing, development of p-values, design of randomized clinical trials). Traditional research is designed to compare the results at time one (e.g., the cholesterol levels of a group of middle-aged men) with the results at time two (typically months after the initial measure). Research conducted in this manner is referred to as *static group comparisons* (Benneyan, Lloyd, and Plsek 2003). The focus is not on how the data varied over time, but rather whether the two sets of results are "statistically different" from each other.

On the other hand, research based on control chart principles takes a very different view of the data, one that is dynamic. Control charts approach data as a continuous distribution that has a rhythm and pattern. In this case, control charts are more like an EKG readout or the pattern of vital signs seen on a telemetry monitor in the ICU. Control charts are plots of data

FIGURE 5.3

Discussion
Questions for
Developing an
Analysis Plan

When data start to arrive in your office, what will be your responses to the following questions?

- Where will the data be physically stored? This is a particular problem if you are collecting survey data. The surveys can start to pile up quickly. Will you save the surveys, put them on microfilm, or recycle them when you are done with your analysis?

- Who will be responsible for receiving the data, logging it into a book, and assigning identification numbers?

- Have you set up a code book for the data? If not, who will do this?

- What plans have you made for entering the data into a computer? Do you even have access to a computer? If you do not have a computer, what is your plan for manual analysis?

- If you do have access to a computer, who will do the actual data entry? Will you verify the data after it has been entered? Did you give any thought to using a professional data-entry service?

- Who will be responsible for actually analyzing the data? (This question applies whether you are performing manual or automated analysis.)

- What computer software will be used? Will you produce descriptive statistical summaries, cross-tabulations, graphical summaries, or control charts?

- Once you have a pile of computer output, who will be responsible for translating the raw data into information for decision making? Will you need to develop a written summary of the results? Do different audiences need to receive the results? Do they have different demands for the formats of the reports?

arranged in chronological order. The mean or average is plotted through the center of the data, and then the upper control limit (UCL) and lower control limit (LCL) are calculated from the inherent variation within the data. These control limits define the amount of variation within the data. The UCL and LCL are basically built around the standard statistical notion of establishing plus and minus 3 standard deviations around the mean. This chapter does not go into further detail on the selection, use, and interpretation of control charts; it merely introduces the key terms. Additional details on control charts can be found in other chapters of this book or in the literature (Benneyan, Lloyd, and Plsek 2003; Carey 2003; Carey and Lloyd 2001; Western Electric Co. 1985; Wheeler 1995; Wheeler and Chambers 1992).

Milestone 7

The final leg of the measurement journey involves taking *action* with the data and the conclusion drawn about the inherent variation in the indicator being tracked. Data without a context for action are useless. Unfortunately, a considerable amount of healthcare data is collected, analyzed, and then not acted on.

In 2000, Don Berwick provided a simple formula for quality improvement. During his keynote address at the National Forum on Quality Improvement in Health Care, he stressed that real improvement results from the interaction of three forces: will, ideas, and execution. Berwick's reference to execution is the same as taking action. Quality improvement requires action. This is the essence of the Plan-Do-Study-Act (PDSA) cycle described in Chapter 4. Without the *action* part, the PDSA cycle is nothing more than an academic exploration of interesting stuff. When Shewhart (Schultz 1994) first identified the components of the PDSA cycle, he did so with the intention of placing data completely within the action context. Data collection should not become the ultimate goal of a team. Action to make things better for those we serve is the ultimate goal.

Yet, it is curious to note the consistent and somewhat bothersome results when groups are asked to evaluate how effective they are with respect to will, ideas, and execution. I have administered the self-assessment shown in Table 5.2 to hundreds of healthcare professionals in the United States and abroad. Where would you place your own organization on each of these three components? If you are like most respondents, you will mark high for will, medium to high for ideas, and low for execution. We seem to give ourselves high marks for good intentions and desires, moderate to high marks for generating ideas on how we can improve things, but low assessments on being able to take action and actually implement change. For many (both within and outside the healthcare industry), this low level of performance on executing change has been a persistent and nagging challenge. There is hope, however, in the simple fact that it is easier to learn how to become more effective at managing and executing change than it is to try to instill good will in people who have none.

Conclusion

While defining indicators and collecting data play key roles in the quality measurement journey, it should be clear by now that indicators and data serve little purpose unless they are used to test theories and make improvements. The milestones reviewed in this chapter and summarized in Table 5.1 can serve as guideposts for your quality journey. They need to be seen,

Key Component	Self-Assessment		
Will	High	Medium	Low
Ideas	High	Medium	Low
Execution	High	Medium	Low

TABLE 5.2
Self-Assessment for Making Quality Improvement a Reality

Note: All three components MUST be viewed together. Focusing on one or even two of the components will guarantee suboptimal performance.

however, not as isolated tasks to be completed but as an integrated way of thinking about how to channel will, ideas, and action into an organizationwide roadmap for improvement. Happy trails!

Study Questions

1. Why have organizations created MDSs? Name an existing MDS and describe its contents and objective(s).
2. Why are operational definitions so important to good measurement? Provide an example of a vague operational definition, and then describe what you would do to make the definition more specific and clear.
3. Explain how stratification differs from sampling. Provide an example of when you would use stratification and when it is appropriate to develop a sampling strategy.
4. Name the two basic approaches to sampling. Which approach is better? Why do you make this conclusion? Select one sampling methodology and describe how you would apply it to a quality improvement initiative.

Acknowledgments

I want to acknowledge the assistance of several colleagues who helped me research information for this section and reviewed initial drafts of the discussion. Specifically, I want to thank Karen Svab, Tina Stiris, Lou Ann Schraffenberger from Advocate Health Care's corporate offices, and Cheryl Meyer from Advocate Health Care's Home Health Care division. Karen did a wonderful job of tracking down information on the MDS topic and the numerous components related to this diverse issue. Tina was able to masterfully cut through the extensive detail surrounding the Joint

Commission Core Indicators and boil it down to a few key points. Lou Ann, who is a nationally recognized expert in the area of coding and medical records, was able to narrow this extremely complex field down into a short history with major data sources (e.g., UHDDS, UB-92, and CMS 1500). Finally, Cheryl was able to summarize the essence of the OASIS initiative into an extremely cogent set of points.

Notes

1. NUBC's web site is www.nubc.org.
2. This form, UB-92, and several other standard forms used by CMS can be found at www.cms.hhs.gov/providers/edi/edi5.asp.
3. Additional information on the RAI MDS can be found at the CMS web site: www.cms.hhs.gov/medicaid/mds20/man-form.asp.
4. Information on the OASIS system can be obtained at the CMS web site: www.cms.hhs.gov/oasis/hhoview.asp.
5. Additional detail on the Joint Commission Core Measures project can be found at www.jcaho.org/pms/core+measure/index.htm.
6. More information on NCQA and HEDIS can be found at www.ncqa.org.
7. Several years ago, I had the opportunity to observe a team that forgot to note when they changed the operational definition of a key indicator. They noticed a dramatic improvement in their indicator and were eager to present their finding to the organization's quality council. The shift in their data was so dramatic that I asked if they had done anything different when they collected their data. Frequently, a change in the operational definition or sampling plan can produce such a large shift in the data. To a person, however, they all said no. As I continued asking the staff if anything was being done differently, I finally found a data analyst who recalled a "slight" modification in the operational definition. Interestingly, this change in the way the indicator was defined coincided with the shift in the results. If the old operational definition had been applied to the more recent data, the results would not have shown a change. Similarly, if the new definition had been applied to the old data, the improved performance would have been observed previously.
8. Wheeler (1993) states this conclusion in a slightly different fashion: "When people are pressured to meet a target value there are three ways they can proceed: (1) they can work to improve the system, (2) they can distort the system, (3) or they can distort the data." Wheeler credits Brian Joiner as the originator of this list.

9. The exception occurs under one or more of the following condi-
    tions: (1) small volume of patients, (2) low response rate, or (3)
    short data collection period. For example, if your hospital has an
    average daily census of 72 patients and you know historically that
    the average response rate to the survey was only 10 percent, you
    would probably send a survey to every patient. Similarly, if you were
    only going to survey one week out of the entire quarter, you would
    want to give a survey to every patient. Remember that sampling is
    an extremely useful tool, but it is not always needed.

10. Do not feel that you have to go out and buy the most recent books
    on sampling or statistical methods. The basic principles behind mod-
    ern sampling techniques have been around since the 1940s. Many of
    the books I have on this subject, for example, are 20 to 30 years old.

REFERENCES

Babbie, E. R. 1979. *The Practice of Social Research.* Belmont, CA: Wadsworth
    Publishing.

Benneyan, J., R. Lloyd, and P. Plsek. 2003. "Statistical Process Control as a
    Tool for Research and Health Care Improvement." *Journal of Quality
    and Safety in Healthcare.*

Berwick, D. 2000. Presented at the National Forum on Quality Improvement in
    Health Care.

Caldwell, C. 1995. *Mentoring Strategic Change in Health Care.* Milwaukee, WI:
    ASQ Press.

Campbell, S. 1974. *Flaws and Fallacies in Statistical Thinking.* Englewood
    Cliffs, NJ: Prentice-Hall.

Carey, R. 2003. *Improving Healthcare with Control Charts.* Milwaukee, WI:
    ASQ Quality Press.

Carey, R., and R. Lloyd. 2001. *Measuring Quality Improvement in Healthcare: A
    Guide to Statistical Process Control Applications.* Milwaukee, WI: ASQ
    Quality Press.

Deming, W. E. 1950. *Some Theory of Sampling.* New York: John Wiley & Sons.

———. 1960. *Sample Design in Business Research.* New York: John Wiley & Sons.

———. 1975. "On Probability as a Basis for Action." *The American Statistician*
    29 (4): 146–52.

———. 1995. *Out of the Crisis.* Cambridge, MA: MIT Press.

Donabedian, A. 1980. *Explorations in Quality Assessment and Monitoring,
    Volume I: The Definition of Quality and Approaches to Its Assessment and
    Monitoring.* Chicago: Health Administration Press.

———. 1982. *Explorations in Quality Assessment and Monitoring, Volume II:
    The Criteria and Standards of Quality.* Chicago: Health Administration
    Press.

Gaucher, E., and R. Coffey. 1993. *Total Quality in Healthcare*. San Francisco: Jossey-Bass.

Hess, I., D. Riedel, and T. Fitzpatrick. 1975. *Probability Sampling of Hospitals and Patients*. Chicago: Health Administration Press.

Huber, D., C. Delaney, J. Crossley, P. Mehmert, and S. Ellerbe. 1992. "A Nursing Management Minimum Data Set." *Journal of the American Nursing Association* 22 (7/8): 35–40.

Institute of Medicine. 2001. *Crossing the Quality Chasm*. Washington, DC: National Academy Press.

Ishikawa, K. 1982. *Guide to Quality Control*. White Plains, NY: Quality Resources.

Joint Commission on Accreditation of Healthcare Organizations. 1993. *The Measurement Mandate*. Oakbrook Terrace, IL: Joint Commission.

Langley, G., K. Nolan, T. Nolan, C. Norman, and L. Provost. 1996. *The Improvement Guide*. San Francisco: Jossey-Bass.

Maddox, B. 1981. "Sampling Concepts, Strategy and Techniques." Pennsylvania Department of Health, State Health Data Center, Technical Report 81-1, July 1.

Nolan, T. 2000. "A Primer on Leading Improvement in Health Care." Presented at the Fifth European Forum on Quality Improvement in Health Care, March 2000, Amsterdam.

Schultz, L. 1994. *Profiles in Quality*. New York: Quality Resources.

Selltiz, C., M. Jahoda, M. Deutsch, and S. Cook. 1959. *Research Methods in Social Relations*. New York: Holt, Rinehart and Winston.

Western Electric Co. 1985. *Statistical Quality Control Handbook*. Indianapolis, IN: AT&T Technologies.

Wheeler, D. 1993. *Understanding Variation: The Key to Managing Chaos*. Knoxville, TN: SPC Press.

———. 1995. *Advanced Topics in Statistical Process Control*. Knoxville, TN: SPC Press.

Wheeler, D., and D. Chambers. 1992. *Understanding Statistical Process Control*. Knoxville, TN: SPC Press.

DATA COLLECTION

John J. Byrnes

Everywhere you turn, everyone wants *data*. But what do they really mean? Where do you get it? Is chart review the gold standard, the best source? Are administrative databases reliable; can they be the gold standard? And what about health plan claims databases—are they even accurate at all? What is the best source for inpatient data that reflect the quality of patient care from both a process and an outcome perspective? When working in the outpatient environment, where and how would you obtain data reflecting the level of quality delivered in physician office practices? These are some of the questions that challenge many healthcare leaders as they struggle to develop quality improvement and measurement programs. This chapter clarifies these issues and some myths commonly held by the industry and provides a practical framework for obtaining valid, accurate, and useful data for quality improvement work.

Categories of Data: Case Example

Quality measurements can be grouped into four categories, or domains: clinical quality (including both process and outcome measures), financial performance, patient satisfaction, and functional status. To report on each of these categories, several separate and distinct data sources may be required. In fact, the challenge is often to collect as many data elements from as few data sources as possible, with the objective of consistency and continuity in mind. For most large and mature quality improvement projects, teams will want to report their performance in all four domains.

A clinical outcome report (COR) from Spectrum Health, a large integrated healthcare system in Grand Rapids, Michigan, illustrates this point. The Spectrum Health system consists of nine hospitals, a 400,000-member health plan, and more than 130 service locations throughout western Michigan. This example provides a complete picture of the care delivered to several distinct patient populations by one of the inpatient hospitalist groups, Michigan Medical, a multispecialty group practice with more than 170 healthcare providers in 30 locations across West Michigan. To produce this COR, a variety of data sources was required, including extracts from the finance and medical record systems. The data were then processed by a third-party vendor who applied a series of rigorous data cleanup algorithms and added severity adjustment and industry benchmarks. The resulting report, or dashboard, contains information for patients with congestive heart failure, ischemic stroke, community-acquired pneumonia, and gastrointestinal bleeding.

The report contains measures of the clinical processes (use of angiotension converting enzyme [ACE] inhibitors, beta-blockers, digoxin, coumadin, natrecor, and echocardiograms), financial performance (length of stay, total patient charges, pharmacy charges, lab charges, X-ray charges, and IV therapy charges), and clinical outcomes (acute renal failure, mortality rate, and readmission within 31 days). The measures were selected by the hospitalist team from more than 200 indicators available in the database as the most important in assessing the quality and cost of care delivered. The measures also include some of the Joint Commission on Accreditation of Healthcare Organizations (Joint Commission) Core Measures.[1] But we still do not have patient satisfaction or functional status measures. For those, the team has to rely on other sources of data.

To obtain patient satisfaction information, the team will use the hospital's patient satisfaction surveys. These surveys are completed by telephone within one week of a patient's discharge by the outbound call center. The results can be reported by nursing unit, are updated quarterly, and can be trended over the last six to eight quarters. In the future, the team hopes to have patient satisfaction information by physician or physician group, such as the Michigan Medical hospitalists group.

To complete the measurement set, the team will need to include the results of the patient's functional status (following their treatment). Many hospital procedures are intended to improve the functional status of the patient. A patient who undergoes a total knee replacement, for example, should experience less knee pain when he or she walks, have a good range of motion of the joint, and be able to perform the activities of daily living that most of us take for granted. For this report, the team will want to examine its patient's functional status before and after hospitalization to demonstrate that the treatments were effective.

In summary, it is important to maintain a balanced perspective of the process of care when designing data collection efforts by collecting data in all four categories: clinical quality, financial performance, patient satisfaction, and functional status. Quality improvement teams who fail to maintain this balance may experience some surprising results of their improvement efforts. For instance, a health system in the Southwest initially reported on a series of very successful quality improvement projects—clinical care had improved, patient satisfaction was at an all-time high, and patient outcomes were at national benchmark status. However, subsequent review of the projects identified that some of the interventions had an untoward effect on the financial outcomes of the process under improvement. Several interventions significantly decreased revenue, and others increased the cost of care unnecessarily. If financial measures had been included in the data collection and reporting process, the negative financial effect could have been minimized and the same outstanding quality improvements would have resulted. In the end, the projects were considered only marginally successful because of the lack of a balanced approach to process improvement and measurement.

Considerations in Data Collection

The Time and Cost of Data Collection

All data collection efforts take time and money. The key is to balance the cost of data collection versus the value of the data to your improvement efforts. In other words, are the cost and time of data collection worth the effort? Will the data have the power to drive change and improvement? Although this cost-benefit analysis may not be quite as tangible as in the world of business and finance, it is still imperative that the value equation be considered. Generally, medical record review and prospective data collection are considered the most time-intensive and expensive forms of data collection. Many reserve these for highly specialized improvement projects or to answer questions that have surfaced following review of administrative data sets. Administrative data[2] are often considered very cost effective, especially as the credibility of administrative databases has improved and continues to improve through the efforts of coding and billing regulations, initiatives,[3] and rules-based software development. Additionally, third-party vendors have emerged that can provide data cleanup and severity adjustment. Successful data collection strategies often combine both code- and chart-based sources into a data collection plan that capitalizes on the strengths and cost effectiveness of each.

The following situation illustrates how the cost effectiveness of an administrative system can be combined with the detailed information available in a medical record review. A data analyst, using a clinical decision support system (administrative database), discovered a higher than expected incidence of renal failure (a serious complication) following coronary artery bypass surgery. The rate was well above 10 percent for the most recent 12 months (more than 800 patients were included in the data set), and had slowly increased over the last six quarters. However, the clinical decision support system did not contain enough detail to explain *why* such a high number of patients were experiencing this complication or whether this was a complication of the coronary artery bypass graft procedure versus a chronic condition present on admission. To get to the "why," the data analyst used chart review to (1) verify that the rate of renal failure as reported in the administrative data system was correct, (2) isolate cases representing postoperative incidence, (3) identify the root cause(s) of the renal failure, and (4) answer additional questions about the patient population that were of interest to the physicians. In this example, the analyst used the administrative system to identify unwanted complications in a large patient population (a screening or surveillance function) and reserved chart review for a much smaller, focused review (80 charts) to validate the incidence and answer why the patients were experiencing the complication. This is an excellent example of the effective use of two common data sources and demonstrates how the analyst is able to capitalize on the strengths of both while using each most efficiently.

Collecting the Critical Few Rather than Collecting for a Rainy Day

Many quality improvement efforts take the approach of collecting every possible data element "just in case we need it." Ironically, the justification for this approach is often based on saving time, as there is a feeling that since the chart has already been pulled, one might as well be thorough. This syndrome of stockpiling just in case versus fulfilling requirements "just in time" has been well studied in supply chain management and proven to be ineffective and inefficient and create quality issues (Denison 2002). Similarly, in terms of data collection, this approach provides little value to the effort and is one of the biggest mistakes quality improvement teams tend to make. Rather than provide a rich source of information, this approach unnecessarily drives up the cost of data collection, slows the data collection process, creates data management issues, and often overwhelms the quality improvement team with too much data.

For all quality improvement projects, it is critical to collect only the data required to be successful. For ongoing data collection efforts, as a rule, you should be able to link every data element collected to a report, thereby ensuring that you do not collect data that are not used (James 2003). In the reporting project discussed above, the hospitalist team was limited to selecting no more than 15 measures for each clinical condition. They also selected the indicators that (1) have been shown by evidence-based literature to have the greatest effect on patient outcomes (e.g., in congestive heart failure, use of ACE inhibitors and beta-blockers, evaluation of left ventricular ejection fraction); (2) reflect areas where significant improvements are needed; (3) will be reported in the public domain (Joint Commission Core Measures); and (4) together, provide a balanced view of the clinical process of care, financial performance, and patient outcomes.

Inpatient Versus Outpatient Data

The distinction between inpatient and outpatient data is an important consideration in planning the data collection process because the data sources and approach to data collection can be quite different.

The case of a team working on a diabetes disease management project and the issues they will need to address illustrates this point. First, disease management projects tend to focus on the entire continuum of care, so they will need data from both the inpatient and outpatient settings. Second, the team will need to identify whether the patients receive the majority of care in one setting or the other and decide whether data collection priorities should be established with this is mind. For diabetes, the setting that has the most influence on patient outcomes is the outpatient setting, so collection of outpatient data would be a priority over the inpatient data. Third, the team must select the measures that reflect the key aspects of care that have the most influence on patient outcomes. Remembering to collect the critical few, the team would consult the American Diabetes Association (ADA) guidelines for expert direction on this issue. Fourth, the team must recognize that the sources of outpatient data are much different than inpatient data, and they tend to be more fragmented and harder to obtain.

To identify outpatient data sources, the team should consider the following questions: Are the physicians in organized medical groups that have an outpatient electronic medical record, which could be a source of data? Will their financial or billing system be able to identify all of the patients with diabetes in their practice? If not, can the health plans in the area supply the needed data by practice site or individual physician? For diabetes, some of the most important measures are based on laboratory testing. Do the physicians have their own lab? If so, do they archive the laboratory data for the needed 12- to 24-month snapshot? If they do not do their own lab testing, do they use a common reference lab that would be able to supply the data? Once these questions are answered, the team will be ready to proceed with data collection in the outpatient setting.

Sources of Data

As discussed above, the sources of data for quality improvement projects are extensive. Some sources are simple to obtain, and others are more complex; some data sources are inexpensive, some are expensive, and some are very expensive. In the average hospital or health system, data sources often include medical records, prospective data collection, surveys of various types, telephone interviews, focus groups, administrative databases, health plan claims databases, cost accounting systems, patient registries, stand-alone clinical databases, and lab and pharmacy databases.

The keys to a successful quality improvement project and data collection initiative are the following:

1. Identify the purpose of the data measurement activity (for monitoring at regular intervals or investigation over a limited period, or one-time study).
2. Identify the most appropriate data sources.
3. Identify the most important measures for collection (the critical few).
4. Design a common-sense data collection strategy that will provide complete, accurate, and timely information.

Together, these steps will provide good value to the team and the information required to drive quality improvements.

Medical Record Review (Retrospective)

Retrospective data collection involves identification and selection of a patient's medical record or group of records *after* the patient has been discharged from the hospital or clinic. Additionally, review generally cannot take place until all medical and financial coding functions are complete because these coded criteria are used as a starting point to identify the study cohort. For many quality improvement projects, medical record review continues to be the mainstay of data collection for several reasons.

First, many proponents of medical record review believe it to be the most accurate method of data collection. They believe that because administrative databases have been designed for financial and administrative purposes rather than quality improvement, they do not contain adequate detail, are fraught with errors, and contain "dirty data," that is, data that make no sense or appear to have come from other sources.

Second, some database projects rely on medical record review because many of the data elements are not available in administrative databases. For example, measures that require a time stamp, such as administration of antibiotics within one hour prior to surgical incision, are not available within most administrative databases.

Third, several national quality improvement database projects, including HEDIS, Joint Commission Core Measures, Leapfrog,[4] and the National Quality Forum's (NQF) Voluntary Consensus Standards for Hospital Care, are dependent on retrospective medical record review for a significant portion of required data elements. Not only do they contain measures requiring a time stamp but some measures also require the data collector to include or exclude patients based on criteria that are not consistently captured in administrative databases. The measure "percent of patients with congestive heart failure who are receiving an ACE inhibitor" is an example of this. The use of ACE inhibitors in this population is indicated in all patients with an ejection fraction of less than 40 percent. The ejection fraction is not part of the typical administrative database. Sometimes this information is contained in a stand-alone database in the cardiology department and is generally inaccessible, or it may only be contained in a transcribed report in the patient's medical record. Hence, accurate reporting of this measure is completely dependent on retrospective chart review, yet it is one of the most critical interventions that a patient with congestive heart failure will receive. A recent consensus document presented to NQF[5] suggested that clinical importance should rate foremost among criteria for "effectiveness" and that measures that score poorly on feasibility[6] because of the burden of medical record review should not be excluded solely on that basis if their clinical importance is high (National Quality Forum Consumer, Purchaser and Research Council Members 2002).

Fourth, focused medical record review is the primary tool for answering the *why* of given situations, as described above. Suffice it to say that medical record review continues to be a key component of many data collection projects, but it needs to be used judiciously because of the time and cost involved.

The approach to medical record review involves a series of well-thought-out steps, beginning with the development of a data collection tool and ending with the compilation of collected data elements into a registry or electronic database software for review and analysis.

Prospective Data Collection, Data Collection Forms, and Scanners

Prospective data collection is also reliant on medical record review, but it is completed during a patient's hospitalization or visit rather than retrospectively. The data collection is commonly completed by nursing staff, dedicated research assistants, or full-time data analysts. The downside to asking nursing staff to perform data collection is that it is an immensely time-consuming task that can distract nurses from their direct patient care responsibilities. The author's preferred approach is to hire research assistants or full-time data analysts who can perform the data collection and be responsible for data entry and analysis. Because this will be their only job, the accuracy of data collection is better; if the staff are also responsible for presenting their work to various quality committees, the data are more likely to be rigorously validated.

Obviously, this method of data collection is expensive, but if the time required for data entry can be minimized, staff can focus on accurate collection and the analysis/reporting functions. One way to accomplish this is by converting the data collection forms into a scannable format. With this approach, data entry can be as simple as feeding the forms into the scanner and viewing the results on the computer screen. The key to success is careful design of the forms and careful completion to ensure that all of the data elements are captured by the scanner.

The most efficient data collection tools follow the actual flow of patient care and medical record documentation whether the data are collected retrospectively or prospectively. The advantages of prospective data collection are many. First, detailed information not routinely available in administrative databases can be gathered. Physiologic parameters can be captured, such as the range of blood pressures for a patient on vasoactive infusions or 24-hour intake and output for patients with heart failure. As discussed earlier, data requiring a time stamp can also be captured. It is clear that timely administration of certain therapies (e.g., antibiotic administration within one hour prior to surgical incision or within four hours of hospital arrival for patients with pneumonia) improves patient outcomes. The timing of administration of "clot busters" for patients with certain types of stroke can mean the difference between full recovery or no recovery, and the window of opportunity for these patients is small, usually within three hours of the onset of symptoms. For patients with acute myocardial infarction, the administration of aspirin and beta-blockers within the first 24 hours is critical to survival.

Prospective chart review also allows the data collection staff to spot patient trends as they develop, rather than getting the information in a retrospective fashion after the patients have been discharged. For instance, an increasing incidence of ventilator-associated pneumonia may be detected sooner, or an increase in the rate of aspiration in patients with stroke may be spotted as it occurs.

Unfortunately, the downside to this data collection approach is cost. Prospective data collection is very costly and time consuming, and it often requires several full-time data analysts. Project IMPACT,[7] a popular critical care data system, requires 3.5 full-time analysts for data collection, entry, analysis, and reporting for approximately 75 beds in the surgical and medical intensive care units at Spectrum Health.

Administrative Databases

Administrative databases are a common source of data for quality improvement projects. *Administrative data* refers to information that is collected, processed, and stored in automated information systems. This includes enrollment or eligibility information, claims information, and managed care encounters. The claims and encounters may be for hospital and other facility services, professional services, prescription drug services, laboratory services, and so on.

Examples of administrative data sources include hospital or physician office billing systems, health plan claims databases, health information management or medical record systems, and registration systems (admission/ discharge/transfer). Ideally, a hospital will also maintain a cost accounting system that not only integrates the previously mentioned systems into one database but also provides the extremely important elements of patient cost. Although each of these sources has its unique characteristics, for the purposes of discussion they will be considered collectively under "administrative databases" (with the exception of health plan claims databases, which will be covered later in the chapter).

Administrative databases are an excellent source of data for reporting on clinical quality, financial performance, and some patient outcomes. In fact, administrative databases provide the backbone for many quality improvement programs, including Spectrum Health's COR described in the beginning of this chapter.

The advantages of administrative databases include the following:

1. They are a less expensive source of data compared to other alternatives such as chart review or prospective data collection techniques.
2. They take advantage of existing transaction systems already required in the daily business operations of a healthcare organization (frequently referred to as "legacy systems").
3. Most of the code sets embedded in administrative databases are standardized,[8] simplifying internal comparison between multifacility organizations and external benchmarking with purchased or government data sets.
4. Most administrative databases are staffed by "super-users" who are skilled at sophisticated database queries.
5. Database architecture and support are provided by expert database administrators in information technology departments.
6. The volume of indicators available is 100 times greater than that available through other data collection techniques.
7. Data reporting tools are available as part of the purchased system or through third-party add-ons or services.
8. Many administrative databases, especially well-managed financial and cost accounting systems, undergo regular reconciliation, audit, and data cleanup procedures that enhance the integrity of their data.

Because of these advantages, Spectrum Health makes extensive use of administrative data systems to supply the primary source data for quality improvement projects. Spectrum Health's COR uses two administrative data sources: the billing system and the medical record system. Information from these sources is extracted and sent to a vendor that provides data processing services. The vendor performs an extensive data cleanup using in excess of 1,500 edits that identify problems with the source data. The vendor also applies severity adjustment, statistical analysis, and benchmarks and returns the data in the form of a clinical decision support system (CDSS PinPoint) within 45 days of submission of the raw data.

The system contains more than 35 of the most common clinical conditions (medical and surgical procedures), with at least 200 measures of clinical quality, financial performance, and patient outcomes for each condition. In all, the decision support system contains more than 7,500 standardized performance measures with the ability to report performance at the system level, by individual hospital, and by individual physician. The database is updated quarterly, and historical data are now archived in the Spectrum Health data warehouse for future quality improvement projects and clinical studies.

The yearly cost to maintain this system for three of Spectrum Health's hospitals is approximately $330,000, or the equivalent of four to five data analysts, yet the system's reporting power far surpasses anything that can be accomplished by five analysts performing chart review. Is such a system a good value proposition? Yes, because the full cost can be repaid with the successful implementation of one or two quality improvement projects carefully selected from the many opportunities identified by the system. In fact, one of the first projects identified by the system was the need to improve blood product utilization in total joint replacements to avoid wasting money by cross-matching blood that is never used. The savings realized as a result of this project alone more than covered the cost of the entire system for the first year.

Some argue that administrative data are less reliable than chart review (Iezzoni et al. 1994). However, in the author's experience, when the administrative data are properly cleaned and validated, the indicator definitions are clear and concise, and the limitations of the data are understood, administrative data can be used just as effectively as chart review. To illustrate this point, the most common measures from the system described above were validated using four approaches: (1) chart review using an appropriate sampling methodology, (2) chart review performed for the Joint Commission Core Measures, (3) comparison to similar measures in stand-alone databases that rely on chart abstraction or prospective data collection strategies (e.g., National Registry of Myocardial Infarction), and (4) face validation performed by physicians with expertise in the clinical condition under study. Results proved the administrative data sources to be extremely reliable.

Patient Surveys: Satisfaction and Functional Status
Patient Satisfaction Surveys

Patient satisfaction surveys have long been a favorite tool of quality improvement professionals, especially teams interested in the perceptions of patients, either in terms of the quality of care or the quality of service provided. But the complexity of the science underlying survey research is often underestimated, resulting in less-than-desirable results. Indeed, there is quite an art (and science) to constructing surveys that produce valid, reliable, relevant information. Likewise, survey validation alone is a time-consuming and complex undertaking. For those interested in survey development and validation, many excellent textbooks on the subject review the concepts of reliability, validity, sampling methodology, and bias; the reader is referred to these sources for an in-depth review of this topic.

Practically speaking, when an organization or quality improvement team is considering the use of surveys, it has several choices on how to proceed. The team can design the survey tool itself, hire an outside expert to design the survey, or purchase an existing survey or survey service that has been well validated. Usually, the fastest and least expensive approach is to purchase existing, well-validated survey instruments or utilize a survey organization to provide a turnkey solution. One such organization is Press Ganey, which currently serves more than 30 percent of all U.S. hospitals.[9]

The frequency with which surveys are conducted and reported to the organization is also extremely important. When patient satisfaction surveys are conducted on a continual basis, using a proper sampling methodology, the organization has the ability to rapidly respond to changes in patients' wants and needs. It also has the ability to rapidly respond to emerging breaks in service.

The ability to report survey results at an actionable level is key to success; in most cases, that means reporting results at the nursing unit or location of service. Furthermore, full engagement at the management and staff levels is important to ensure that the results are regularly reviewed and action plans are developed.

One of the most successful patient satisfaction survey projects the author observed was the "Point of Service Patient Satisfaction Surveys" at Lovelace Health Systems in the late 1990s. In that program, any patient who received care within the system had an opportunity to comment on the quality of the care and service they experienced. The survey forms were short (one page), concise, and easy to read, and they took only a few minutes to complete. The most important determinants of satisfaction (as determined by the survey research staff) were reflected in the questions, and patients were also given an opportunity to provide comments at the end of the survey. The surveys were collected and reviewed on a daily or weekly basis by the unit manager so that emerging trends could be identified and quickly corrected. Survey results were tabulated monthly and posted on the units for all to see, including the patients who visited the clinics and inpatient areas. The results were also reviewed on a unit-by-unit basis by the senior management team each month.

Functional Status Surveys

The measurement of functional status following a medical treatment is the fourth category of data collection for clinical quality improvement projects. As a general rule, medical treatments and hospital procedures are intended to improve the functional status or quality of life experienced by the patient. For example, a patient hospitalized for congestive heart failure should be able to walk farther, have more energy, and experience less shortness of breath following a "tune-up" in the hospital. A patient who undergoes a total knee replacement should have less knee pain when he or she walks, experience a good range of motion of the joint, and be able to perform the activities of daily living most of us take for granted, such as walking several miles, dancing, doing yard work, and performing normal household chores.

Functional status is usually measured before and at several points following the treatment or procedure. For some surgical procedures, such as total joint replacement, it is common to obtain a baseline assessment prior to the procedure and then assessments at regular intervals following surgery, often at 1, 3, 6, and sometimes 12 months postoperative. The survey can be collected by several means including mail or telephone and, most recently, on the Internet.

The most widely recognized early pioneer of functional status surveys is John Ware, Ph.D., the principal developer of the SF-36, SF-12, SF-8, and disease-specific health outcome surveys.[10]

Health Plan Databases

Health plan databases can be an excellent a source of data for quality improvement projects, particularly projects that have a population health management focus. For many years, health plans have used a variety of means to collect data to report on their performance, track the management of the care received by their members, and direct programs in disease management and care management. Because of this experience, health plan data have become more and more reliable. In fact, most health plans now have sophisticated data warehouses and a staff of expert data analysts.

Why are health plan databases so valuable? Because they contain detailed information on *all of the care* received by health plan members. How is this accomplished? All services provided to a patient generate a bill (or claim). When the bill is submitted to the health plan for payment, it is captured in a claim-processing system. As a result of this process, all of the care received by an entire population of patients, including hospitalizations, outpatient procedures, physician office visits, lab testing, prescriptions, anything billed to and paid for by the health plan, is contained in the health plan claims database.

Why is this so important? From a population management perspective, the health plan claims database is often the only source for *all* information on the care received by a patient and, for that matter, an entire population of patients. It is therefore an excellent source of data for disease management programs where the goal is to improve the health for a specific population of patients. Not only does it provide a comprehensive record of patient activity but it can also be used to identify and select patients for enrollment into disease management programs. An excellent tracking tool for examining the entire continuum of care, claims databases are also the only externally available source of information for describing physician office practice. In essence, a claims database is the single best source of information on the total care received by a patient. Several examples follow to illustrate these points.

Health plan databases are commonly used to identify patients who have not received needed preventive services such as mammograms, colon cancer screening, and immunizations. They can identify patients who are not receiving the appropriate medications for many chronic medical conditions such as heart failure or asthma. They can also be used to support physicians in their office practices. Figure 6.1 is an example of a report developed at Spectrum Health[11] for a systemwide diabetes disease management program. It provides participating physicians with a quarterly snapshot of (1) the percentage of their patients who are receiving all of the treatments and tests recommended by the ADA guidelines, (2) how the physician's performance compares to that of his or her peers, and (3) all of the patients who have fallen outside the ADA standards in the last quarter and are in need of recommended tests or treatments.

What are the limitations of health plan databases? Many of the same considerations covered under hospital administrative databases apply to health plan databases, including questions associated with accuracy, granularity, and timeliness. Users of health plan claims databases must also keep in mind that changes in reimbursement rules (and the provider's response to those changes) may affect the integrity of the data over time. Historical

FIGURE 6.1

Diabetes
Provider
Support
Report

Rolling Calendar Year July 1, 2001–June 30, 2002   PCP:
                                                                                   Provider Group:

I. Provider-Specific Data

Criteria	ADA Standards	Points	Tested	In Standard	Percent
Education	1 / 2 year	48	42	42	88
Eye exams	Annual	48	30	30	63
GlycoHb ordered	Annual	48	45	45	94
GlycoHb level	≤ 7.0	48	45	37	82
Microalbumin ordered	Annual	48	31	31	65
Microalbumin > 30	Rx filled	10	10	5	50
LDL ordered	Annual	48	42	42	88
LDL level	< 100	48	42	31	73

* Patients in this report have had at least two diagnoses of diabetes.

II. Percent of Patients Within Standard

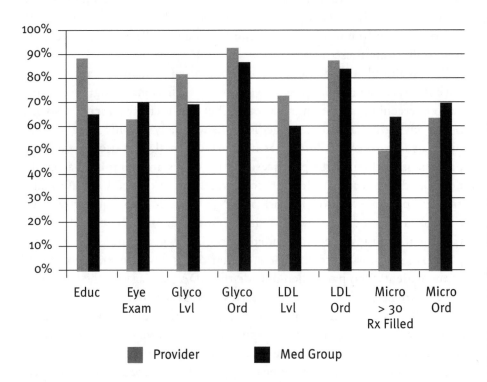

FIGURE 6.1
(continued)

III. High-Risk Patient Detail—Patients Outside ADA Standards in Current Quarter

Criteria for inclusion—one or more of the following: (1) no education in last two years; (2) no eye exam in last one year; (3) GlycoHb > 7.0 or no GlycoHb ordered in last year; (4) no microalbumin in last one year; (5) microalbumin > 30 and no ACE/ARB filled; or (6) LDL ≥ 100 or no LDL ordered in last year.

Name	MR No.	Education	Eye Exam	Glycohemaglobin Ordered	Glycohemaglobin Level	Microalbumin Ordered	Microalbumin > 30, Rx Filled	Lipids Ordered	Lipids Result
Patient	100-319-xxx		7/21/99	7/15/99	6.7	5/28/99	N	2/29/00	120
Patient	100-427-xxx					2/22/00		2/22/00	118
Patient	100-587-xxx								
Patient	100-595-xxx	8/12/99		8/21/99	7.0				
Patient	100-623-xxx			2/2/00	10.8			1/21/00	142
Patient	100-666-xxx	7/14/99		12/15/99	10.7				
Patient	100-782-xxx	2/12/00		11/27/99	11.0				
Patient	100-847-xxx	2/12/00		3/12/99	7.0				
Patient	100-849-xxx	12/27/99		8/1/99	6.1			5/24/99	118
Patient	100-882-xxx	10/15/98		8/31/99	6.8			3/21/00	132
Patient	100-882-xxx	4/25/99		4/23/00	6.3				
Patient	100-893-xxx	7/31/98		9/19/99	12.4			8/25/99	123
Patient	100-901-xxx	6/15/99		6/2/00	6.3				
Patient	100-901-xxx	1/15/00		1/23/00	12.0			9/19/99	98
Patient	100-902-xxx	1/18/00		5/15/99	12.4			7/31/99	92
Patient	100-909-xxx							2/15/00	145
Patient	100-944-xxx	12/27/99		10/10/99	11.9			10/6/99	150
Patient	100-914-xxx			2/4/00	10.8			4/14/00	92
Patient	100-919-xxx			4/29/00	6.2			6/1/00	89
Patient	100-809-xxx	6/13/00	6/15/00	6/2/00	6.9	4/2/00	N	2/11/00	126
Patient	100-914-xxx	1/15/00	12/20/99	12/12/99	11.2	12/12/99	N	1/16/00	132
Patient	100-917-xxx	1/18/00	2/13/00	1/18/00	6.9	1/15/00	N	11/21/99	160
Patient	100-929-xxx	7/22/99	8/1/99	7/21/99	10.0	7/21/99	N	12/5/99	98

Note: ADA = American Diabetes Association.
Source: Spectrum Health, Grand Rapids, MI.

issues of up-coding may make some historical data inaccurate, especially as they relate to tracking and trending of complication rates and the categorization of certain types of complications. Finally, health plan databases track events, the type of procedure performed, or that a lab test was completed. They do not contain detailed information on the outcomes of care or the results of tests (e.g., lab tests, radiology examinations, results of biopsies). Nevertheless, health plan claims data are inexpensive to acquire, available electronically, and typically encompass large populations across the continuum of care. When properly utilized, they are a rich source of data for population management, disease management, and quality improvement projects.

Patient Registries

For a variety of reasons, many organizations establish condition-specific patient registries for their more sophisticated quality improvement projects. Why? Perhaps they do not have a reliable source of clinical information, available data are not timely enough, or they wish to collect patient outcome information over several months following a hospitalization or procedure. Often, the desire to develop a patient registry involves all of the above considerations, and the registry includes data collected using all of the aforementioned approaches. Given the detailed nature of patient registries, they can be an extremely powerful source of quality improvement data, and their design is very straightforward. Most commonly, the registries are specialty or procedure specific. Acute myocardial infarction, total joint replacement, coronary artery bypass graft, and congestive heart failure are common examples of procedure- or condition-specific registries

The advantages of patient registries include the following:

1. They are a rich source of information because they are customized.
2. They can collect all of the data that the physicians or health system determines are most important.
3. They can be used for quality improvement and research purposes.
4. They are not subject to the shortcomings of administrative or health plan databases.
5. A multitude of data sources and collection techniques can be combined to provide a complete picture of the patient experience, including the quality of care that was provided and long-term patient outcomes (often up to a year following the procedure).

Patient registries are versatile and flexible because just about any reliable data source or collection methodology can be used to populate the registry. This includes administrative data, outbound call centers, prospective data collection, retrospective chart review, and a variety of survey instruments, particularly for patient satisfaction and functional status. However, with all customized database projects, particular attention must be given to balancing the volume of data collected and the insight it will provide or the change it will drive versus the cost of the data collection. To ensure a successful registry project, the oversight team must commit to collecting only the necessary data elements required for success of its project.

An orthopedic patient registry illustrates how the considerations outlined above were addressed. First, an oversight team including the service line director, medical director, and physicians was established. The inclusion of physicians from the beginning of the project created a tremendous level of physician involvement, to the point that the physicians felt great pride of ownership in the project. Second, the scope of data collection was narrowed to focus only on total knee and hip replacements. Third, the purpose and use of the registry was clearly outlined; the registry was limited to identifying clinical issues and improving the quality of patient care. No other use was allowed, and a nonpunitive environment was established. Fourth, the number of data elements was restricted to the critical few—those most important to assessing patient outcomes and the integrity of the patient care processes—which also meant they would be reported and reviewed regularly by the oversight team (see Table 6.1).

Data collection was accomplished through several means, as illustrated in Table 6.1 and Figure 6.2. Patients were identified through the administrative database. Data collection was completed prospectively during the hospitalization, and any missing elements were captured by retrospective chart review. All data were collected on scannable forms to ease the data-entry burden. Longitudinal outcomes were tracked through the outbound call center using a variety of patient interview tools and survey instruments, with calls made at 1, 3, 6, and 12 months following the primary procedure. Ultimately, the data were combined in a commonly available database product and audited for completeness and accuracy.

Case Study in Clinical Reporting

So far, the different categories of data, considerations for data collection, and six data sources have been covered, so let us pull all of this together in a current hospital setting.

Earlier, the COR system in use at Spectrum Health was briefly introduced. The COR system consists of two databases (assembled from a variety of data sources), two reporting engines,[12] and many types of predefined production reports.

Two databases are actually assembled from the raw data sources described throughout this chapter. The first database contains 40 clinical

TABLE 6.1
Orthopedic
Patient
Registry
Data Elements

Orthopedic Database Characteristics	
Total Data Elements	329
Manual Data Elements	216
Electronic Data Elements	113
No. of Patients (monthly)	106
Data Sources	
• Patient	
• Case managers	
• OR system	
• Billing/cost accounting system	
• Call center	

Number of Data Elements by Category	
Patient History	32
Demographic	56
Functional Status	42
Procedures/OR	26
Complications	3
Devices/Equipment	13
Postoperative	45
Follow-up	28 (x 4) = 112

Number of Data Elements by Source	
Patient	35
Case Manager	69
OR System	48
Billing/Cost Accounting System	65
Call Center	112

Source: Spectrum Health, Grand Rapids, MI.

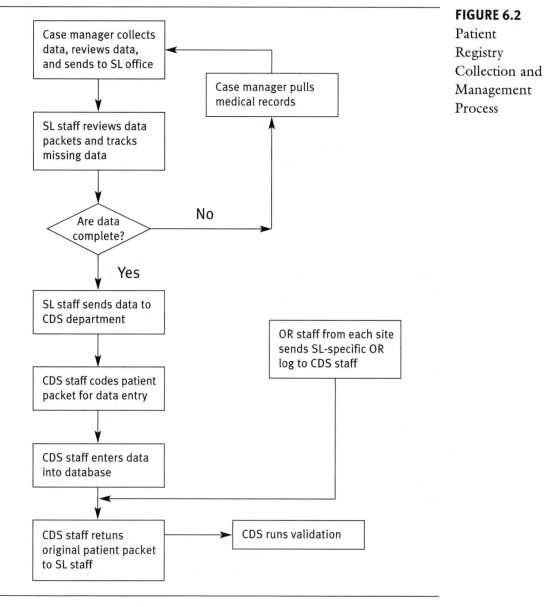

FIGURE 6.2
Patient
Registry
Collection and
Management
Process

Note: CDS = clinical decision support; OR = operating room; SL = service line.

conditions with 200 measures per condition. The data are extensively cleaned and severity adjusted based on clinical criteria specific to each of the 40 conditions.[13] The second database contains the edited data (from the first database) after they have passed through the data cleanup process. However, these data are not subdivided into 40 clinical conditions, but remain in an open architecture used primarily for ad hoc queries that fall outside the 40 conditions.

Data for the system are obtained from several sources, including the financial system, medical record system, and manual chart review, both retrospective and prospective. The system was first populated with an extract of the finance and medical record system with two years of historical data. These 24 months of data provided a good overview of care delivered in the past and served as the baseline measurement set for many of the projects. Data extracts are completed quarterly to update the database. The chart review required for a subset of measures, most commonly the Joint Commission Core Measures, is completed on a monthly basis.

The most commonly used reports include (1) an executive dashboard with health system– and hospital-level data, (2) physician-level reports, and (3) a surveillance report.

The executive dashboard, shown in Figure 6.3, contains hypothetical measures of clinical quality for lower joint replacement. The executive dashboard is reviewed quarterly by the executive leadership team and medical directors. It is also shared with the quality committee of the board of directors, the system quality committee, and each of the teams working on improvements in the ten highest-volume conditions. In addition to the spreadsheet-like display of the dashboard, the COR includes trended displays for each measure representing the last 18 months (see Figure 6.4).

The physician-level reports can contain any of the indicators in the database, including those generated for the executive dashboard. The physician-level information is shared at medical staff or professional standards committees and is peer-review protected. The physician-level data are also severity adjusted so they clearly identify which patients can be considered "sicker" at the time of presentation to the hospital. The presentation format is similar to the executive dashboard.

The surveillance report is an extremely useful tool supplied by the vendor (MEDai, Inc.). This quarterly report provides a list of all measures outside the severity-adjusted expected value for each clinical condition. The report ensures that each measure in the database is screened on a quarterly basis and, if outside of the severity-adjusted expected value, flagged for review. An example of this report is shown in Figure 6.5.

Conclusion

As you can see, many data sources and data collection approaches are available to choose from. Rarely does one method serve all purposes, so it is important to understand the advantages and disadvantages of all. For this reason, the case above, like all successful quality improvement initiatives, uses a combination of data and data collection techniques, thus capitaliz-

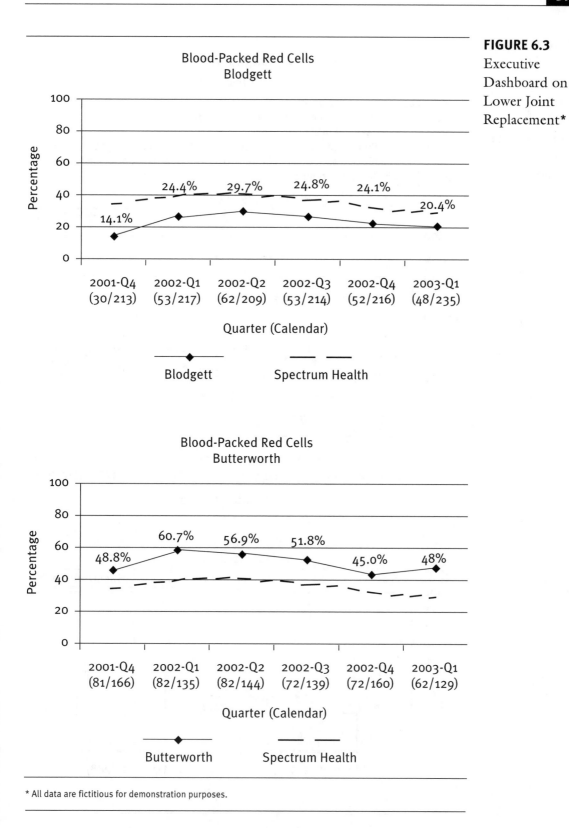

FIGURE 6.3
Executive
Dashboard on
Lower Joint
Replacement*

* All data are fictitious for demonstration purposes.

FIGURE 6.4

Clinical
Outcome
Report:
Example of
Trended Data
Over Six
Quarters*

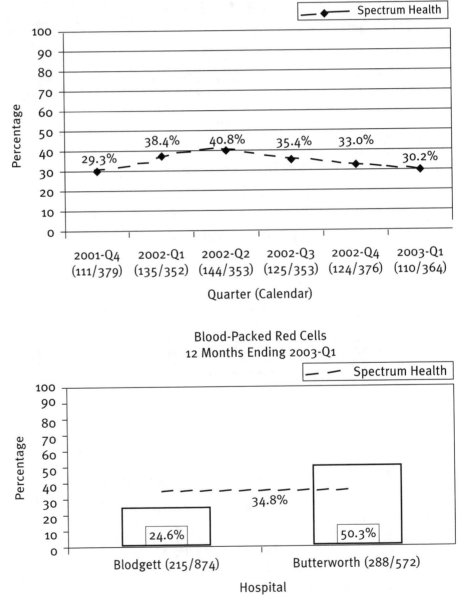

Lower Joint Replacement

Indicator: Blood-Packed Red Cells

Time Frame:	October 1, 2001–March 31, 2002
Numerator:	Presence of a match in the charge detail description reflecting usage of packed red cells
Denominator:	Primary procedure code reflecting total replacement of the hip, knee, or ankle joint or revision of an existing prosthesis
Target:	To be determined

Blood-Packed Red Cells

Spectrum Health

29.3%   38.4%   40.8%   35.4%   33.0%   30.2%

Percentage

2001-Q4   2002-Q1   2002-Q2   2002-Q3   2002-Q4   2003-Q1
(111/379) (135/352) (144/353) (125/353) (124/376) (110/364)

Quarter (Calendar)

Blood-Packed Red Cells
12 Months Ending 2003-Q1

Spectrum Health

34.8%

24.6%   50.3%

Blodgett (215/874)   Butterworth (288/572)

Hospital

* All data are fictitious for demonstration purposes.

Cholecystectomy   **Total patients: 455**

- Accidental Operative Puncture or Laceration value of 2.5% is significantly higher than the expected value of 0.4%.
- Lap Procedure to Open value of 8.3% is significantly higher than the expected value of 3.1%.
- Cholecystectomy Open value of 12.5% is significantly higher than the expected value of 5.7%.
- Clindamycin value of 10.5% is significantly higher than the expected value of 1.2%.

Large Intestinal Resection   **Total patients: 350**

- Probable Hospital-Acquired Infection Present value of 15.2% is significantly higher than the expected value of 9.2%.
- Length of Stay value of 8.87 is significantly higher than the expected value of 7.85%.
- Sepsis Documented as Secondary Diagnosis value of 8.3% is significantly higher than the expected value of 4.0%.
- Wound Infection value of 5.3% is significantly higher than the expected value of 2.3%.
- Postoperative Infections value of 7.3% is significantly higher than the expected value of 2.3%.
- Antibiotic Resistant Drugs value of 1.5% is significantly higher than the expected value of 0.2%.
- Clindamycin value of 7.9% is significantly higher than the expected value of 4.2%.

* All values are fictitious and for demonstration purposes only.

Source: Courtesy of MEDai, Inc. Reprinted with permission.

FIGURE 6.5
Surveillance Report Showing Measures Outside the Severity Adjusted Expected*

ing on the strengths and minimizing the weaknesses. With this knowledge comes the ability to increase your effectiveness and efficiency in the use of data and measurement for the purpose of clinical quality improvement.

Study Questions

1. What are the salient advantages and disadvantages of the quality of data coming from medical records versus administrative sources?
2. Give two examples of areas where you can identify a balanced set of measures.
3. Will electronic medical records make data collection better? Why or why not?

Acknowledgments

Special thanks go to Lori Anderson for her diligent review, suggestions, and contributions to this chapter, as well as to Monica Carpenter for her editorial assistance.

Notes

1. The Joint Commission Core Measures are an initial attempt to integrate outcomes and other performance measurement into the accreditation process by requiring hospitals to collect and submit 25 measures distributed across five initial core measurement areas.
2. Administrative data generally reflect the content of discharge abstracts (e.g., demographic information on patients such as age, sex, zip code; information about the episode of care such as admission source, length of stay, charges, discharge status; diagnostic and procedural codes). Namely, the Uniform Hospital Discharge Data Set and the Uniform Bill (UB-92) of the Centers for Medicare and Medicaid Services (CMS), formerly known as the Health Care Financing Administration (HCFA) provide specifications for the abstraction of administrative/billing data.
3. Examples include the Health Insurance Portability and Accountability Act (HIPAA) of 1996 (Public Law 104-191); *International Classification of Diseases, Ninth Revision* (ICD-9), developed by the World Health Organization (WHO) and transitioned to ICD-10-CM; Systematized Nomenclature of Medicine (SNOMED) project; and the Unified Medical Language System (UMLS).
4. The Leapfrog Group is a coalition of more than 140 public and private organizations that provide healthcare benefits. It was created to help save lives and reduce preventable medical mistakes by mobilizing employer purchasing power to initiate breakthrough improvements in the safety of healthcare and by giving consumers information to make more informed hospital choices.
5. NQF is a private, not-for-profit membership organization created to develop and implement a national strategy for healthcare quality measurement and reporting. Its mission is to improve U.S. healthcare through endorsement of consensus-based national standards for measurement and public reporting of healthcare performance data that provide meaningful information about whether care is safe, timely, beneficial, patient centered, equitable, and efficient.

6. *Feasibility* infers that the cost of data collection and reporting is justified by the potential improvements in care and outcomes that result from the act of measurement.

7. The Project IMPACT data set was created by and for ICU practitioners in a multiyear effort by nearly 100 Society of Critical Care Medicine multidisciplinary critical care experts in conjunction with Tri-Analytics, Inc. For additional information, please see the project's web site: www.projectimpacticu.cc/research.html.

8. The Uniform Hospital Discharge Data Set and UB-92 provide specifications for the abstraction of administrative/billing data, providing standardization for admission source; charges (national revenue codes); discharge status; and diagnostic and procedural codes in the form of ICD-9, CPT-4, NCD, and HCPCS codes.

9. For more information, see www.pressganey.com

10. For more information on Ware's work and a description of available surveys, please visit www.qualitymetric.com.

11. This report was developed as part of a systemwide Spectrum Health Diabetes Collaborative. The collaborative has representation from all nine Spectrum Health hospitals, Spectrum's 400,000-member health plan, several physician groups, the continuing care division, the Visiting Nurse Association, and long-term care. The original design was first developed at Lovelace Health System in Albuquerque, New Mexico, as part of the Episode of Care Disease Management program.

12. One reporting engine is provided by a third-party vendor, MEDai, Inc., in Orlando, Florida, and the second was developed internally for data trending and automation of COR production.

13. The clinical criteria for the severity adjustment are specific to each condition. Therefore, the list of criteria for chronic obstructive pulmonary disease is substantially different than the criteria for coronary artery bypass graft, and so forth. The severity adjustment is also based on the patient's status at the time of admission, rather than at discharge, and does not include complications and procedures, as these are characteristics of the physician, not the patient.

REFERENCES

Denison, D. C. 2002. "On the Supply Chain, Just-in-Time Enters New Era." *Boston Globe* May 5.

Iezzoni, L. I., J. Daley, T. Heeren, S. M. Foley, J. S. Hughes, E. S. Fisher, C. C. Duncan, and G. A. Coffman. 1994. "Using Administrative Data to Screen Hospitals for High Complication Risk." *Inquiry* 31: 40.

National Quality Forum Consumer, Purchaser and Research Council Members. 2002. "Hospital Performance Measurement Project. Proposal to NQF." Washington, DC: National Quality Forum.

James, B. 2003. *Designing Data Systems*. Advanced Training Program in Health Care Delivery Research. Salt Lake City, UT: Intermountain Health Care.

Suggested Reading

2001. "The Leader's Perspective: Concepts, Tools and Techniques in Opportunity Analysis." *Disease Management & Quality Improvement Report* 1 (6).

Anderson, L. 2001. "Using Administrative Data for Quality Improvement." Presented at the Second Annual Symposium on Disease Management, American Governance and Leadership Group, 7–8 May, La Jolla, CA.

Byrnes, J. 1998. "Demonstrating the Value of Integrated Healthcare Through Outcome Measurement and Disease Management Systems." *Integrated Healthcare Report,* 6–10.

———. 2001. "A Revolutionary Advance in Disease Management: Combining the Power of Disease Management Programs, Evidence Based Medicine, Electronic Medical Records, and Outcome Reporting Systems to Drive Quality in Health Care." *Disease Management & Quality Improvement Report* 1 (1): 1–9.

Byrnes, J. J., and L. B. Anderson. 2001. "Hardwiring Quality Improvement into the Core of Our Business by Emulating the Financial Model of Accountability and Reporting." *Disease Management & Quality Improvement Report* 1 (4): 1–8.

Carey, R. G., and R. C. Lloyd. 2001. *Measuring Quality Improvement in Healthcare: A Guide to Statistical Process Control Applications.* Milwaukee, WI: ASQ Quality Press.

Eddy, D. M. 1998. "Performance Measurement: Problems and Solutions." *Health Affairs (Millwood)* 17 (4): 7–25.

Fuller, S. 1998. "Practice Brief: Designing a Data Collection Process." *Journal of the American Health Information Management Association* 70 (May): 12–16.

Gunter, M., J. Byrnes, M. Shainline, and J. Lucas. 1996. "Improving Outcomes Through Disease Specific Clinical Practice Improvement Teams: The Lovelace Episodes of Care Disease Management Program." *Journal of Outcomes Management* 3 (3): 10–17.

Iz, P. H., J. Warren, and L. Sokol. 2001. "Data Mining for Healthcare Quality, Efficiency, and Practice Support" *34th Annual Hawaii International Conference on System Sciences (HICSS-34),* 6, 3–6 Jan.

Joint Commission on Accreditation of Healthcare Organizations. 2003. *2003 Hospital Accreditation Standards.* Oakbrook Terrace, IL: Joint Commission.

Lucas, J., M. J. Gunter, J. Byrnes, M. Coyle, and N. Friedman. 1995. "Integrating Outcomes Measurement into Clinical Practice Improvement Across the Continuum of Care: A Disease-Specific EPISODES OF CARE Model." *Managed Care Quarterly* 3 (2): 14–22.

Micheletti, J. A., T. J. Shlala, and C. R. Goodall. 1998. "Evaluating Performance Outcomes Measurement Systems: Concerns and Considerations." *Journal of Healthcare Quality* 20 (2): 6–12.

Mulder, C., M. Mycyk, and A. Roberts. 2003. "Data Warehousing and More." *Healthcare Informatics* 1 (March): 6–8.

Reader, L. 2001. "Applications of Computerized Dynamic Health Assessments: The Move from Generic to Specific." *Disease Management & Quality Improvement Report* 1 (8).

Slater, M. A., and L. B. Anderson. 2001. "The Power of Data to Drive Clinical Quality Improvement and Optimal Disease Management." *Disease Management & Quality Improvement Report* Jan.

STATISTICAL TOOLS FOR QUALITY IMPROVEMENT

Kwan Y. Lee, Linda S. Hanold, Rick G. Koss, and Jerod M. Loeb

Fundamentals of Performance Measurement

Purpose of Measurement

Performance measurement is undertaken to meet multiple internal and external needs and demands. Internal quality improvement literature identifies three fundamental purposes for conducting performance measurement: (1) assessment of current performance, (2) demonstration and verification of performance improvement, and (3) control of performance.

These purposes of measurement are designed to complement and support internal performance-improvement activities. The first step in a structured performance-improvement project is to assess current performance. This assessment assists in the identification of the strengths and weaknesses of the current process, thereby helping to identify areas for intervention. It also provides the baseline data against which future measurement data will be compared after interventions have been implemented. The comparison of postintervention measurement data to baseline data will demonstrate and verify whether the intervention was an improvement. Measurement for control of performance is intended to provide an early warning and correction system that will highlight any undesirable changes in process operations. This is critical to sustaining the improvements that have been realized through process-improvement activities.

Performance measurement is also undertaken to meet external needs and demands, including healthcare provider accountability, decision making, public reporting, organizational evaluation, and support for national performance-improvement goals and activities. Healthcare purchasers and payers are demanding that providers demonstrate their ability to provide high-quality patient care at fair prices. Specifically, they are seeking objective evidence that hospitals and other healthcare organizations manage their costs well, satisfy their customers, and have desirable outcomes. Consumers are interested in care-related information for selection purposes. That is, information is used to identify where they believe they will have the greatest probability of a good outcome for treatment of their given condition. Evaluators, such as the Joint Commission on Accreditation of Healthcare Organizations (Joint Commission), the National Committee on Quality Assurance, and others, factor this information into their evaluation and accreditation activities. Performance-measure data can fulfill these needs, provided that the measure construct is sound, the data analyses/data interpretations are scientifically credible, and the data are reported in an easily understood and usable format.

Generally, the benefits of effective performance measurement include the following (Joint Commission 2000):

- Provides factual evidence of performance
- Promotes ongoing organization, self-evaluation, and improvement
- Illustrates improvement
- Facilitates cost-benefit analysis
- Helps to meet external requirements/demands for performance evaluation
- May facilitate the establishment of long-term relationships with various external stakeholders
- May differentiate the organization from competitors
- May contribute to the awarding of business contracts
- Fosters organizational survival

Framework for Measurement

Performance improvement can most accurately be thought of as a philosophy. The organizationwide application of this philosophy comprises the organizational framework for measurement. Healthcare organizations that are committed to ongoing performance improvement have incorporated this philosophy or framework into their overall strategic planning process. Performance-improvement projects are not undertaken in isolation but rather as part of a cohesive performance-improvement program. Such a program comprises a performance-improvement process, plan, and projects (Joint Commission 2000).

The *performance-improvement process* is a carefully chosen, strategically driven, values-based, systemic, organizationwide approach to the achievement of specific, meaningful, high-priority organizational improvements. The performance-improvement plan is then derived from this overall context.

The *performance-improvement plan* consists of a detailed strategy for undertaking specific projects to address improvement opportunities. This plan should include (1) the identified and prioritized opportunities for improvement, (2) the staff needed to coordinate and conduct the improvement project, (3) expected time frames, and (4) needed financial and material resources. It is helpful to integrate the performance-improvement plan with the organizationwide strategic plan so that the performance-improvement priorities are viewed as equally important as other organizational priorities and so that they are given equal consideration in the allocation of resources and in the short- and long-term planning processes.

Performance-improvement projects evolve from the establishment and articulation of the performance-improvement plan. Projects are the diverse, individual, focused initiatives into which hospitals invest to achieve clearly defined, important, and measurable improvements.

Other components that support successful implementation of the performance-improvement program and attainment of the stated project goals and objectives include the following (Joint Commission 2000):

- *Leadership commitment*—Leaders must create the setting that demands and supports continuous improvement. Leaders affect how staff works, which in turn affects how patients experience the care and services delivered. The literature identifies leadership by senior management as the most critical success factor for organizational performance improvement

- *Staff understanding and participation*—Another critical component for successful performance improvement is staff involvement. Each employee is responsible for an organization's performance and, therefore, for the improvement of that performance. Thus, employees must understand the healthcare organization's mission, vision, and values and the contribution of their work to achieving that vision. They need to understand the value of continuous organizational improvement and their role in this context. Finally, they must become familiar with principles, tools, and techniques of improvement and become adept at using these implements to measure, assess, and improve.

- *Establishment of partnerships with key stakeholders*—Establishment of such partnerships will provide an understanding of each of your stakeholders' specific and unique performance data and information needs. This will allow your organization to produce customized, meaningful performance reports that present the information in the most easily understood and informative format for various external audiences.

- *Establishment of a performance-improvement oversight body*—This group oversees all aspects of the healthcare organization's performance-improvement process, including determining improvement priorities, integrating performance-improvement efforts with daily work activities, initiating and facilitating performance-improvement projects, providing performance-improvement education, developing performance-improvement protocols, monitoring the progress of improvement efforts, quantifying resource consumption for each project, communicating improvement internally and externally, and ensuring that process improvements are sustained.

- *Selection and use of a performance-improvement methodology*—Using a single improvement methodology across all improvement initiatives is critical to facilitating a cohesive and consistent approach to improvement within the organization. Improvement methodologies may be internally developed or may be adapted or adopted from external sources such as the Joint Commission's FOCUS-PDCA method or Ernst & Young's IMPROVE method.

- *Development of performance-improvement protocols*—Performance-improvement protocols describe how the organization implements its performance-improvement process. Protocols typically describe the purpose and responsibilities of the oversight body, the process for proposing improvement projects, the process for reviewing and selecting projects, methods for convening project teams, the roles and responsibilities of team members, the selected performance-improvement method and how to implement it, and reporting and communication requirements.

- *Identification and response to performance-improvement resource needs*—Performance improvement requires investment and support, including an expert resource person, employee resources who are allocated dedicated time to work on the project, education, information and knowledge, equipment, and financial resources.

- *Recognition and acknowledgment of performance-improvement successes and efforts*—Acknowledging improvement successes builds organizational momentum for future successes, engenders a sense of meaningful contribution in individual employees, and bonds the organization in celebration. In-house and/or public recognition of improvement successes rewards teams by respecting and appreciating their unique talents, skills, and perspectives. In turn, this fosters employee dedication and loyalty.

- *Continuous assessment of the effectiveness of improvement efforts*—Healthcare organizations are not static, nor are the functions performed in these organizations. Thus, improvement efforts must be routinely reviewed to determine that successes are sustained in the rapidly changing healthcare environment that defines today's healthcare organization.

Selecting Performance Measures

Numerous opportunities for improvement exist in every healthcare organization. However, not all improvements are of the same magnitude. Improvements that are powerful and worthy of organization resources include those that will positively affect a large number of patients, eliminate or reduce instability in critical clinical or business processes, decrease risk, and ameliorate serious problems. In short, it may be most appropriate to focus on high-risk, high-volume, problem-prone areas to maximize your performance-improvement investment.

Because performance measurement lies at the heart of any performance-improvement process, it is imperative that performance measures be selected in a thoughtful and deliberate manner. Performance measures may be internally developed or adopted from a multitude of external resources. However, regardless of the source of performance measures, each measure should be considered against certain characteristics to help ensure a credible and beneficial measurement effort. Critical performance measure characteristics include the following (Joint Commission 2000, 1998):

- *Relevance*—Selected measures should directly relate to your organization's improvement goals and should be linked to your organization's mission, vision, values, and strategic goals and objectives.
- *Reliability*—Reliability refers to data constancy and consistency. Reliable measures accurately and consistently identify the events they were designed to identify across multiple healthcare settings.
- *Validity*—Valid measures identify opportunities for improvement (i.e., events that merit further review) relative to the services provided and the quality of the healthcare results achieved. Valid measures raise good questions about current processes and therefore underlie the identification of opportunities for improvement.
- *Cost effectiveness*—Performance measurement requires resource investment and therefore implies that the ultimate value of the measurement activity should justify the related expenditure of resources. Some measurement activities are simply not worth the investment necessary to collect and analyze the data. Thus, it is necessary to consider the cost versus the benefit (i.e., value) of all measurement activities.
- *Provider control*—There is little value in collecting data on processes or outcomes over which the organization has little or no control. You must be able to influence the processes and outcomes (i.e., implement interventions) tracked by any performance measure that is used.

- *Precise definition and specification*—Performance measures and their data elements must be precisely defined and specified to ensure uniform application from measurement period to measurement period and/or to ensure comparability across organizations. Precisely defined and specified measures ensure that the measures will be collected and calculated in the same way each time and/or in each organization.
- *Interpretability*—Interpretability refers to the extent to which the measure rationale and results are easily understood by users of the data/information.
- *Risk adjustment or stratification*—This refers to the extent to which the influences of factors that differ among groups being compared can be controlled or taken into account.

While the presence or absence of some of these characteristics may not be obvious prior to implementation, pilot testing will help with this determination. Pilot testing may disclose that a particular measure is not appropriate before significant resources have been invested in the activity.

Finally, your performance measure selection process should consider the various types of performance measures. As first described by Avedis Donabedian (1966), there are three components of quality: structure, process, and outcome. Meaningful measures can be developed for each of these components. *Structures* describe hospital characteristics such as organization structure, specialty services provided, and patient census. *Processes* include the components of clinical care (i.e., how care and services are provided) such as assessment and evaluation, diagnosis, and therapeutic and/or palliative interventions. *Clinical outcomes* are multidimensional and describe how the delivered care affects the patient's health, health status, functionality, and well-being. Structure, process, or outcome measures can be further defined as continuous-variable measures or rate-based measures as follows:

- *Continuous-variable measures*—Each value of a continuous-variable measure is a precise measurement that can fall anywhere along a continuous scale. An example is the number of days from surgery to discharge of patients undergoing coronary artery bypass graft (CABG) procedures.
- *Rate-based measures*—The value of a measurement of a rate-based measure reflects the frequency of an event or condition and is expressed as a proportion or a ratio. A **proportion** shows the number of occurrences over the entire group within which the occurrence could take place (e.g., patients delivered cesarean section over

all deliveries). A **ratio** shows occurrences compared with a different, but related, phenomenon (e.g., ventilated patients who develop pneumonia over inpatient ventilator days).

Statistical Process Control

Statistical process control (SPC) can be simply defined as the use of numbers and data to study the things we do in order to make them behave the way we want (McNeese and Klein 1991). In other words, SPC is a method of using data to track processes (the things we do) so that we can improve the quality of products and services (make them behave the way we want). SPC uses simple statistical tools to help us understand any process that generates products or services.

Statistical process control evolved from work done by Walter Shewhart in the 1920s at Bell Labs in New York. Developed as a quality control tool in manufacturing, SPC was only introduced into healthcare about 20 years ago. During World War I, Shewhart had been assigned to design a radio headset for the military. One of the key pieces of information he had to have to design a headset was the width of people's heads. So Shewhart went out and measured them and discovered not only that head width varied but also that it varied *according to a pattern*. It turned out that the size of most people's head fell within a relatively narrow range, but some people had heads that were larger or smaller than the norm, and a few heads were much larger or smaller than average. Shewhart found that this pattern of variation, what is now known as the normal distribution (or bell-shaped curve), was present in many manufacturing processes as well (McNeese and Klein 1991).

Later, Shewhart developed a *control chart* based on this pattern of variation. Control charts, one of the SPC tools discussed later in this chapter, are used to track and analyze variation in processes over time. They were not widely used until World War II, when they assisted in the production of wartime goods.

After the Second World War, statistical process control began to be used extensively in Japan to improve the quality of its products as it was rebuilding its economy. Japanese industry underwent massive statistical training because of the influence and efforts of Shewhart, W. Edwards Deming, and J. M. Juran. Statistical process control did not really catch on in the West until the 1980s, by which time the United States and Europe were scrambling to catch up with the standard for quality set by Japanese manufacturers.

The theory behind SPC is quite straightforward. It requires a change in thinking from error detection to error prevention. In manufacturing, once a product is made, correcting errors is wasteful, time consuming, and expensive. The same is true in healthcare. It is better and more cost effective to make the product, or provide the service, right the first time.

Statistical process control changes the approach toward producing a product or service. The approach moves from inspecting the product or evaluating the service after it is produced to understanding the process itself so that it (the process) can be improved. Any problems should be identified and resolved *before* the product is produced or the service provided. This requires monitoring how the process is performing through routine, selective measurements of the process.

All processes, whether in manufacturing or healthcare, produce data. Statistical process control uses data generated by the process to improve the process. Process improvement, in turn, leads to improved products and services. Figure 7.1 illustrates how a process that generates a product or service simultaneously generates data that can be used to continuously improve itself when analyzed using SPC tools.

In summary, the use of statistical process control in healthcare has a number of benefits. Among these are (1) increased quality awareness on the part of healthcare organizations and practitioners; (2) increased focus on patients; (3) the ability to base decisions on data; (4) implementation of predictable healthcare processes; (5) cost reduction; (6) fewer errors and increased patient safety; and (7) improved processes, which result in improved healthcare outcomes and better quality care.

Control Chart Analysis

Every process varies. For example, it would be highly improbable that a healthcare organization (HCO) would have the same number of patient falls every month.

However, not every process will vary in the same way. For example, let us suppose that in a given year the number of patient falls averaged 20 per month and ranged between 17 and 23 per month. This would suggest a stable process because the variation was predictable within given limits. In SPC terminology, this type of variation is called *common cause variation*. Common cause variation does not imply that the process is functioning either at a desirable or undesirable level; it only describes the nature of variation, namely that it is stable and predicable within given limits.

Next, let us suppose that during the following year, the HCO saw the average number of falls stay the same, but in one month 35 falls occurred. This change in variation would be described as *special cause variation*. The process has changed and is no longer predictable within limits. In this case, the special cause would be a negative finding. One should not

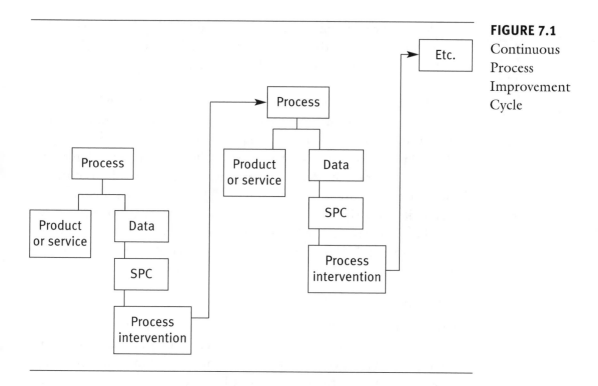

FIGURE 7.1

Continuous Process Improvement Cycle

make any change in the fall-prevention protocols until the cause of the special cause is identified and eliminated.

On the other hand, if the observed variation were only common cause variation (as in the first case), then it would be appropriate to try to improve the process by introducing a new fall-prevention program. If after introducing a fall-prevention program the number of falls in the second year decreased to, say, an average of 17 per month with a range of 14 to 19, this change would be a special cause that was positive. The special cause signaled the success of the intervention.

In summary, the control chart will tell an HCO whether the observed variation is due to common or special causes and will help them determine how to approach improving a process. If there is a special cause, one should investigate it and eliminate it, not change the process. If there is common cause variation, it is appropriate to change the process to improve it. A control chart will subsequently reveal whether or not the change was effective.

Elements of a Control Chart

A control chart is a line graph with the addition of a centerline representing the overall process average (or mean). It shows the flow of a process over time, as distinguished from a distribution, which is a collection of data regardless of the order in which they were collected. A control chart is a dynamic presentation of data, a distribution a static presentation. The measure of the process being monitored or evaluated will appear on the vertical axis.

A control chart also has an upper and lower control limit. The control limits are not the same as confidence limits of a distribution. The control limits describe the variability of a process over time and are usually set at three standard deviations (or sigmas), while the confidence limits of a distribution describe the degree of certainty that a given point is different from the average score, that is, an "outlier." Data falling outside the three-sigma limits are a signal that the process has significantly changed. This data point is properly referred to as a special cause, not an outlier. However, the three-sigma rule is only one test to detect special cause variation. (See Figure 7.2.)

Tests for a Special Cause

There are two errors (or mistakes) that we can make in trying to detect a special cause. First, we can conclude that there is a special cause when one is not present (Type I error). Second, we can conclude that there is no special cause when in fact one is present (Type II error). Walter Shewhart, who developed the control chart, recommended that using three-sigma control limits offered the best balance between making either the first or second mistake.

Other tests were developed by Shewhart's disciples at Western Electric, for example, observing eight consecutive points either above or below the mean, four of five consecutive points beyond one sigma, or two of three consecutive points beyond two sigmas. (See Figure 7.3.)

A *trend* is defined as six consecutive data points incrementally increasing or decreasing. There is a tendency for those unfamiliar with control charts to see "trends" with fewer than six points. This will often result in identifying common cause patterns as special causes.

Number of Data Points

Shewhart recommended that 20 to 25 data points be used to evaluate the stability of a given process. If a process with 25 points has only common cause variation, one can be reasonably certain that a process is "in control." One can then estimate the capability of the process, that is, how it is likely to perform in the near future. Even with less than 25, it is still useful to examine a process for the presence of special causes. However, with less than 25 points it is usually best to refer to the upper and lower control limits as "trial limits." If one observes a special cause with, for example, only 12 points, one should take the time to investigate it. However,

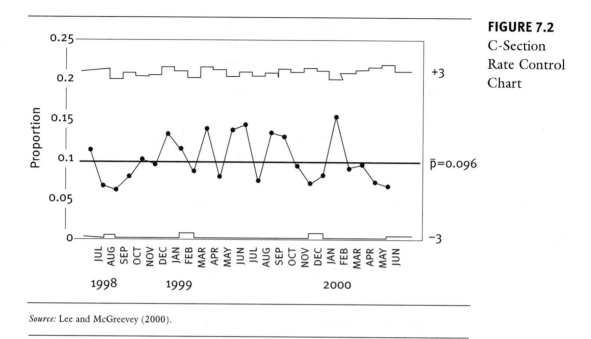

FIGURE 7.2
C-Section
Rate Control
Chart

Source: Lee and McGreevey (2000).

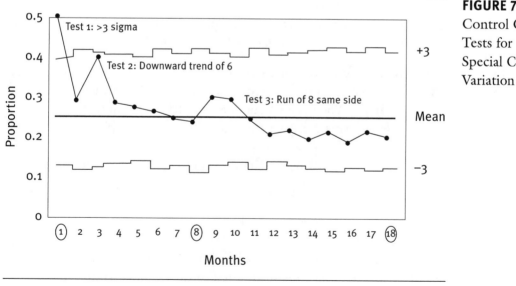

FIGURE 7.3
Control Chart
Tests for
Special Cause
Variation

Source: Lee and McGreevey (2000).

with only 12 data points, there is a higher probability of missing a special cause when it is present (Type II error). Nor can one confidently estimate process capability with only 12 data points.

Choosing the Correct Control Chart

There are many different control charts. However, for its initial efforts, the average facility can manage well with the four that follow:

1. p-chart
2. u-chart
3. Individual values and moving range chart (XMR chart)
4. X-bar and S chart

The first two are for analyzing what are called *attributes* data. The second two are for analyzing *variables* data.

Attributes Data

Attributes data are discrete whole numbers, not continuous measurements. They are counts of unacceptable outcomes. One can keep score of these counts in the following two ways:

1. The number of *defectives*, where an outcome is either good or bad. For example, the patient either fell or did not fall during his or her stay.
2. The number of *defects*, or unacceptable events, for example, the total number of patient falls.

When one is counting defectives, one would choose a p-chart for the analysis. The number plotted on a chart would be either a proportion or a percentage. When one is counting total defects—for example, the number of falls per patient day each month—then one will plot this ratio on a u-chart.

Examples of attributes data to be plotted as percentages on p-charts follow:

*   Percentage of patients who died
*   Percentage of C-sections
*   Percentage of scripts that had one or more medication errors
*   Percentage of patients readmitted to the hospital within 30 days

Examples of attributes data to be plotted as ratio data on u-charts follow:

*   Total number of patient falls per patient day
*   Total number of medication errors per total number of scripts

- Total number of surgical complications divided by the total number of surgeries

Variables Data

Variables data are measurements that are plotted on a continuous scale. They are either whole numbers or expressed in terms of decimals. Variables data are plotted either on an X-bar and S chart or an individuals chart (XMR chart).

Examples of variables data follow:

- Length of stay data
- Number of prescriptions filled
- Number of surgeries performed
- Length of intubation time
- Average door-to-drug time for thrombolytics for acute myocardial infarction patients

An individual's chart will be used when there is only one measurement for each time period.

The X-bar and S chart is a paired chart; that is, the X-chart will reveal whether there is a special cause across months, while the S-chart will reveal whether there are special causes within each month.

To interpret the X-bar chart successfully, the S-chart must be free of any data points beyond the upper control limit (the only test used on the S-chart.) If the S-chart does have a data point beyond three standard deviations from the mean, that data point or points should be investigated for a special cause. A special cause on the S-chart must be identified and eliminated before the X-bar chart can be interpreted accurately (Lee and McGreevey 2000).

Comparison Chart Analysis

The objective of comparison analysis is to evaluate whether individual healthcare organizations' performance is different from the expected level derived from other organizations' data. This is an interorganizational analysis because analysis is performed based on data from multiple organizations. This is also a cross-sectional analysis because comparisons are made at a specific point in time (e.g., month). When an organization's performance level is statistically significantly different from the expected level, it is called an *outlier performance*. An outlier performance may be either favorable or unfavorable depending on the direction of improvement of the measure.

The use of comparison analysis in addition to the control chart can be a powerful approach. The two analyses are alike in that an organization's actual (or observed) performance level is evaluated against a comparative norm, but they are fundamentally different as to how such a norm is established. In control chart analysis, the norm is determined from an organization's own historic data (i.e., process mean) so that one may assess the organization's internal process stability. On the other hand, in comparison analysis, the norm is obtained based on several organizations' performance data to evaluate an organization's relative performance level. Therefore, the two analyses evaluate an organizational performance in two distinct perspectives and as a result can provide a more comprehensive framework to assess overall performance level.

Because of different focuses of the analysis, however, the control and comparison analyses may portray different pictures about an organization's performance. For example, an organization's control chart may show a favorable pattern (i.e., in control), but the comparison chart could be unfavorable (i.e., a bad outlier). This may happen when an organization's performance is consistently lower than that of other organizations and may suggest implementing a new process to achieve a performance improvement. On the other hand, an organization without an outlier performance in the comparison analysis may show an out-of-control pattern in the control chart. In this case, the organization needs to investigate any presence of special cause variation in the process before making any conclusions about its performance level. In general, the control chart analysis is done before the comparison analysis to ensure the process stability so that the observed performance data truly represent the organization's performance capability.

Statistical Assumptions About Data

Statistical analyses differ depending on what assumptions are made about data. For instance, if a normal distribution is assumed for a data set, comparison analysis is performed using a Z-test. Different assumptions are made depending on the type of measures (i.e., proportion, ratio, or continuous variable) as described below.

- *Proportion measures:* It is assumed that the proportion measures follow a binomial distribution. This is the probability distribution of the number of successes (i.e., numerator) in a series of independent trials (i.e., denominator), each of which can result in either a success or a failure with a constant probability. For example, for a proportion measure cesarean-section rate, each individual is assumed to have an equal probability of delivering from a cesarean section under the binomial assumption. Under certain circumstances (e.g., large sample size), a binomial distribution can be approximated using a normal distribution to simplify statistical analysis.

- *Ratio measures:* The ratio measures are similar to the proportion measures in that both are based on count (or attribute) data but differ in that the numerator and denominator address different attributes. An example is the number of adverse drug reactions (ADRs) per 1,000 patient days. For this type of measure, the probability of a success (e.g., an ADR) is very small, while the area of opportunity (e.g., patient days) is usually large. For ratio measures, a Poisson distribution is assumed. Like binomial distribution, a Poisson can be approximated by a normal distribution.
- *Continuous-variable measures:* The continuous-variable measures deal with interval scale data and are generally not restricted to particular values. Examples are CABG length of stay or the number of minutes before administration of antibiotics. An appropriate distributional assumption for this type of measure is a normal distribution (or t distribution for small sample size).

What Data Are Compared?

The comparative norm (e.g., expected rate) in the comparison analysis is the predicted rate if the measure is risk adjusted and the comparison-group mean if the measure is not risk adjusted. Because the comparative data are developed by performance-measurement systems and only summary-level data are received by the Joint Commission, the accuracy of comparison analysis will depend on the quality of data submitted by individual measurement systems. Whenever appropriate, risk-adjusted data are preferable as a comparative norm rather than the summary data from comparison group. This is because organization- or patient-level variability (e.g., different levels of severity of illness) could be reduced through a valid and reliable risk-adjustment procedure. In this case, the comparison data are customized for individual organizations, and hence more fair and accurate performance comparisons can be made.

How to Determine Statistical Outlier

In comparison analysis, an underlying hypothesis (i.e., null hypothesis) about an organization's performance is that the observed performance is not different statistically from the expected level. By applying a set of statistical procedures (i.e., hypothesis testing) to actual performance data, one determines whether the null hypothesis is likely to be true for individual organizations. If it is not true, the performance is called an outlier. In general, statistical outliers can be determined using two approaches: one is based on the P-value, and the other is based on the expected range. These two approaches always result in the same conclusion about the outlier status.

- *Outlier decision based on P-value:* A P-value is the probability of obtaining the same or more extreme data than that observed when the null hypothesis is true (i.e., when the organization's actual performance was not different from the expected). Hence, if the P-value is very small (e.g., less than 0.01), it will indicate that the actual performance is likely to be different from the expected level. In this case, the null hypothesis is rejected and an outlier is determined. A P-value is calculated based on an assumption about the probability distribution of data. If a normal distribution is assumed, a P-value less than 0.01 is equivalent to a Z-score greater than 2.576 or less than –2.576 for a two-sided test. (See Figure 7.4.)
- *Outlier decision based on expected range:* An expected range (also called the acceptance interval) is an interval having upper and lower limits that represents the set of values for which the null hypothesis is accepted. Usually, the midpoint of the interval is the expected rate (or value) for the organization. When the observed data are outside the expected range, an outlier is determined. The expected range can be useful for displaying an organization's outlier status in a chart.

Comparison Chart Construction

A comparison chart is a graphical summary of comparison analysis. It displays tabular information from the comparison analysis into a standardized graphical format so that a visually intuitive assessment may be made about an organization's performance.

A comparison chart consists of actual (or observed) rates, expected rates, and expected ranges (i.e., upper and lower limits) for a given time frame. Unlike control charts, which require at least 12 data points (e.g., months) for a meaningful interpretation, comparison charts can be created with a single valid data point because of its cross-sectional nature. The comparison chart will depict rolling 24 data points.

To create a comparison chart, one must calculate the expected range. An expected range is obtained using a two-step process.

- *Step one:* Calculate confidence limits for the observed rate (or value) using the formulas given in Appendix 2, which appears at the end of the book. (Here, the observed rate is considered as a random variable, while the expected rate is assumed to be a constant value.) If the confidence interval includes values outside the allowable range, the interval must be truncated. For proportion measures, the values must be between 0 and 1. For ratio measures, the values must be 0 or any positive numbers. Continuous variable measures may include any positive or negative numbers.
- *Step two:* Convert the confidence interval into the expected range.

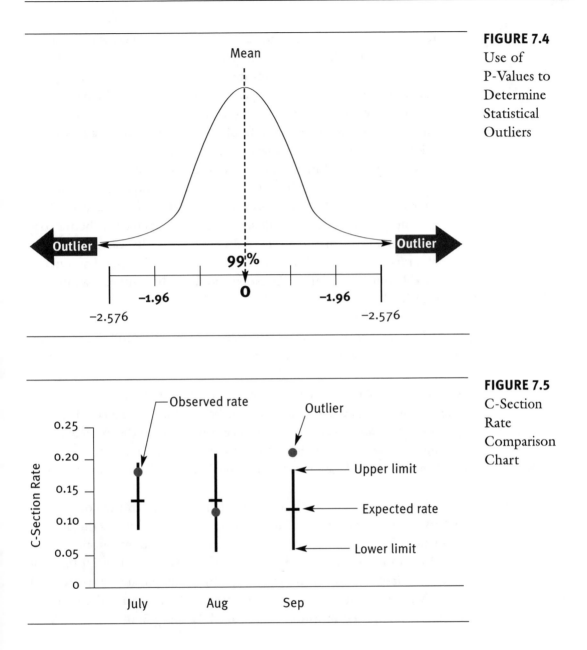

FIGURE 7.4
Use of
P-Values to
Determine
Statistical
Outliers

FIGURE 7.5
C-Section
Rate
Comparison
Chart

Comparison Chart Interpretation

Depending on the direction of improvement of a measure, outlier interpretations are different. A performance measure is positive, negative, or
neutral depending on the direction of improvement.

- *Positive measures:* A rate increase signals improvement. In other
  words, a larger rate is better than a smaller rate. An example is the
  immunization rate measures. For these measures, an observed rate

above the expected range indicates a favorable outlier, while a rate below the range indicates an unfavorable outlier.

- *Negative measures:* A rate decrease signals improvement; that is, a smaller rate is better than a larger rate. An example is the mortality rate measures. For these measures, an observed rate above the expected range indicates an unfavorable outlier, whereas a rate below the range indicates a favorable outlier.

- *Neutral measures:* Either an increase or decrease in rate could be a signal of improvement. In other words, there is no clear direction of improvement for these measures. For example, it is difficult to determine whether a cesarean-section rate of 5 percent is better (or worse) than or equal to a rate of 95 percent. In this case, an observed rate either above or below the expected range is an unfavorable outlier. For these measures, no favorable outliers can be identified.

The comparison analysis will result in one of the following scenarios regardless of the type of measures.

No outlier—actual performance is within the expected range,
Favorable outlier—actual performance is better than the expected,
Unfavorable outlier—actual performance is worse than the expected,
Incomplete data—data are not analyzable because of data error, or
Small sample size—data are not analyzable because of small sample size.

Data are incomplete if any data elements used in the comparison analysis are missing or invalid. Small sample sizes are defined as the denominator cases less than 25 for proportion measures; the numerator cases less than 4 for ratio measures; and the number of cases less than 10 for continuous variable measures. In addition, a small sample size is triggered if fewer than ten organizations are represented in the comparison group data for non-risk-adjusted measures (Lee and McGreevey 2000).

Using Data for Performance Improvement

Once collected, performance measure data require interpretation and analysis if they are going to be useful for improving the processes and outcomes of healthcare. There are a number of ways to use data for improvement purposes, all of which involve comparison. Data can be used to compare (1) an organization's performance against itself over time, (2) the performance of one organization to the performance of a group of organizations collecting data on the same measures in the same way, and (3) an organization's performance against established benchmarks or guidelines.

As a first step, an organization needs to determine if the process it is measuring is in control. To improve a process it must first be understood. Processes that are characterized by special cause variation are unstable, unpredictable, and therefore difficult to understand. Control charts should be used to determine if processes are stable and in statistical control or if special-cause variation exists. If special cause variation does exist it must be investigated and eliminated. Once any special cause variation has been eliminated, organizations can be confident that the data accurately reflect performance.

Consider a hypothetical situation in which a hospital measures its C-section rates using a control chart. The control chart shown in Figure 7.6 indicates existence of special cause variation on time 8 as the observed rate deviates from the upper control limit. Suppose that the hospital conducted a root cause analysis after time 8 to identify the source of special cause and found that there was a serious problem in the hospital's coding practice. The hospital then implemented an intervention plan at time 10, and the hospital's rates came under control (time 11–20). In addition, the process mean (i.e., centerline) has shifted from 0.42 to 0.15 after the intervention. The hospital should continue to monitor its C-section rates using the new process mean as part of a continuous quality improvement plan.

Control charts, however, only tell us about the stability of the process; they do not speak to the quality of care. After determining that the process of interest is stable and in control, organizations need to use other SPC tools and data-analytic techniques to determine if they are performing as they want to perform. One way to measure if a healthcare organization is performing up to its goals and targets is to compare its performance against itself over time. By consistently tracking the same measures on an ongoing basis, an organization can spot trends, cycles, and patterns, all of which will help determine if it is meeting its preset targets and if its performance is improving or declining. Importantly, healthcare organizations will also be able to monitor the impact of any quality-improvement interventions they may have implemented and track the sustainability of those improvements.

Another way to use data for improvement purposes is to compare the performance of one organization to the performance of a group of organizations collecting data on the same measures in the same way. This way the healthcare organization can track how they are performing compared to other organizations providing the same services. These comparisons can be local, regional, national, or based on any number of other strata. Statistical analyses can pinpoint whether a healthcare entity is per-

FIGURE 7.6
Control Chart
Reflecting a
Change in
Process

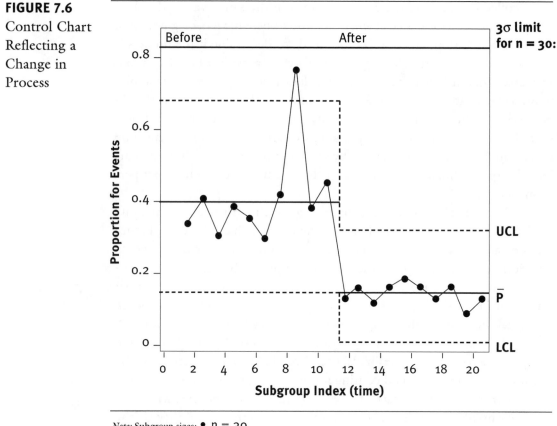

Note: Subgroup sizes: • n = 30

forming in a way that is comparable to other organizations or if it is at a level that is, statistically speaking, significantly above or below others in the comparison group. Discovering that you are performing at a level that is significantly below that of your peers is often a powerful incentive to improve.

A third method of comparing performance is through benchmarking. There are a variety of definitions of benchmarking but, generally speaking, it compares an organization's performance in relation to a specified service or function with that of industry leaders or exemplary-performing organizations. Benchmarking is goal directed and promotes performance improvement by doing the following:

- Providing an environment amenable to organization change through continuous improvement and striving to match industry-leading practices and results

- Creating objective measures of performance that are driven by industry-leading targets instead of by past performance
- Providing a customer/external focus
- Substantiating the need for improvement
- Establishing data-driven decision-making processes (Czarnecki 1994).

In healthcare, professional societies and expert panels routinely develop scientifically based guidelines of patient care practices for given treatments or procedures. The goal of these guideline-setting efforts is to provide healthcare organizations with tools that, if appropriately applied, can help raise their performance to the level of industry leaders. Performance measure data can be used to track how often, and how well, organizations comply with the guidelines.

Study Questions

1. What are common data quality problems in healthcare performance measurement? How should the sufficiency of data quality be evaluated? What are the threats associated with poor quality data in the use of data?
2. When sample data are used in performance measurement, how can appropriate sample sizes be determined, and how can it be ensured that the sample data represent the entire population? How should small sample sizes be handled in the analysis and use of control and comparison charts?
3. How does the rigorous use of control and comparison charts for performance management and improvement contradict, if at all, the art of medicine philosophy that each patient is unique?

REFERENCES

Donabedian, A. 1966. "Evaluating the Quality of Medical Care." *The Milbank Quarterly* 44: 166–203.

Czarnecki, M. T. 1994. *Benchmarking Strategies for Health Care Management.* Gaithersburg, MD: Aspen Publishers, Inc.

Joint Commission on Accreditation of Healthcare Organizations. 2000. *A Guide to Performance Measurement for Hospitals.* Oakbrook Terrace, IL: Joint Commission on Accreditation of Healthcare Organizations.

———. 1998. *Attributes of Core Performance Measures and Associated Evaluation Criteria.* Oakbrook Terrace, IL: Joint Commission on Accreditation of Healthcare Organizations.

Lee, K. Y., and C. McGreevey. 2000. *Mining ORYX Data 2000—A Guide for Performance Measurement Systems.* Oakbrook Terrace, IL: Joint Commission on Accreditation of Healthcare Organizations.

McNeese, W. C., and R. A. Klein. 1991. *Statistical Methods for the Process Industries.* Milwaukee, WI: American Society for Quality Press.

PHYSICIAN AND PROVIDER PROFILING

David B. Nash and Adam Evans

This chapter examines how physician profiles can improve physician performance in the context of continuous quality management and value-based purchasing of healthcare. It also discusses the issues with developing profiles and the factors that affect their implementation in healthcare organizations. Finally, a case where physician profiles have been used successfully to improve the quality of care is presented.

Background and Terminology

The Centers for Medicare & Medicaid Services (CMS) has forecasted annual healthcare spending to increase from 14.1 percent of the gross domestic product in 2001 to 17.7 percent of the gross domestic product in 2012 (CMS 2003). With the increased spending on healthcare, many Americans are beginning to question whether they are receiving increased quality and value for their healthcare dollars. The Institute of Medicine (IOM) detailed that anywhere from 44,000 to 98,000 people die each year from preventable medical errors (IOM 2000). Increased reports like this one, which detail problems with medical errors and adverse events, have the government, employers, and the public all demanding more affordable healthcare and improved quality.

The Physician's Role in Improving Quality

Physicians' actions have been noted to compromise a significant majority of outcomes in healthcare (Royer 1999). Unexplained clinical variation leads to increased healthcare costs, medical errors, patient frustration, and poor clinical outcomes. With the increase in information being collected on physician practice patterns, widespread variations in practice have begun to be noted. In healthcare, variation has been noted to exist among providers by specialty, geographical region, and practice setting. Unexplained clinical variation is present among treatment options for patients with various conditions. While variation can lead to similar outcomes, it often can lead to problems with care. Since one agreed-on medical treatment does not always exist, unexplained clinical variation continues. Therefore, if significant improvements are to be made in the healthcare system, they must come from changing physician behavior to reduce practice variation.

In response to the public's demand for more accountability on the part of physicians, initial attempts to change physician behavior resulted in the development of physician report cards (Ransom 1999). However, these report cards have been met with criticism from the medical community. Complaints center largely on the gauges of quality used to measure physician performance and the inconsistencies in risk-adjustment methods to compare outcomes between physicians (University Health System Consortium 2003). As an alternative to report cards, creating physician profiles to measure performance will help to minimize variations in healthcare.

Physician Profiling

Physician profiling is an attempt to gather data to analyze physician practice patterns, utilization of services, and outcomes of care (Black and Massanari 1997). The goal of physician profiling is to improve physician performance through accountability and feedback and to decrease practice variation through adherence to evidence-based standards of care. By establishing consistent treatment methods for physicians, it is hoped that high-quality, low-cost healthcare will be achieved. Profiling will allow physicians' performance to be measured against that of colleagues on a local, state, and national level. The idea is that physicians, being highly driven, goal-oriented individuals, will be motivated to increase their performance in areas in which they do not currently rank the highest. Examples of categories in which physicians would be evaluated include patient satisfaction and amount of resources utilized (Gevirtz and Nash 2000).

Numerous studies have highlighted differences between what physicians think they do and what they actually do in practice (Gevirtz and Nash 2000). Since many physicians tend to overrate their performance, developing profiles will allow a physician's treatment pattern to be recorded. Profiling will enable providers' actions to be compared to the current evidence-based best practices in medicine and help to reduce practice variation. With this information, physicians would then be able to make changes to improve wasteful or unproductive practice patterns to better satisfy their patients. Development of profiles will also provide a future framework for evaluating physicians and improving quality.

Establishing measures to assess physician performance will lead to greater accountability and performance by physicians. Since the dissemination of IOM's 2001 report *Crossing the Quality Chasm*, which detailed the problems with processes of care and unexplained clinical variation in the U.S. healthcare system, employers, consumers, and the public are demanding information on which to base healthcare and provider choices. Publishing information on the strengths and weaknesses of physicians will provide purchasers of healthcare with greater information to make decisions based on quality. As physicians continue to decrease variation and improve outcomes in response to increased feedback and measurement of performance, the question of whether purchasers of healthcare are willing to pay for improved performance arises.

Scope and Use of Profiling in Healthcare

Value-Based Purchasing

The government, large employers, and the public are concerned about whether high-quality care is provided at an affordable cost. Since many employees receive health insurance through their employers, employers have a vested interest in purchasing high-quality care. Employers recognize that workers who are satisfied with their health benefits will have a greater desire to remain with a company and will be more productive.

Evidence is growing that purchasers of healthcare are beginning to use value-based purchasing to make healthcare decisions. In addition to cost, employers are interested in incorporating outcomes and value into their decisions when selecting which providers to contract with. Efforts to determine quality measures for hospitals and health plans are now being expanded to include physicians (*Consumer Driven Healthcare* 2003). Common strategies employers use to compare quality among physicians include collecting data on physicians, selective contracting with high-quality providers, partnering with providers to improve quality, and rewarding or penalizing providers to improve quality (Maio et al. 2003). These strategies will have a significant effect on physician practice patterns and decision making. Being armed with information regarding higher-quality providers will enable employers to make objective decisions regarding higher-quality care that is in the best interest of their employees. In addition, collecting reliable and accurate data on physician performance will provide purchasers with greater leverage in contract negotiations with physicians. In some situations, such data could facilitate a working relationship between purchasers of healthcare and providers to improve the quality of care individuals are receiving. Measuring physician performance could lead to the development of continuous quality management programs that will improve various aspects of patient care and clinical outcomes. Financially rewarding physicians who meet the highest standards of performance would encourage greater participation from physicians as well.

Profiling as Part of Continuous Quality Improvement

Physicians realize that a problem with quality exists in the United States but resent those current efforts to improve quality that have centered on them, primarily because of intrusive efforts into examining physician medical records and outcomes with minimal, if any, physician input (Nash 2000). Physicians have dismissed conclusions on their performance on the basis of inaccurate data. This finger pointing fails to establish the delivery of healthcare as a systemic process that encompasses a wide variety of individuals.

These efforts have resulted in the development of a continuous quality improvement strategy in many healthcare organizations that recognizes a systems solution to improving healthcare. Continuous quality improvement integrates structure, process, and outcomes of care into a management system that allows processes to be analyzed over time and outcomes to be improved (see Chapter 5). *Structure* relates to the array of organizational resources in place to provide healthcare to patients. *Process* measures interactions between individuals in the healthcare system. *Outcomes* include both the patient response to the treatment and how it affected their quality of life (Gevirtz and Nash 2000). This approach involves everyone in an organization and focuses on process failures, not failures of individuals. Through understanding problems in processes, the factors that contribute to poor quality can be identified and improved on.

As part of their continuous total quality management strategies, healthcare organizations make use of several tools for maintaining the most competent physician staffs. These tools, described briefly here, include credentialing, outcomes management, physician report cards, benchmarking, and clinical pathways (Nash 2000).

Credentialing

Credentialing refers to the process of hiring a well-qualified medical staff that is able to deliver the highest-quality care. Physicians are offered certain positions based on a variety of criteria such as peer review, board certification, and hours spent in continuing medical education. By developing standards for competency, the hospital is able to maintain the highest level of quality among the physicians within its system.

Outcomes Management

Outcomes management is the relationship between outcomes in clinical research and patient satisfaction. Besides measuring morbidity and mortality, outcomes management takes into account the quality of healthcare received from the patient's perspective (Nash 2000).

Physician Report Cards

Physician report cards compare physicians on outcomes related to things such as patient satisfaction and cost utilization patterns. This information can be effective in encouraging changes in physician behavior because physicians typically are very competitive people. If ranked against their peers, physicians who do not perform well will likely take steps to improve their performance. This will serve to eliminate future liabilities to both the physician and the hospital. At this point, report cards have not been well received by providers (Brian and May 1997). Many providers have criticized report cards because too much variation exists in the methodologies used to evaluate provider outcomes (Dews and Myers 2000). Report cards also do not explain variation among providers' outcomes and therefore make improving processes of care problematic. Another criticism is that they do not provide feedback to physicians enabling them to improve their performance.

Benchmarking

Benchmarking encompasses the use of quantitative measures of best practices to compare individuals' performance. When compared to the best accepted practices within the hospital and at other organizations, physicians might be more willing to change if they see that their behavior negatively affects the system. For example, postoperative complications after hysterectomies could be compared for several different institutions. If one institution was found to have a longer length of stay than others, an investigation into the factors contributing to increased length of stay could be performed in that institution. Based on this, efforts could be made to decrease the length of stay so that it more closely resembles the norms in the area.

Clinical Pathways

Clinical pathways involve selection of conditions known to have wide variations in treatment and then developing processes to decrease variation. By combining physician input with evidence-based medicine, new treatment pathways are developed to increase quality, improve outcomes, and decrease costs.

Use in Healthcare Organizations

Physician profiling is one of the many tools used in continuous quality improvement and will result in added value to purchasers of healthcare and help educate physicians for the future. Because unexplained clinical variation can lead to poorer outcomes for patients, measuring the difference between what physicians think they do and what they actually do in practice is an essential part of improving physicians' performance and the overall processes of care for an organization. Although physicians typically do not like to examine their own performance, numerous studies have documented that, when armed with information on their performance relative to that of their colleagues, physicians will change their behavior to meet a specified outcome (National Health Information 2003a).

The most effective profiles should be able to document variations in provider performance on an individual, local, and national basis. Physicians by nature are competitive people. If shown how they perform versus a group of peers, physicians will be more likely to improve on the areas where they rank low in the group. Profiles should be easy to understand and provide specific suggestions. If a physician's strengths and weaknesses are laid out in an easy-to-understand manner, he or she may be more likely to make changes in behavior.

The use of physician profiles can be a valuable educational tool in healthcare organizations (Royer 1999). While doing things correctly the first time will yield the lowest costs, this is not always possible in medicine. The development of physician profiles will provide physicians with the information to determine what conditions they are treating appropriately, how they compare to their peers, and what areas they can improve on. Profiling will enable physicians to understand the current trends among physicians in a specialty and learn the most cost-effective practices. Based on this, quality improvement plans can be developed to help educate physicians on how to improve their performance.

The creation of an information technology infrastructure to analyze the performance of all physicians in a healthcare system can be useful in identifying what disease groups the hospital treats most. Clinical pathways can then be developed to treat these conditions, and processes of care can be improved.

Patients can also benefit from the creation of physician profiles. A healthcare organization interested in increasing patient satisfaction would find physician profiles extremely valuable. Through a survey, patients could evaluate things such as physician bedside manner, amount of time spent in the waiting room, and amount of time spent with the physician. These data could be analyzed and conveyed to physicians with suggestions for improvement. This commitment to improving customer service on the part of physicians would serve to increase both patient care and patients' confidence in the healthcare they receive. Patient enrollment with the physicians in the healthcare organization would increase, and this could bring more profit to the system.

Clinical and Operational Issues

Accepted best standards of practice are always evolving in healthcare with new medicines and treatment options. Physician profiles can be helpful in comparing various processes to help determine the most efficient, cost-effective way to practice medicine. In addition, the development of ongoing measurements to evaluate physicians will encourage physicians to stay abreast of the latest trends in medicine.

Before encouraging the use of profiles, the organization and its physicians must adopt a commitment to continuous quality improvement. This entails issues such as improving patient satisfaction, drafting an agreement to work with the physicians on staff at the hospital, and developing agreed-on quality indicators.

Listed below are a number of concerns in the creation of physician profiles (Gevirtz and Nash 2000).

- What do you want to measure, and why is this important?
- Are these the most appropriate measures for quality improvement?
- How will you measure performance? (What, if any, is the gold standard?)
- How and when will the measures be collected?
- How reliable are the profiles you are creating?
- What are the most appropriate measures of physician performance?
- Can you measure these variables? (How will you collect the data?)
- What is the appropriate design (e.g., measuring percentages, means)?
- How will you interpret the results (e.g., risk adjust, acceptable results)?
- How will these findings influence change?

The implementation and use of profiles should be part of a continuous quality improvement process. The most effective approach for profiling consists of a step-by-step approach. An approach that goes slowly and involves a diverse group of members of the healthcare organization will be more likely to gain support and produce change within the system.

Choosing Which Measures to Profile

Within a healthcare organization, an infinite number of areas lend themselves to quality improvement, such as appropriate prescription of antibiotics, surgical outcomes, patient safety, patient satisfaction, and decreased costs. The committee should identify the areas most appropriate for profiling and the areas in which it wants to improve quality. It must be accepted that not all medical conditions are appropriate for profiling. Only diseases for which evidence-based guidelines exist for treatment should be profiled. This information could come from nationally recognized practice guidelines or other practice parameters. Using guidelines gives the team a checklist of objectives with which to compare its actions. Without guidelines, the team cannot be sure that all the components included in the process of care are always being satisfied. This emphasis on rational decision making will produce greater support from the physicians in the organization and be more likely to lead to improved performance.

Collecting the Data

The committee should then identify what techniques it will use to gather and disseminate the data. The information should be able to be gathered without interfering with the daily operations of patient care. Traditional methods of data collection have relied on medical records and claims data. In situations where these methods are not available or the most appropriate, direct observation or surveys can be used. The gathering of data for either method can be difficult, and the committee must assesses what data are most applicable for measuring performance. The committee should also identify how much data will need to be gathered to have statistically valid results.

Interpreting the Results

Once the data are gathered, it is essential to develop an objective and appropriate way to interpret the results. The physician's performance should be compared relative to the accepted national goals for the disease or whatever the quality committee decides is an appropriate target. Some areas where physicians can be of help in constructing profiles include diseases where there is potential for improved processes and outcomes, agreement on benchmarks and gauges of quality, and encouraging other physicians to participate in the quality improvement process. From this information, statistically significant and clinically significant outcomes can be determined. Profiles should only be gathered on physicians who have a large volume of patients with the disease. A physician who sees 200 patients with a condition is more likely to value the data on his or her performance than a physician who sees 20 patients with the same condition.

The data must also be risk adjusted to compensate for the diverse populations of patients that physicians encounter. Risk adjusting will provide validity to the results the physician is receiving and prevent physicians from arguing that their patients are sicker.

Communicating the Results

Once the profile has been developed, the format in which the profile will be of most value to the physician must be determined. Graphical representations of data are the easiest to understand and will allow physicians to see their progress over a specific time period. The information conveyed to the physician must be kept simple. Physicians are busy individuals; if given too much information, they may become overwhelmed and their efforts to improve quality might decrease. Figure 8.1 illustrates an example of a physician profile (National Health Information 2003a).

In addition, it should be decided whether the information distributed will be blinded or nonblinded. Some physicians may resent having their performance publicly available for other physicians to see, especially if they rank lower in certain areas. Ideally, nonblinded data will allow physicians to seek out other physicians who have better outcomes and learn ways to improve. Also, those physicians who rank lower will want to improve because they will not want to be continuously seen as performing at a lower level than their peers. For this part of the process, physician buy-in is crucial.

Meetings should be implemented on a monthly, weekly, or quarterly basis in which physicians have the opportunity to provide input on how the profiling system is working. In addition, this will allow time for the physicians to obtain feedback on their performance and discuss ways in which they can improve.

Keys to Successful Implementation and Lessons Learned

Implementation

Administrators or quality improvement teams who wish to develop profiles should be encouraged to work closely with physicians. At the start of the project, physician leaders who identify themselves as interested in quality improvement should be approached. Having physicians on the committee team who are open to change, respected by their peers, and knowledgeable about quality will increase the chance that other physicians in the organization will participate.

Different specialties require different levels of information and different methodologies to analyze outcomes. In their use of physician profiles, individuals at Providence Medical Center in Seattle found that surgeons were more prone to focus on conclusions, whereas cardiologists were often interested in statistical significance (Bennett, McKee, and Kilberg 1996). Incorporating physicians from many specialties into the quality process will result in greater validity of the data and improved physician participation.

After the development of a profile, a time frame should be determined for all physicians to review it and submit any complaints before it becomes an official tool of the organization. Remember, if physicians are

FIGURE 8.1

Example of a Physician Profile

Prescribed Medication Use
Prescriber: Jane Doe MD
Peer Group: Internal Medicine

Report Period: April–June, 2003

# of Your Regence patients who filled your prescription: 175   **All Oregon prescription card claims**

Your Average Cost per Rx

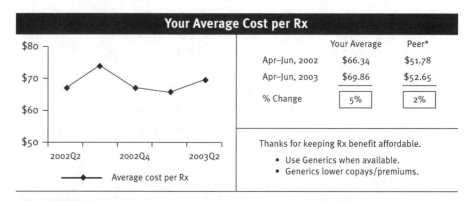

	Your Average	Peer*
Apr–Jun, 2002	$66.34	$51.78
Apr–Jun, 2003	$69.86	$52.65
% Change	5%	2%

Thanks for keeping Rx benefit affordable.
- Use Generics when available.
- Generics lower copays/premiums.

───── Average cost per Rx

Prescribed Medication Opportunities

Use more generics in these drug classes:

Drug Class	Your Generic %	Peer* %	Consider these alternatives:
Antidepressants	11%	38%	Use *fluoxetine*
Hypotensives–ACE Inhibitors/ARBs	13%	59%	Use *cuptopril, enalapril, listinopril, moexipril*
Lipid Lowering Agents	0%	17%	Use *lovastatin*

Use preferred drugs in place of these non-preferred drugs:

Non-preferred Drug	Rxs	Avg$/Rx	Consider these alternatives:
Non-preferred: ZOCOR	34	$159	Use *lavastatin (Mevacor), Lescol/XL, Lipitor*
Non-preferred: DIOVAN HCT	23	$79	Use *lisinopril + HCTZ, enalapril + HCTZ*
Non-preferred: AMBIEN	25	$70	Use *generic sedative-hypnotics*
Non-preferred: ADVIR DISKUS	12	$144	Use *Azmacort/Flovent/Pulmlcort + Serevent/ Foradil*
Non-preferred LEXAPRO	12	$97	Use *fluaxetine (Prozac)*

Class Overview: Lipid Lowering Agents

Drug Name		Rxs		Drug Cost	Avg$/Rx
LIPITOR		57	54%	$5,975	$105
ZOCOR	NP	34	32%	$5,402	$159
PRAVACHOL	NP	3	3%	$709	$236
LESCOL XL		9	9%	$634	$70
OTHER		2	2%	$182	$92
Total: This Class		**105**	**100%**	**$12,901**	**$123**

NP = non-preferred

Generic lovastatin (Mevacor®) has similar LDL reduction to Pravachol® at less cost.

Lipitor® has highest LDL reduction per cost.

% Preferred Rxs in Class

	Q2 '02	Q3 '02	Q4 '02	Q1 '03	Q2 '03
Your Rate	64%	57%	62%	61%	63%
Peer Rate*	95%	94%	94%	93%	92%

* The peer comparator is statistically derived at the 70th percentile of Oregon Internal Medicine prescribers.

Source: David Clark, The Regence Group, Blue Cross Blue Shield of Oregon. Reprinted with permission.

offered the opportunity to participate in the development of profiles, they may be more likely to accept them. Once the reviews have been submitted, the committee on profiling should meet to finalize the profile and set a time frame to begin using the profiles.

After the profile has been in use for a defined period, multiple educational sessions should be organized. The message sent to physicians needs to consistently indicate that this is a program designed for quality improvement. Changing physician behavior is a process that will happen over time, and physicians need to be constantly reassured that they are following the best treatment protocols to help their patients. Providing physicians with incentives to improve their performance, such as bonuses or award recognition, will also result in greater improvements in quality.

Profiling may connote a negative feeling for the physician in much the same way criminal profiling has angered many drivers. If physician profiles are to be successful in improving healthcare outcomes, they must be seen by the physician as nonpunitive and used primarily for educational purposes. Physicians have to believe that this is a quality improvement initiative designed to help them improve their weaknesses and target patients who may need more closely monitored care. They cannot be made to feel threatened by the profiling system.

Lessons Learned

There are many critiques of the use of profiling. For one, no consensus exists as to what constitutes a profile, what it should measure, and the groups to which the information should be targeted (Dews and Myers 2000). Employers and consumers want different levels of information with which to make healthcare decisions. Employers are interested in differences in quality and outcomes across providers. Consumers want to know how providers perform with respect to their specific condition (*Consumer Driven Healthcare* 2003).

Many physicians are also skeptical of profiling; they feel that because they see their patients on a regular basis they know what is best for them. Encouraging physicians to adhere to generally accepted guidelines might not be the most appropriate for the population of patients they care for.

Another critique surrounds individuals with chronic conditions who might see several doctors for their condition. Examining the practice pattern of a physician and related outcomes in this case might not be accurate. Also, because many patients constantly switch providers, developing profiles over a meaningful period may be difficult (Gevirtz and Nash 2000).

Physicians might also be skeptical of an employer's calculation of their outcomes. Physicians who treat a low volume of patients with a specific condition might resent being compared to other physicians who treat a larger volume of patients with the same condition. Proper risk adjusting for the severity of the patient population for which a physician cares will provide greater credibility to the data. Considering these circumstances, many physicians will be anxious over the accuracy of the data used to evaluate them.

Agreeing on the best treatment for a particular medical condition is also a difficult task. The emergence of new technologies, drugs, and payment schemes on a yearly basis significantly affects a physician's practice and makes reaching consensus on a specific treatment challenging. For these reasons, some physicians may be reluctant to accept national treatment guidelines.

Another issue that physicians have with profiles is that a patient's outcome is partly due to patient compliance. The profile has to recognize a level where the physician's efforts to improve quality are at their maximum; beyond this mark, efforts to improve outcomes are largely the result of actions of the patient. Future attempts at profiling will have to take patient compliance into account.

Case Study

This section highlights a successful program that developed physician profiles to improve the quality of care. Touchpoint Health Plan in Appleton, Wisconsin, achieved the top performance in Health Employer Data and Information Set measures in 2002 concerning beta-blocker treatment after myocardial infarction, eye exams and cholesterol control for enrollees with diabetes, and breast cancer screening. Eight years prior to this award, the organization began to collect information on physician performance and began displaying information in graphical, nonblinded formats that compared the performance of individual physicians to that of their colleagues (National Health Information 2003b). A sample of the type of data that physicians received on performance is shown in Figure 8.2. (References to specific physicians are not provided in this example to protect the privacy of those physicians.)

Graphics similar to the one shown in Figure 8.2 enabled physicians to see if they were performing up to the best standards and how they compared to the rest of their peers. While some physicians did not like being compared to their peers and having their results shown publicly, Touchpoint emphasized that this report was meant to be nonpunitive and was aimed at continuous quality improvement. After developing a quality plan, Touchpoint then started a bonus plan with incentives to encourage improvements in quality (National Health Information 2003b).

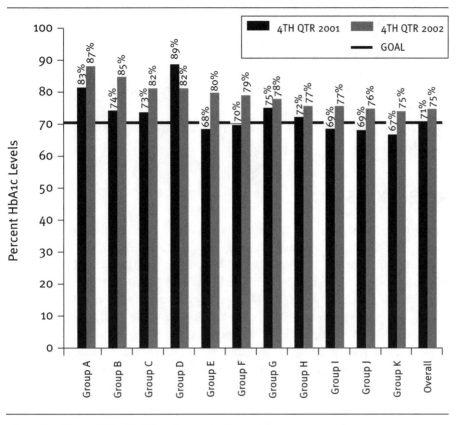

FIGURE 8.2
Touchpoint
Health Plan:
Comparison
of Diabetes
HbA1c Levels
Across
Providers

Source: Dean Gruner, M.D., ThedaCare. Reprinted with permission.

Physicians who met targeted quality measures would receive increased compensation. In addition, physicians who did not meet those measures would not be penalized. A database was also developed for diabetes, cholesterol management, mammography, and childhood immunization. This improved information technology enabled physicians to keep better track of how their patients were being managed (e.g., lab results, patient education). As a result of these improvements in quality, complications of various diseases decreased, costs to the system decreased, and three of the associated hospitals in the health system were ranked among the top 100 hospitals in the United States (National Health Information 2003b).

Touchpoint's success is a good example of how fostering a culture of quality in an organization can enhance the delivery of healthcare. Developing incentives to improve physician performance and investing in information systems are valuable tools that will help to improve outcomes and make processes of care more efficient.

Study Questions

1. What challenges might an administrator who attempts to measure physician performance encounter?
2. Describe the relationship between continuous quality management and physician profiling.
3. Describe the strengths and weaknesses of the profiles discussed in this chapter.

REFERENCES

Bennett, G., W. McKee, and L. Kilberg. 1996. "Physician Profiling in Seattle: A Case Study." In *Physician Profiling and Risk Adjustment*, edited by N. Goldfield and P. Boland, 317–31. Gaithersburg, MD: Aspen Publishers.

Black, S., and D. Massanari. 1997. "The Physicians' Approach to Quality in Managed Care." In *Models for Measuring Quality in Managed Care: Analysis and Impact. Vol. 1*, edited by J. Seltzer and D. B. Nash, 171–82. Washington, DC: Faulkner & Gray.

Brian, C., and J. May. 1997. "How Employers Can Promote Clinical Practice Improvement Among Providers." In *Clinical Practice Improvement Methodology: Implementation and Evaluation. Vol. 2*, edited by S. D. Horn, 23–33. Washington, DC: Faulkner & Gray.

Centers for Medicare & Medicaid Services. 2003. National Health Accounts. [Online information; retrieved 8/19/03.] http://cms.hhs.gov/statistics/nhe/default.asp.

Consumer Driven Healthcare. 2003. [editorial]. *Consumer Driven Healthcare* 2 (7): 99–100.

Dews, P., and W. A. Myers. 2000. "The Employer Perspective on Quality and Outcomes Measurement." In *Enhancing Physician Performance: Advanced Principles of Medical Management*, edited by S. Ransom, W. Pinsky, and J. Tropman, 179–93. Tampa, FL: American College of Physician Executives.

Gevirtz, F., and D. B. Nash. 2000. "Enhancing Physician Performance Through Practice Profiling." In *Enhancing Physician Performance: Advanced Principles of Medical Management*, edited by S. Ransom, W. Pinsky, and J. Tropman, 91–116. Tampa, FL: American College of Physician Executives.

Institute of Medicine. 2000. *To Err Is Human: Building a Safer Health System*. Washington, DC: National Academy Press.

———. 2001. *Crossing the Quality Chasm: A New Health System for the 21st Century*. Washington, DC: National Academy Press.

Maio, V., N. I. Goldfarb, C. T. Carter, and D. B. Nash. 2003. "Value-Based Purchasing: A Review of the Literature." *The Commonwealth Fund Report* No. 636 (May). [Online information; retrieved 11/03.] www.cmwf.org/publist/publist2.asp?CategoryID=3.

Nash, D. B. 2000. "The Elements of Medical Quality Management." In *Fundamentals of Medical Quality Management*, edited by J. Hammons, 259–69. Tampa, FL: American College of Physician Executives.

National Health Information. 2003a. "Wrestle Down Drug Costs with Profiling, Education." In *Physician Profiling and Performance: Changing Practice Patterns Under Managed Care. Vol. II*, 29–32. Atlanta, GA: National Health Information.

———. 2003b. "Touchpoint Docs Respond to Feedback Data." In *Physician Profiling and Performance: Changing Practice Patterns Under Managed Care. Vol. II*, 4–7. Atlanta, GA: National Health Information.

Ransom, S. 1999. "Enhancing Physician Performance." In *Clinical Resource and Quality Management*, edited by S. Ransom and W. Pinsky, 139–69. Tampa, FL: American College of Physician Executives.

Royer, T. 1999. "Measuring Physician Performance." In *Clinical Resource and Quality Management*, edited by S. Ransom and W. Pinsky, 129–37. Tampa, FL: American College of Physician Executives.

University Health System Consortium. 2003. "Health Care Report Cards: Too Soon for a Passing Grade." White Paper, University Health System Consortium, July.

MEASURING AND IMPROVING PATIENT EXPERIENCES OF CARE

Susan Edgman-Levitan

As stated in *Through the Patient's Eyes* (Gerteis et al. 1993),

> Quality in health care has two dimensions. Technical excellence: the skill and competence of health professionals and the ability of diagnostic or therapeutic equipment, procedures, and systems to accomplish what they are meant to accomplish, reliably and effectively. The other dimension relates to the subjective experience, and in health care, it is quality in this subjective dimension that patients experience most directly—in their perception of illness or well-being and in their encounters with health care professionals and institutions, i.e., the experience of illness and healthcare *through the patient's eyes.* Health care professionals and managers are often uneasy about addressing this "soft" subject, given the hard, intractable, and unyielding problems of financing, access, and clinical effectiveness in health care. But the experiential dimension of quality is not trivial. It is the heart of what patients want from health care—enhancement of their sense of well-being, relief from their suffering. *Any* health care system, however it may be financed or structured, must address both aspects of quality to achieve legitimacy in the eyes of those it serves.

Patient satisfaction or patient experience-of-care surveys are perhaps the most common method used to evaluate quality through the eyes of the patient. In the past few decades, there has been a strong push to develop surveys that measure the processes of care that matter most to patients and their families, in lieu of older instruments that tended to focus on processes of care or departments that healthcare managers had some control over or decided on their own were important (e.g., food services, housekeeping, admitting). These departments and services all contribute to a positive experience, but they may or may not be at the core of what matters most to patients and their families.

In 1987, the Picker/Commonwealth Program for Patient-Centered Care set out to explore patients' needs and concerns, as patients themselves define them, to inform the development of new surveys that could be linked to quality improvement efforts to enhance the patient's experience of care. Through extensive interviews and focus groups with a diverse group of patients and their families, the research program defined the following eight dimensions of patient-centered care that could be measured:

1. Access to care;
2. Respect for patients' values, preferences, and expressed needs;
3. Coordination of care and integration of services;
4. Information, communication, and education;
5. Physical comfort;
6. Emotional support and alleviation of fear and anxiety;
7. Involvement of family and friends; and
8. Transition and continuity.

These dimensions of care were further explored and enhanced through the work of the Picker Institute and were used as the basis of the definition of patient centeredness in the 2001 Institute of Medicine (IOM) report *Crossing the Quality Chasm.*

An important design feature of these survey instruments is the use of a combination of *reports* and *ratings* to assess patients' experiences within important dimensions of care, their overall satisfaction with services, and the relative importance of each dimension in relation to satisfaction. In focus groups of healthcare managers, physicians, and nurses to facilitate the design of "actionable" responses, complaints about the difficulty of interpreting *ratings of satisfaction* came up repeatedly. Clinicians and managers expressed well-founded concern about the inherent bias in ratings of satisfaction and asked for more objective measures describing what did and did not happen from the patient's perspective. The end result has been the development of questions that enable patients to *report* about their experiences with care. For example, a report-style question asks, "Did you doctor explain your diagnosis to you in a way you could understand?" instead of, "Rate your satisfaction with the quality of information you got from your doctor."

Regulatory and Federal Patient Survey Initiatives

Measuring patient experiences of care is routinely done in some fashion in most healthcare organizations and settings in the United States. The National Committee for Quality Assurance requires that all health plans submit Consumer Assessment of Health Plans (CAHPS) data as part of their Health

Employer Data and Information Set submission for accreditation. The Centers for Medicare & Medicaid Services (CMS) use CAHPS to collect data from all Medicare beneficiaries in both managed care plans and fee-for-service settings, and approximately half of the state Medicaid programs collect CAHPS data from Medicaid recipients. The Joint Commission on Accreditation of Healthcare Organizations (Joint Commission) requires that every accredited organization perform surveys to evaluate patients' or members' experiences of care, but it does not mandate a particular survey; however, the Joint Commission supports the National Quality Initiative that is using the Hospital CAHPS (H-CAHPS).

The CAHPS study is a multiyear initiative funded by the Agency for Healthcare Research and Quality. *CAHPS* refers to a comprehensive and expanding family of survey instruments designed to capture the experiences of consumers and patients with a range of healthcare products and services. By providing consumers with standardized data and presenting them in a way that is easy to understand and use, CAHPS is intended to help people make decisions that support better healthcare and better health. This emphasis on the consumer's point of view differentiates CAHPS reports from other sources of information about clinical measures of quality. The CAHPS program is also working to integrate CAHPS results into the quality improvement programs of sponsors and healthcare providers. It is anticipated that hospitals will begin to report data from H-CAHPS through the National Health Quality Initiative to CMS and the public in 2005. CMS and the CAHPS team also published *The CAHPS Improvement Guide* in 2003 (Edgman-Levitan et al.) to help health plans and group practices improve their performance on the surveys. All CAHPS products are in the public domain, free, and available for use by anyone.[1]

CAHPS has been tested more completely than any previously used consumer survey (Hays et al. 1999). Surveys and consumer reports are now completed to measure and report the experience of care with health plans for the commercially insured, Medicare and Medicaid populations, and behavioral health services. Work is underway to complete surveys to evaluate patient experiences in a group practice or clinic; with an individual clinician; and in hospitals, nursing homes, and renal dialysis centers by the end of 2004. Many of these instruments are being developed with additional funding from CMS as part of its plan to publicly report results to consumers to foster quality improvement and help consumers improve their decision making about choice of plan, hospital, or provider.

The value of national efforts such as CAHPS lies in the development of standardized surveys and data collection protocols that enable rigorous comparisons among organizations and the creation of trustworthy, accurate benchmark data. Standardized surveys also allow healthcare organizations to share effective improvement strategies that are known to improve scores and enable consumers to make better choices of plans and clinicians when the data are publicly reported. Publicly reported quality measures also prove to be a powerful stimulant to internal quality improvement efforts and frequently result in increased budgets for quality improvement work.

Collecting patient experience-of-care data is also becoming a standard evaluation measure in the education and certification of medical, nursing, and allied health students. The American College of Graduate Medical Education has incorporated extensive standards into its requirements for residency training that focus on the doctor-patient relationship, and the American Board of Internal Medicine is piloting patient experience-of-care surveys for incorporation into the recertification process for board-certified physicians.

Using Patient Feedback for Quality Improvement

Although nationally standardized instruments and comparative databases are essential for public accountability and benchmarking, measurement for the purposes of monitoring quality improvement interventions does not necessarily require the same sort of standardized data collection and sampling. Many institutions prefer more frequent feedback of results (e.g., quarterly, monthly, weekly), with more precise, in-depth sampling (e.g., at the unit or clinic level) to allow targeted improvement. Staff are usually eager to obtain data frequently, but the cost of administration and the response burden on patients must be weighed against the knowledge that substantial changes in scores usually take at least a quarter, if not longer, to appear in the data.

Survey Terminology

Familiarity with terms describing the psychometric properties of survey instruments and methods for data collection can help improve the ability to choose a survey that will provide the organization with credible information for quality improvement. Some of the basic terms are described briefly below.

There are two different and complementary approaches to assessing the reliability and validity of a questionnaire: (1) cognitive testing, which bases its assessments on feedback from interviews with people who are asked to react to the survey questions; and (2) psychometric testing, which bases its assessments on the analysis of data collected using the questionnaire. Although many existing consumer questionnaires about healthcare have been tested primarily or exclusively using a psychometric approach, many survey researchers view the combination of cognitive and psychometric approaches as essential to producing the best possible survey instruments. Consequently, both methods have been included in the development of CAHPS and other instruments (Fowler 1995, 2001).

The cognitive testing method provides useful information on respondents' perceptions of the response task, how respondents recall and report events, and how they interpret specified reference periods. It also helps identify words that can be used to describe healthcare providers accurately and consistently across a range of consumers (e.g., commercially insured, Medicaid, fee-for-service, managed care; lower socioeconomic status, middle socioeconomic status; low literacy, higher literacy) and helps explore whether key words and concepts included in the core questions work equally well in English and Spanish. For example, in the cognitive interviews to test CAHPS, researchers learned that parents did not think pediatricians were primary care providers. They evaluated the care they were receiving from pediatricians in the questions about specialists, not primary care doctors. This discovery resulted in changing the language to ask about "your personal doctor," not your primary care provider (Fowler 1992).

Validity

In conventional use, the term *validity* refers to the extent to which an empirical measure adequately reflects the real meaning of the concept under consideration (Babbie 1995). In more practical language, validity refers to the degree to which the measurement made by a survey corresponds to some true or real value. For example, a bathroom scale that always reads 185 pounds is reliable. Although the scale may be reliable and consistent, however, it is not valid if the person does not weigh 185 pounds.

The different types of validity are as follows:

- *Face validity* is the agreement between empirical measurers and mental images associated with a particular concept. Does the measure look valid to the people who will be using it? A survey has face validity if it appears on the surface to measure what it has been designed to measure.
- *Construct validity* is based on the logical relationships among variables (or questions). Valid questions should have answers that correspond to what they are intended to measure. Since there is no objective way of validating answers to the majority of the questions in surveys, validity of reports can be assessed only by their correlations with other answers a person gives. Construct validity refers to the extent to which a scale measures the construct, or theoretical

framework, it is designed to measure. Satisfaction is an example of a construct. Researchers measure construct validity by testing the correlations between different items and other established constructs. We would expect high *convergent validity*, or strong correlation, between survey items such as waiting times and overall ratings of access. We would expect *discriminant validity*, or little correlation, between patient reports about coordination of care in the emergency room and the adequacy of pain control on an inpatient unit.

- *Content validity* refers to the degree to which a measure covers the range of meanings included within the concept. A survey with high content validity would represent topics related to satisfaction in appropriate proportions. For example, we would expect an inpatient survey to have a number of questions about nursing care, but we would not expect a majority of the questions to ask about telephone service in the patient's room.

- *Criterion validity* refers to whether a newly developed scale is strongly correlated with another measure that has already been demonstrated to be highly reliable and valid. Criterion validity can be viewed as how well a question measures up to a gold standard. For example, if you wanted to ask patients about the interns and residents who took care of them, you would want to be sure patients could distinguish between staff and trainee physicians. You could measure the criterion validity of questions that ask about the identity of physicians by comparing patients' answers to hospital records.

- *Discriminant validity* is the magnitude of difference between survey results when the scales are applied in different settings. That is, survey scores should reflect differences among different institutions, where care is presumably different. Discriminant validity is the extent to which groups of respondents who are thought to differ in what is being measured do in fact differ in their answers (Fowler 2001).

Reliability

In the abstract, *reliability* is a matter of whether a particular technique applied repeatedly to the same object yields the same results each time. The reliability of a survey instrument is initially addressed within the questionnaire development phase. Questions that use ambiguous words, words with many different meanings, or words that are not universally understood will yield unreliable results. Using simple, short words that are widely understood is a sound approach to questionnaire design, even with well-educated samples (Fowler 1995). An instrument is reliable if consistency across respondents exists (i.e., the questions mean the same thing to every respondent). This will ensure that differences in answers can be attributed to differences in respondents or their experiences.

Instrument reliability, or the reliability of a measure, refers to the stability and equivalence of repeated measures of the same concept. In other words, instrument reliability is the reliability of the answers people give to the same question when they are asked it at different points in time, assuming no real changes have occurred that should cause them to answer the questions differently. Reliable survey questions always produce the same answers from the same respondents when answered under similar circumstances. Reliability is also the degree to which survey questions are answered consistently in similar situations. Inadequate wording of questions and poorly defined terms can compromise reliability. The goal is to ensure (through pilot testing) that questions mean the same thing to all respondents.

The *test-retest reliability coefficient* is a method to measure instrument reliability. Using this method, one measures the degree of correspondence between answers to the same questions asked of the same respondents at different points in time. If there is no reason to expect the information ought to change (and the methodology for obtaining the information is correct), one should expect the same response both times. If answers vary, the measurement is unstable and thus unreliable.

Internal consistency is the intercorrelation among a number of different questions intended to measure (or reflect) the same concept. The internal consistency of a measurement tool may be assessed using *Cronbach's alpha reliability coefficient*. Cronbach's alpha is a test for a model's or survey's internal consistency. Sometimes called a *scale reliability coefficient*, Cronbach's alpha assesses the reliability of a rating summarizing a group of test or survey answers that measure some underlying factor (e.g., some attribute of the test taker) (Cortina 1993; Cronbach 1951).

Readability of Survey Instruments

The readability of survey questions has a direct effect on the reliability of the instrument. Unreliable survey questions use ambiguous words and words that are not universally understood. No simple measure of literacy exists. The Microsoft Word program comes with a spelling and grammar checker that will produce a statistical analysis of a document. The spelling/grammar checker will calculate a Flesch-Kincaid index for any document, including questionnaires. The Flesch-Kincaid index (Flesch 1948) is a coarse formula that uses sentence length (words per sentence) and complexity, along with the number of syllables per word, to derive a number corresponding to grade level. Documents containing shorter sentences with shorter words have lower Flesch-Kincaid scores.

Weighting Survey Results

Weighting of scores is frequently recommended if members of a (patient) population have unequal probabilities of selection into the sample. If necessary, weights are assigned to the different observations made to provide a representative picture of the total population. Basically, the weight assigned to a particular sample member should be the inverse of its probability of selection.

Most weighting questions arise when an unequal distribution of patients exists by discharge service, nursing unit, or clinic. When computing an overall score for a hospital or a group of clinics with an unequal distribution of patients, weighting by probability of selection is appropriate. The probability of selection is estimated by dividing the number of patients sampled by the total number of patients. When the probability of selection for patients from different services or units is equal, this implies that patients from different services or units will be represented in the sample in the same proportion as they occur in the population. If the probability of selection for patients from different hospitals or medical groups is the same, this implies that the sample size for different hospitals or medical groups will vary according to the number of total discharges from each hospital.

Similarity—presenting the results stratified by service, unit, or clinic—provides an accurate and representative picture of the total population. For example, the most straightforward method for comparing units to an overall score would be to compare medical units to all medical patients, surgical units to all surgical patients, and childbirth units to all childbirth patients.

The weighting issue also comes up when hospitals or clinics are being compared within a system. If the service case mix is similar, we can compare by hospital without accounting for case-mix difference. If service case mix is not similar across institutions, scores should be weighted before between-hospital comparisons are made. Alternatively, comparisons should be made at the service level.

Response Rates

The response rate for mailed surveys is calculated by dividing the number of useable returned questionnaires by the number of patients who were mailed questionnaires. Adjustments are made to the denominator to exclude ineligible cases—"undeliverables" and patients who should not have been sent a questionnaire, such as deceased patients.

The calculation is different for telephone surveys. The following cases are often removed before calculating rates: nonworking numbers, numbers that were never answered or were answered by a machine, patients who were too ill or confused to be interviewed, and patients the interviewer determined were ineligible for some other reason.

When response rates are low, the internal validity of the sample is compromised. Survey results based on response rates of 30 percent or less may not be representative of patient satisfaction (at that institution). Although a representative sample is mailed, certain population groups are more likely to self-select out of the survey process. An expected (and typical) response bias is seen in all mailed surveys. For example, young people and Medicaid patients are less likely to respond to mailed surveys.

An optimal response rate is necessary to have a representative sample; therefore, boosting response rates should be a priority. Methods to improve response rates include the following:

- Making telephone reminder calls for certain types of surveys;
- Using the Dillman (1978) method, a three-wave mailing protocol designed to boost response rates;
- Ensuring that telephone numbers or addresses are drawn from as accurate a source as possible; and
- Offering incentives appropriate for the survey population (e.g., drugstore coupons, free parking coupons).

Survey Bias

Bias refers to the extent that survey results do not accurately represent a population. It is impossible to conduct a perfectly unbiased survey. By considering the sources of bias during the survey design phase, its effect can be minimized. It is always helpful to consider the potential biases in survey results.

Sampling Bias

All patients who have been selected to provide feedback should have an equal opportunity to respond. Any situation that results in certain patients being less likely to be included in a sample leads to bias. For example, patients whose addresses are outdated or whose phone numbers are obsolete or incomplete in the database are less likely to be reached. Up-to-date patient lists are essential. It is also important for a survey vendor to eliminate sampling bias through probability sampling. That is, giving all patients who meet the study criteria an opportunity to be included in the sample.

Nonresponse Bias

In every survey, some people agree to be respondents but do not answer every question. Although nonresponse to individual questions is usually low, occasionally it can be high and can have a real effect on estimates. Three categories of patients are selected to be in the sample who do not actually provide data, as follows:

1. Those the data collection procedures do not reach, thereby not giving them a chance to answer questions
2. Those asked to provide data who refuse to do so (do not respond to the survey)
3. Those asked to provide data who are unable to perform the task required of them (e.g., people who are too ill to respond to a survey or whose reading and writing skills preclude their filling out self-administered questionnaires)

Regardless of the representativeness of the sampling frame, bias is almost always introduced by the fact that not all people contacted choose to respond to the survey. By gathering demographic information on all patients in the sample pool, the size and type of nonresponse bias can be estimated. It is important to look at the profile of respondents and non-respondents by demographic variables that are important to you (e.g., age, gender, payer, or discharge service).

Administration Method Bias or Mode Effects

The way a survey is administered inevitably introduces bias of one sort or another. When comparing data that have been collected using different modes of administration (e.g., mail and telephone), differences may be real or they may be the result of different modes of administration. An instrument that produces comparable data whether they are collected by mail or telephone has no bias caused by mode effect. For example, in mail surveys, patients who are not literate or do not have a mailing address are excluded from the survey. In telephone surveys, bias is introduced by not being able to query people who do not have phones. In face-to-face interviews, interviewers can influence respondents simply by their body language and facial expressions. In surveys conducted at the clinic or hospital, respondents may be reluctant to answer questions candidly. Combining methods such as phone follow-up of mailed surveys or making phone interviews available to low-literacy patients can reduce some of these biases.

A major concern about comparability is that telephone interviews often collect more favorable responses (or answers that reflect more positively on respondents) than do mail surveys. CAHPS testing showed that the majority of the differences could be linked to the way question skips were handled. The telephone interview used explicit screening questions, whereas the mail version asked respondents to check an "inapplicable" box when the question did not apply. The explicit screening question identified many more people to whom questions did not apply than were reflected in the mail data.

Proxy-Response Bias

Studies comparing self-reports with proxy reports do not consistently support the hypothesis that self-reports are more accurate than proxy reports (U.S. Department of Health and Human Services 1987). However, the conclusions drawn from studies in which responses were verified using hospital and physician records show that, on average, (1) self-reports tend to be more accurate than proxy reports, and (2) health events are generally underreported in both populations. In terms of reporting problems with care, most studies comparing proxy responses to patients responses show that proxies tend to report more problems with care compared to patients (vom Eigen et al. 1999). Therefore, the percentage response by proxy needs to be taken into consideration in the interpretation of survey results.

Recall Bias

Typically, patients receive questionnaires from two weeks to four months after discharge from the hospital. This sometimes raises concern about the reliability of the patient's recall. Studies of memory have shown that the greater the effect of the hospitalization and the nature of the condition, the greater the ability to recall health events. Studies also suggest that most people find it difficult to recall precise details, such as minor symptoms or the number of times a specific event occurred. For ambulatory surveys, patients should be surveyed as close to the visit or event as possible.

Case-Mix Adjustment

Case-mix adjustment accounts for the different types of patients that are cared for in institutions. Adjustments should be considered when hospital survey results are being released to the public. The characteristics commonly associated with patient reports on quality of care are (1) patient age (i.e., older patients tend to report fewer problems with care) and (2) discharge service (i.e., childbirth patients evaluate their experience more favorably than do medical or surgical patients, with medical patients reporting the most problems with care) (Hargraves et al. 2001).

Scope and Use of Patient Experiences in Healthcare

Customer Service and Patient Satisfaction

The ability of healthcare organizations to deliver high-quality, patient-centered care to their members and patients depends in part on their understanding of basic customer service principles and their ability to integrate these principles into clinical settings.

Healthcare organizations should pay attention to customer service for several reasons. First, better service translates into higher satisfaction for the patient and, subsequently, for the employer who pays most of the bills. Second, as in any other service industry, a satisfied (and loyal) member or patient creates value over the course of a lifetime. In the context of healthcare, this value may manifest itself in the form of repeat visits, trusting relationships, and positive word of mouth. A dissatisfied member or patient, on the other hand, generates potential new costs. Many health plans, for example, have found that the cost of replacing members lost to disenrollment can be high. Patients who are not involved in decision making the way they want to be; who cannot get an appointment with their clinician when they are sick; or who are not treated with respect and dignity by their hospital, plan, or clinician may not follow clinical advice, can develop worse outcomes, and frequently share their negative stories with friends and family members. Third, existing patients and members are an invaluable source of information that can help healthcare organizations understand how to improve what they do and reduce waste by eliminating services that are unnecessary or not valued (Heskett et al. 1994).

Finally, poor customer service raises the risk of a negative "grapevine effect." More than 50 percent of people who have a bad experience will not complain openly to the plan or the medical group. But research shows that nearly all (96 percent) are likely to tell at least ten other people about their bad experiences. Through several years of experience in collecting CAHPS data, it has become apparent that even patient surveys do not adequately capture the full story about problems because, contrary to what many staff and clinicians think, the angriest patients are often the least likely to respond to patient surveys.

Word-of-mouth reputation is important because studies continue to find that the most trusted sources of information for people choosing a health plan, medical group, doctor, or hospital are close family, friends, and work colleagues. When a survey asked people whom they would go to for this kind of information, more than two-thirds of respondents said they would rely on the opinions of family members and friends (Kaiser Family Foundation and Agency for Healthcare Research and Quality 2000). In a study conducted by General Electric, "The impact of word-of-mouth on a customer's purchase decision was twice as important as corporate advertising" (Goodman 1987).

Healthcare organizations also need to pay attention to customer service because service quality and employee satisfaction go hand in hand. It is almost impossible to find an organization with satisfied patients when the employee satisfaction is low. Employees often are frustrated and angry about the same things that bother patients and members: chaotic work

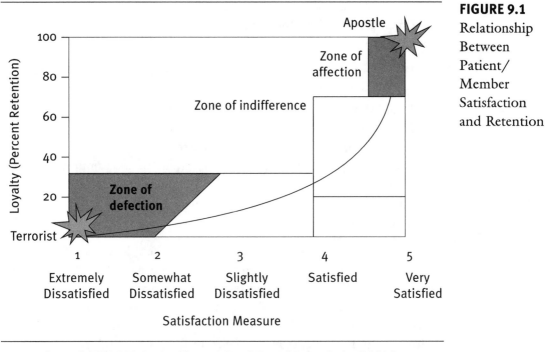

FIGURE 9.1
Relationship
Between
Patient/
Member
Satisfaction
and Retention

Source: Heskett et al. (1994, 167). Reprinted by permission of *Harvard Business Review*: Exhibit from "Putting the Service-Profit Chain to Work" by Heskett, J. L., T. O. Jones, G. Loveman, E. Sasser, Jr., and J. A. Schlesinger, 167 (Mar./Apr.) 1994. Copyright © 1994 by the Harvard Business School Publishing Corporation, all rights reserved.

environments, poor systems, and ineffective training. No amount of money, signing bonuses, or other tools currently used to recruit hard-to-find staff will offset the negative effect of these problems on staff. The real cost of high turnover may not be the replacement costs of finding new staff, but the expenses associated with lost organizational knowledge, lower productivity, and decreased customer satisfaction.

Achieving Better Customer Service

The most successful service organizations pay attention to the factors that ensure their success: investing in people with an aptitude for service, technology that supports frontline staff, training practices that incorporate well-designed experiences for the patient or member, and compensation linked to performance. In particular, they recognize that their staff members value being able to achieve good results, and they equip the staff to meet the needs of members and patients. For health plans, this could mean developing information systems that allow staff to answer members' questions and settle claims quickly and easily; for provider organizations, this could mean providing the resources and materials that clinicians need to provide high-quality care in a compassionate, safe environment.

Experts on delivering superior customer service suggest that healthcare organizations adopt the following set of principles (Leebov, Scott, and Olson 1998):

1. **Hire service-savvy people.** Aptitude is everything; people can be taught technical skills.
2. **Establish high standards of customer service.**
3. **Help staff hear the voice of the customer.**
4. **Remove barriers so staff can serve customers.**
5. **Design the processes of care to reduce patient and family anxiety to increase satisfaction.**
6. **Help staff cope better in a stressful atmosphere.**
7. **Maintain a focus on service.**

Many customer service programs have been developed for companies outside healthcare. Although the strategies are similar, Leebov, Scott, and Olson (1998) have adapted this work for healthcare settings in ways that increase its credibility and buy-in, especially from clinical staff. Their books and articles include practical, step-by-step instructions about how to identify and solve customer service problems through the healthcare delivery system (Leebov, Afriat, and Presha 1998).

"Listening Posts" to Incorporate Patient and Family Perspective into Quality Improvement Work

Patient satisfaction and patient experience-of-care surveys are the most common *quantitative* measures used by healthcare organizations, but other important *qualitative* methods, or listening posts, can be used to obtain important information from patients and their families to guide improvement work. Although patient satisfaction surveys provide extremely useful data, they are not the best source of information for innovative ideas about improving the delivery of care. Also, even healthcare organizations with high satisfaction scores often have many opportunities to improve services, which may not be revealed by survey data.

Quality improvement activities that focus on the needs and experiences of customers (i.e., members and patients) can only succeed in an environment that emphasizes the concepts and responsibilities of customer service. One critical element of effective customer service is the capacity to elicit detailed, constructive feedback in a way that assures people that someone is really listening to them. When this is done well, members and patients are more likely to report a positive experience. At the very least, the organization should not be surprised by any negative reports.

However, this hands-on approach can be a major challenge for healthcare organizations that are not accustomed to communicating with their members or patients in this way. Many assume they understand how to fix the problem and do not probe beneath the surface of complaints and survey responses. For example, complaints about unhelpful office staff in a practice could stem from many sources, such as the following:

- Not being given clear instructions about how to get to the practice;
- Not being able to get an appointment when they needed it;
- Being put on hold in the middle of a medical emergency; or
- Real rudeness and disrespect during a visit or on the phone.

The solutions to these problems vary tremendously. Without digging deeper with patients or members to understand the true problem, a healthcare organization or quality improvement team could waste a great deal of money on the wrong fixes.

The term *listening posts* refers to a variety of ways to learn about the experiences of patients and staff and involve them in the improvement process. Most already exist in some form in most health plans or clinical practices. The most difficult issue related to listening posts is building a system to routinely synthesize all of the feedback received from these different source into a coherent picture of what they reveal about the way care is delivered. Once this system is in place, root-cause analyses can be performed to identify problems, such as a particular staff member or medical group that accounts for many of your problems, versus problems that are systemic to your delivery of care, such as an antiquated manual appointment system.

Listening post strategies include:

- Focus groups
- Walkthroughs
- Complaint/compliment letters
- Patient and family advisory councils

Surveys

Analyzing data from CAHPS and other patient satisfaction or patient experience-of-care surveys can be beneficial, as can more frequent, small-scale use of individual questions to monitor a specific intervention.

Focus Groups

Staff or patients can be brought together in a moderator-led discussion group to collect more precise information about a specific problem and new ideas for improvement strategies. A focus group allows for more in-depth exploration of the drivers of dissatisfaction and can provide excellent ideas for reengineering services. In addition, videotapes of focus groups can be very effective at changing the attitudes and beliefs of staff members because the stories participants tell often bring to life the emotional effect of excellent service as well as service failures (Bader and Rossi 2001; Krueger and Casey 2000).

Walkthroughs

A walkthrough may be the easiest way to give staff the patient's perspective and the fastest way to identify system, flow, and attitude problems, many of which can be fixed almost overnight. Performing a walkthrough is an effective way of recreating for staff the emotional and physical experiences of being a patient or family member. Walkthroughs provide a different perspective and bring to light rules and procedures that may have outlived their usefulness. This method of observation was developed by David Gustafson, Ph.D. (unpublished), at the University of Wisconsin in Madison and adapted by the author to incorporate the staff perspective.

During a walkthrough, one staff member plays the role of the patient and another accompanies him or her as the family member. They go through a clinic, service, or procedure exactly as a patient and family do. They do everything patients and families are asked to do, and they abide by the same rules. They do this openly, not as a mystery patient, and throughout the process ask staff members a series of questions to encourage reflection on the processes or systems of care and identify improvement opportunities.

The staff conducting the walkthrough take notes to document what they see and how they feel during the process. They then share these notes with the leadership of the organization and quality improvement teams to help develop improvement plans. For many conducting walkthroughs, it is the first time they have ever entered their clinics, procedure rooms, or labs as the patient and family do. Clinicians are routinely surprised at how easy it is to hear staff comments about patients from public areas and waiting rooms. Walkthroughs usually turn up many problems with flow, signage, and wasteful procedures and policies that can be fixed almost immediately.

As an alternative to a walkthrough, a similar technique called *patient shadowing* can be used. A staff member asks permission to accompany a patient through the visit and take notes on the patient's experience. Since this approach does not require taking a slot away from a real patient, it can be useful in settings where visits are at a premium.

Complaint/Compliment Letters

Reviewing these letters systematically can often provide a better picture of where more background research is needed with staff and patient focus groups or a walkthrough versus when a manager should be involved to address a personnel problem.

Patient and Family Advisory Councils

For some patients and health plan members, the issue is not a concern about being heard. Rather, their dissatisfaction with their healthcare experience reflects frustration with a system that does not involve them in decisions that will affect the design and delivery of care. From their perspective, the system is superficially responsive: It acknowledges that a problem with service or care exists, but it does not bother to investigate whether a proposed solution will really address the problem from the patient's or member's point of view.

A patient and family advisory council is one of the most effective strategies for involving families and patients in the design of care (Webster and Johnson 2000). First designed and advanced by the Institute for Family-Centered Care, these councils are composed of patients and families who represent the constituencies served by the plan or medical group. It is important to involve both families and patients because they see different things and each have an important perspective to consider.

The goal of the councils is to integrate patients and families into the healthcare organization's evaluation and redesign processes to improve the experience of care and customer service. In addition to meeting regularly with senior leadership, council members serve as listening posts for the staff and provide a structure and process for ongoing dialog and creative problem solving between the organization and its patients and families. The councils can play many roles, but they do not function as boards, nor do they have fiduciary responsibility for the organization.

Council responsibilities may include input into or involvement in

- Program development, implementation, and evaluation;
- Planning for major renovation or the design of a new building or service;
- Staff selection and training;
- Marketing plan or practice services;
- Participation in staff orientation and in-service training programs; and
- Design of new materials or tools that support the doctor-patient relationship.[2]

These councils help overcome a common problem that most organizations face when they begin to develop patient- and family-centered processes: They do not have direct experience of illness or the healthcare system. Consequently, healthcare professionals often approach the design process from their own perspective, not those of patients or families. Improvement committees with the best of intentions may disagree about who understands the needs of the family and patient best. But family members and patients rarely understand professional turf boundaries. Their suggestions are usually inexpensive, straightforward, and easy to implement because they are not bound by the usual rules and sensitivities.

In general, when starting a patient and family advisory council, it is best to start with members recommended by staff. Depending on the size of the organization, most councils have between 12 and 30 patient or family members and 3 or 4 members from the staff of the organization. The council members are usually asked to commit to one 2- to 3-hour meeting a month, usually over dinner, and participation on one committee. Most councils start off with one-year terms for all members to allow for graceful departures in case a member is not well suited for the council.

Look for people who can listen and respect different opinions. They should be supportive of the institution's mission as well as constructive with their input. Staff members frequently describe good council members as people who know how to provide constructive critiques. Council members also need to be comfortable speaking to groups and in front of professionals.

Keys to Successful Implementation and Lessons Learned

Avoid Failure by Establishing Clear Goals

Collecting feedback from patients and their families will provide rich information for quality improvement work. For these efforts to be successful, it is important to consider the following questions:

1. What is your aim for improvement?
2. What types of information from patients, families, and your staff will help you achieve your aim?
3. How frequently do you need to measure your performance to achieve your aim?
4. Who will review the data?
5. What is your budget?

Once you know the answers to these questions, you can plan your data collection strategy.

What Is Your Aim for Improvement?

If you are trying to improve overall satisfaction with care, willingness to recommend your organization to family members and friends, or both, you will need to focus your measurement efforts on all of the dimensions of care that matter to patients. You will need to choose a survey that accurately measures these dimensions. If you are trying to improve a specific dimension of the patient's experience of care or the performance of a specific unit (e.g., emergency room, surgical unit, outpatient clinic), you will need to think carefully about what type of survey will meet your needs.

Be sure to understand the strongest drivers of overall satisfaction as measured by the survey you are using. You might want to focus your initial improvement work on the drivers that are stronger drivers of overall satisfaction. In general, many studies document the importance of access to care, doctor-patient communication, and respect for patient preferences; however, you may decide that preparing patients for discharge from the hospital is so important to clinical outcomes that it will take precedence over the other dimensions.

What Types of Information Will Help You Achieve Your Aim?

Match the type of feedback you are collecting to your aim. If you are trying to improve overall satisfaction with care, you may need a combination of survey data, focus group information, and information from compliment/complaint letters. If you are trying to improve a specific unit, you may need a combination of survey data, focus group information, and the results of a walkthrough or information from a targeted patient and family advisory council.

Choose a survey instrument that measures the processes of care that matter most to your patients. Make sure it is a validated instrument and that the comparative data are truly comparable. Find out how many organizations like yours are in the database and whether the data can be broken out to give you customized benchmarks. For example, a community hospital near a ski resort measuring patient experiences of care with its emergency room is probably more interested in benchmarks from other emergency rooms that see lots of orthopedic problems than from large urban emergency rooms with many trauma victims.

Pick a survey that has a mode of administration that suits your patient population, and make sure the questions have been tested for administration in that mode. For example, if you have a patient population with low literacy, you might want to choose a telephone survey or a survey that is administered using interactive voice recognition (i.e., "push 1 for yes, 2 for no").

How Frequently Do You Need to Measure Your Performance?

Plan your data collection carefully. Avoid oversurveying patients or appearing to be uncoordinated in your efforts to improve care. If you are trying to improve overall satisfaction with care, quarterly surveys are appropriate;

it would be unusual to see any changes in the data with increased frequency of data collection. If you are testing a specific intervention, you will want to try small tests of change; more frequent measuring will be required to determine if your improvement interventions are effective or how they need to be modified. You will need to develop a sampling strategy by service, unit, or condition depending on your aim. You may determine that continuous sampling is important versus a one-time snapshot in a quarter or that you need to survey or interview five patients every Monday, ten patients a week, or all of the patients seen in a specific clinic.

Never underestimate the potential for response bias when surveying patients about their experiences. Many people are very concerned that negative responses will jeopardize the quality of care they receive in the future. Make sure that the surveys are administered in a way that provides anonymity and confidentiality. Also, make sure that the measures are done at a time when the person can really evaluate his or her experiences. For example, many vendors try to get surveys to recently discharged patients as quickly as possible. Sending them too early may mean that the person has not recovered enough to know whether they got all the information they needed to help them manage their condition going forward or if they have the information they need about when they can drive, return to work, or perform other activities of daily living.

Who Will Review the Data?

Make sure you understand the needs and perspectives of your audience for the data. Include open-ended comments, stories, and anecdotes wherever possible in reports. These are always powerful motivators for behavior change, and most staff enjoy reading them. In studies done by Richard Nisbett at the University of Michigan, data by itself were found to be the least persuasive motivator of culture or behavior change; stories combined with data were moderately persuasive; and stories alone were the most persuasive (e.g., Nisbett and Borgida 1975). Consider how you can combine stories from your walkthroughs, focus groups, and patient family advisory councils to enrich the understanding your staff will have about the experiences of care, both positive and negative. If you are trying to get the attention of senior leaders or clinicians, the scientific rigor of the data collection will be important, and comparative data are usually essential to clarify whether the myths about the organization's performance measure up to the reality.

It is also important to think about how the reports are formatted and presented to different audiences. Web-based reports support widespread and rapid dissemination of data. Some audiences need sophisticated graphical presentations; others are most interested in open-ended comments.

What Is Your Budget?

Do everything you can to create a budget that supports the type of data collection necessary to achieve your goals. If you are reporting patient experience-of-care data to the public, you need to maximize the rigor of the data collection to ensure excellent response rates and sampling, and you may need to spend more money to accomplish that goal. If you are collecting the data primarily for quality improvement purposes, you need to consider vendors that can supply the data via the Internet using reporting formats that facilitate quality improvement such as putting the results into control charts. All of these features have different budget implications that need to be considered before putting together a request for proposal.

Be careful not to include any in-house data collection activities (postage, printing the surveys and mailing them) or analyses as "free." Sometimes organizations actually spend more money by choosing a lower-cost vendor that requires a lot of in-house support and in-kind contributions that do not get factored into the overall cost of the data collection. Most healthcare organizations are not sophisticated about these issues, and their internal staff often take far longer to accomplish the same tasks a good survey vendor could get done correctly and much more economically. For example, vendors will sometimes drop the cost of postage and mailing the surveys out of their overall budget for a project, expecting the healthcare organization to pick up these costs. These tactics can falsely lower a project bid and need to be carefully screened.

Lessons Learned, or "The Roads Not to Take"

Honest criticism is hard to take, particularly from a relative, a friend, an acquaintance, or a stranger.

—*Franklin P. Jones*

Resistance to lower-than-expected results is common and completely reasonable. It is not necessarily a sign of complacency or lack of commitment to high-quality, patient-centered care. Most healthcare clinicians and staff are working harder than they ever have, and the systems they are using to deliver care are not necessarily designed to give patients or staff a positive experience. The expectations of patients and families have also risen over the last decade in response to greater access to clinical information and excellent service experiences in other industries such as banking, financial services, retail stores, and web-based retailers.

Getting feedback from patients that their clinical care falls short of expectations is frustrating and demoralizing for healthcare clinicians and employees. With this in mind, it is important to present both positive and negative results from patient surveys or listening posts and, whenever possible, to include strategies and systematic supports that make it easier for staff to perform at the levels they desire. Executives, senior clinicians, and managers need to be prepared to respond effectively to the common arguments clinical and administrative staff use to deny the validity of feedback from patients. Most of this resistance comes in two forms: *people resistance*, arguments about a patient's ability to accurately judge his or her interactions with healthcare clinicians and staff or the importance of such perceptions; and *data resistance*, arguments that attempt to undermine the scientific credibility of the data.

How to Address People Resistance

- "No one comes here for a good time." They certainly do not, and patients and family members will be the first to agree. They want patient- and family-centered care, designed to meet their needs, and they are looking for compassion and healing whenever possible. Most people want to have as little contact with the healthcare system as possible, but when they need care, they want it delivered in a compassionate, considerate manner.

- "But I was very nice." *Nice* is not necessarily what quality care is about. Patients and their families have clearly articulated needs with respect to the care they receive. If these needs are ignored or not met, the people they encounter can be extremely nice but nevertheless ineffective. Usually, staff emphasize this point when "being nice" was their only recourse to redress other important service failures (e.g., they were apologizing for delays in care, the absence of equipment that the patient needed, missing lab work or X-rays). The solution is to make sure staff have the resources, systems, and training they need to meet the needs of patients.

- "This patient/family is very difficult or dysfunctional." Sometimes it is helpful to ask staff to describe patients or families they like and do not like. They usually like patients and families who are grateful or people from the same culture or who speak the same language, but beyond that the attributes of popular patients and families become pretty grim. The most popular patients never ring their call lights, never ask for help, never ask questions or challenge their nurses and doctors, and never, ever read medical books or use the Internet for help. Their families are not present, and they do not have friends. In fact, they are as close to dead as possible.

  Many people who work in healthcare forgot how anxiety provoking any encounter with the healthcare system is, from finding a parking spot to concern over hearing bad news. For most patients and families, a visit to the doctor or hospital is more akin to visiting a foreign country or going to jail than it is to a positive, healing experience. We do not speak the same language, and few helpful guidebooks exist to show patients the way.

We also do everything we can to force people to comply with our rules and regulations, no matter how outdated or meaningless they are, and then we are surprised when they react in anger or dismay. Why should a heart patient have to use a wheelchair to enter the hospital when he or she has been walking around the community for months and then be required to walk out the door only a few days after surgery? Why is it a surprise when families fight over chairs or sofas in an ICU waiting room when we only provide a fraction of the chairs or couches necessary to let at least two family members be present for each patient? Patients are often characterized as difficult when they get angry that they are forced to go to an emergency room for a simple acute problem after office hours.

It is often helpful to point out the effect of these unspoken beliefs and rules and to remind everyone that the patients who are least likely to get better are the ones we like. Passive patients rarely do as well in the long run as activated, assertive patients who want to learn as much as possible about how to improve their health or be more autonomous.

- "How can the patient rate the skill of the doctor/nurse?" Patient and family surveys and the other listening posts described here are not designed to evaluate the technical skills of clinicians, and patients are the first to acknowledge they do not know how to do that. Patients are asked to evaluate the processes of care and the components of doctor- and nurse-to-patient communication, the aspects of care that they and only they can evaluate. Chart documentation about patient education is worthless if the patient did not understand what was being taught to them.

How to Address Data Resistance

- "The sample size is too small—you can't tell anything from it." Interestingly, doctors and other clinical staff trained in statistical methods are often the first to say they will not believe survey data until every last patient has been interviewed. Sampling methodology in the social sciences and for survey research is no different from the sampling used in diagnostic and laboratory tests clinicians trust every day. Remind people that no one draws all of someone's blood to check their hematocrit; a teaspoon or two is plenty!
- "Only angry people respond to surveys." This is often not the case. Patients may be afraid that negative responses to surveys will affect

the quality of care they receive—a sad indictment of the trust they have in their healthcare providers—and we never hear from patients we know are likely to have problems, such as those who are discharged to nursing homes, those who speak foreign languages, and those who die. In fact, the data most people see are likely to represent their happiest patients. This is also an important reason to draw samples that are as representative as possible of the patient population.

- "You really can't determine where something went wrong." Well-designed survey tools that measure things patients care about can provide a pretty good picture of where to start looking. Also, remember to use the other listening posts to get a better picture of the source of the problems, from the perspective of staff and patients, and how to fix it.

- "It's not statistically significant." Again, if you pay attention to the reliability and validity of your survey tools; the sampling strategy, doing everything you can to increase response rates; and the quality of your vendor's comparative database, you will have an excellent idea about the confidence intervals of your data and the statistical significance of trends over time and comparative benchmarks.

- "These aren't my patients, and my patients are different." Everyone thinks their patients are different and that all survey data come from someone else's service or patient panel. Looking at stratified results and comparative data can answer some of these complaints. Here, a synthesis of other sources of data can be helpful. If survey data reveal problems in the same areas addressed by complaint letters or staff, it is easier to obtain buy-in that the problems are real.

Other Reasons for Failure

- "We only survey because we have to." Organizations that only survey because they are required to by an outside entity will never be successful in their efforts to become truly patient centered. Surveying is a waste of time and money until leadership takes the importance of patient- and family-centered care seriously.

- "Our bonuses are based on the results. We have to look good whether we are or not." When the incentives are aligned to reward people for appearing to be excellent instead of for collecting honest feedback and working to improve it, improvement efforts will never be successful. As with efforts to improve patient safety, rewarding people for continuing the status quo or hiding problems will never work.

- "The report sits on the shelf." Reports have to be user friendly and easily accessible. Fortunately, most survey results are now available on the Internet, allowing for easy dissemination across an organization and customization of results to meet the needs of different audiences. The chief of primary care probably does not care about the results of the orthopedic clinic, and doctors want to see results about the dimensions of care important to them, not the dimensions that evaluate other disciplines or things over which they have no control (e.g., the claims processing service in a health plan).

- "Patient experience-of-care data do not appear credible to clinicians and senior leaders." If data and stories collected from patients and their families focus on issues that have relevance to clinicians and meet rigorous scientific standards, clinicians and senior leaders are more likely to take them seriously. The more the information is perceived to have relevance to clinical outcomes, reducing pain and suffering, and improving a person's ability to manage his or her ongoing health problems, the more valued it will be across the organization. If feedback is only collected about "safe" issues (e.g., food and parking), it will be hard to get buy-in to use it for improvement. Involve all of the end-users of the data in the process of selecting survey instruments and vendors. Have them participate in other listening post activities. Videotape focus groups, and have clinical staff do walkthroughs or attend patient and family advisory council meetings.
- "Patient satisfaction is valued more than employee and clinical satisfaction." Again, patient satisfaction will never be high unless staff and clinicians feel nurtured and supported by the organization as well. Patient and staff satisfaction go hand in hand, and acknowledgment of that will help reinforce and motivate improvement efforts in both arenas.

Case Study

A walkthrough is an excellent method to use at the start of a quality improvement project because it is a simple and low-cost but powerful way to provide clinicians and other staff with insights about the experience of care. Walkthroughs always yield ideas for improvement, many of which can be implemented quickly. Walkthroughs also build support and enthusiasm for redesigning care, through the eyes of the patient, much more rapidly than do data or admonitions from managers to "be nice to patients."

As you do the walkthrough, ask questions of staff you encounter. The following questions have been designed to incorporate the staff's perspective about their own work improvement opportunities into the process:

- What made you mad today?
- What took too long?

- What caused complaints today?
- What was misunderstood today?
- What cost too much?
- What was wasted?
- What was too complicated?
- What was just plain silly?
- What job involved too many people?
- What job involved too many actions?

Keep careful notes, and you will have a long list of things you can fix the next day!

Several years ago, the medical director and head nurse of a public community hospital emergency room joined an Institute for Healthcare Improvement Service Excellence Collaborative to improve the care in their emergency room. At the start of the collaborative, they did a walkthrough where the doctor played a patient with asthma and the nurse was his family member. They had several surprises along the way, and their experience ultimately guided a redesign of the emergency room physical environment and processes of care. One realization came as they began the walkthrough— the "patient" and the "family member," both clinical leaders of the emergency room, realized that they had *never* entered the emergency room through the patient's entrance, even after years of working there.

When the patient called the hospital number (from his office) and told the operator he was having an acute asthma attack, he was put on hold without any explanation for several minutes. His call was actually transferred to the emergency department, but his anxiety increased because he did not understand what was happening.

When he was finally connected to the emergency room, his family member took the phone to get directions to the entrance from an address in the neighborhood. The person was incapable of helping them and finally got someone else to give her directions. After this delay, as they followed the directions, they discovered they were wrong.

As they drove up to the hospital, they realized that all of the signage to the emergency room entrance was covered with shrubs and plants. They had no idea where to park or what to do.

The emergency room entrance and waiting area were filthy and chaotic. All of the signage was menacing and told them what *not* to do, rather than where they could get help. They felt like they had arrived at the county jail.

As the patient was gasping for air, they were told to wait and to not ask for how long. At this point in the walkthrough, the doctor described his anxiety as so intense he was worried he was really going to need care!

When the family member used the restroom, it was so dirty she had to leave; she realized that this simple but important thing made her lose all confidence in the clinical care at the emergency room. If staff could not keep the bathroom clean, how could they do a good job with more complicated clinical problems?

Perhaps the most painful part of the walkthrough occurred when the nurse told the patient to take his clothes off and he realized there was no hook, no hanger, no place to put them except the floor. For years, he had judged his patients negatively because of the way they threw their clothes on the floor, only to discover it was, in essence, his fault.

The story could go on and on. Perhaps most important, many of the problems the medical director and head nurse experienced were relatively easy to fix quickly: providing standardized, written directions to the emergency department in different languages for staff to read, changing the signage in the waiting areas and outside the hospital, and paying attention to housekeeping and other comfort issues like placing clothes hooks in the exam areas. Other problems will take longer to redress, but one simple walkthrough helped refocus the hospital's improvement aims and its perspective on the importance of the patient's experience of care.

Conclusion

Apart from the obvious humane desire to be compassionate toward people who are sick, improving the patient experience of care results in better clinical outcomes, reduced medical errors, and increased market share. The leadership, focus, and human resource strategies required to build a patient-centered culture also results in improved employee satisfaction because we cannot begin to meet the needs of our patients until we provide excellent training and support for our clinical staff and all employees. Improving the patient's experience of care could well be the key to transforming the health-care system that we all search for.

Study Questions

1. What is the difference between patient *reports* about experiences with care and patient *ratings* of satisfaction?
2. What criteria should you use when selecting a patient survey?
3. List four methods other than surveys to acquire feedback from patients and families to help improve care.
4. What are four arguments for the importance of collecting feedback from patients and families about their experiences with care?

Notes

1. The CAHPS Survey and Reporting Kit 2002 contains everything necessary to conduct a CAHPS survey, including the CAHPS 3.0 questionnaires in English and Spanish. To learn more about CAHPS, access a bibliography of publications about the CAHPS products, or order a free copy of the kit, go to www.cahps-sun.org.
2. For example, the Peace Health Shared Care Plan, available at www.peoplepowered.org.

REFERENCES

Babbie, E. R. 1995. *Survey Research Methods, 2nd ed.* Belmont, CA: Wadsworth Publishing.

Bader, G. E., and C. A. Rossi. 2001. *Focus Groups: A Step-by-Step Guide, 3rd ed.* San Diego, CA: The Bader Group.

Cortina, J. M. 1993. "What Is Co-Efficient Alpha? An Examination of Theory and Applications." *Journal of Applied Psychology* 78: 98–104.

Cronbach, L. J. 1951. "Coefficient Alpha and the Internal Structure of Tests." *Psychometrika* 16: 297–334.

Dillman, D. A. 1978. *Mail and Telephone Surveys: The Total Design Method.* New York: John Wiley & Sons.

Edgman-Levitan, S., D. Shaller, K. McInnes, R. Joyce, K. Coltin, and P. D. Cleary. 2003. *The CAHPS Improvement Guide: Practical Strategies for Improving the Patient Care Experience.* Baltimore: CMS.

Flesch, R. F. 1948. "A New Readability Yardstick." *Journal of Applied Psychology* 32: 221–33.

Fowler, F. J., Jr. 1992. "How Unclear Terms Affect Survey Data." *Public Opinion Quarterly* 56 (2): 218–31.

———. 1995. *Improving Survey Questions: Design and Evaluation.* Thousand Oaks, CA: Sage Publications.

———. 2001. *Survey Research Methods.* Thousand Oaks, CA: Sage Publications.

Gerteis, M., S. Edgman-Levitan, J. Daley, and T. Delbanco. 1993. *Through the Patient's Eyes.* San Francisco: Jossey-Bass.

Goodman, J. 1987. "Setting Priorities for Satisfaction Improvement." *Quality Review* Winter.

Hargraves, J. L., I. B. Wilson, A. Zaslavsky, C. James, J. D. Walker, G. Rogers, and P. D. Cleary. 2001. "Adjusting for Patient Characteristics when Analyzing Reports from Patients About Hospital Care." *Medical Care* 39 (6): 635–41.

Hays, R. D., J. A. Shaul, V. S. Williams, J. S. Lubalin, L. D. Harris-Kojetin, S. F. Sweeny, and P. D. Cleary. 1999. "Psychometric Properties of the CAHPS 1.0 Survey Measures. Consumer Assessment of Health Plans Study." *Medical Care* 37 (3 Suppl.): MS22–31.

Heskett, J. L., T. O. Jones, G. Loveman, E. Sasser, Jr., and J. A. Schlesinger. 1994. "Putting the Service-Profit Chain to Work." *Harvard Business Review* 167 (Mar./Apr.).

Institute of Medicine. 2001. *Crossing the Quality Chasm: A New Health System for the 21st Century.* Washington, DC: National Academy Press.

Kaiser Family Foundation and Agency for Healthcare Research and Quality. 2000. *Americans as Health Care Consumers: An Update on the Role of Quality Information, 2000.* Washington, DC: Agency for Healthcare Research and Quality.

Krueger, R. A., and M. A. Casey. 2000. *Focus Groups: A Practical Guide for Applied Research.* Thousand Oaks, CA: Sage Publications.

Leebov, W., S. Afriat, and J. Presha. 1998. *Service Savvy Healthcare: One Goal at a Time.* San Francisco: Jossey-Bass/AHA Press.

Leebov, W., G. Scott, and L. Olson. 1998. *Achieving Impressive Customer Service: 7 Strategies for Healthcare Managers.* San Francisco: Jossey-Bass.

Nisbett, R., and E. Borgida. 1975. "Attribution and the Psychology of Prediction." *Journal of Personality and Social Psychology* 32: 932–43.

vom Eigen, K. A., J. D. Walker, S. Edgman-Levitan, P. D. Cleary, and T. L. Delbanco. 1999. "Carepartner Experiences with Hospital Care." *Medical Care* 37 (1): 33–38.

Webster, P. D., and B. Johnson. 2000. *Developing and Sustaining a Patient and Family Advisory Council.* Bethesda, MD: Institute for Family-Centered Care.

Suggested Reading

Charles, C., M. Gauld, L. Chambers, B. O'Brien, R. B. Haynes, and R. Labelle. 1994. "How Was Your Hospital Stay? Patients' Reports About Their Care in Canadian Hospitals." *Canadian Medical Association Journal* 150 (11): 1813–22.

Cleary, P. D. 2003. "A Hospitalization from Hell: A Patient's Perspective on Quality." *Annals of Internal Medicine* 138 (1): 33–39.

Cleary, P. D., and S. Edgman-Levitan. 1997. "Health Care Quality. Incorporating Consumer Perspectives." *Journal of the American Medical Association* 278 (19): 1608–12.

Cleary, P. D., S. Edgman-Levitan, J. D. Walker, M. Gerteis, and T. L. Delbanco. 1993. "Using Patient Reports to Improve Medical Care: A Preliminary Report from 10 Hospitals." *Quality Management in Health Care* 2 (1): 31–38.

Coulter, A., and P. D. Cleary. 2001. "Patients' Experiences with Hospital Care in Five Countries." *Health Affairs (Millwood)* 20 (3): 244–52.

Delbanco, T. L., D. M. Stokes, P. D. Cleary, S. Edgman-Levitan, J. D. Walker, M. Gerteis, and J. Daley. 1995. "Medical Patients' Assessments of Their Care During Hospitalization: Insights for Internists." *Journal of General Internal Medicine* 10 (12): 679–85.

Edgman-Levitan, S. 1996. "What Information Do Consumers Want and Need?" *Health Affairs (Millwood)* 15 (4): 42–56.

Frampton, S., L. Gilpin, and P. Charmel. 2003. *Putting Patients First.* San Francisco: Jossey-Bass.

Fremont, A. M., P. D. Cleary, J. L. Hargraves, R. M. Rowe, N. B. Jacobson, and J. Z. Ayanian. 2001. "Patient-Centered Processes of Care and Long-term Outcomes of Myocardial Infarction." *Journal of General Internal Medicine* 16 (12): 800–808.

Fremont, A. M., P. D. Cleary, J. L. Hargraves, R. M. Rowe, N. B. Jacobson, J. Z. Ayanian, J. H. Gilmore, and B. J. Pine II. 1997. "The Four Faces of Mass Customization." *Harvard Business Review* 75 (1): 91–101.

Goodman, J. 1999. "Basic Facts on Customer Complaint Behavior and the Impact of Service on the Bottom Line." *Competitive Advantage: ASQ Newsletter* 8: 1.

Homer, C. J., B. Marino, P. D. Cleary, H. R. Alpert, B. Smith, C. M. Crowley Ganser, R. M. Brustowicz, and D. A. Goldmann. 1999. "Quality of Care at a Children's Hospital: The Parent's Perspective." *Archives of Pediatric and Adolescent Medicine* 153 (11): 1123–29.

Larson, C. O., E. C. Nelson, D. Gustafson, and P. B. Batalden. 1996. "The Relationship Between Meeting Patients' Information Needs and Their Satisfaction with Hospital Care and General Health Status Outcomes." *International Journal of Quality in Health Care* 8 (5): 447–56.

Leebov, W., and G. Scott. 1994. *Service and Quality Improvement: The Customer Satisfaction Strategy for Health Care.* Chicago: American Hospital Publishing.

Roth, M. S., and W. P. Amoroso. 1993. "Linking Core Competencies to Customer Needs: Strategic Marketing of Health Care Services." *Journal of Health Care Marketing* 13 (2): 49–54.

Seelos, L., and C. Adamson. 1994. "Redefining NHS Complaint Handling— The Real Challenge." *International Journal of Health Care Quality Assurance* 7 (6): 26–31.

Seybold, P. B. 2001. "Get Inside the Lives of Your Customers." *Harvard Business Review* 79 (5): 80–89, 164.

Veroff, D. R., P. M. Gallagher, V. Wilson, M. Uyeda, J. Merselis, E. Guadagnoli, S. Edgman-Levitan, A. Zaslavsky, S. Kleimann, and P. D. Cleary. 1998. "Effective Reports for Health Care Quality Data: Lessons from a CAHPS Demonstration in Washington State." *International Journal of Quality in Health Care* 10 (6): 555–60.

Wasson, J. H., M. M. Godfrey, E. C. Nelson, J. J. Mohr, and P. B. Batalden. 2003. "Microsystems in Health Care: Part 4. Planning Patient-Centered Care." *Joint Commission Journal of Quality and Safety* 29 (5): 227–37.

DASHBOARDS AND SCORECARDS: TOOLS FOR CREATING ALIGNMENT

Michael D. Pugh

This chapter discusses the application of scorecards and dashboards in healthcare organizations. The focus is to examine the use of measurement by senior leadership to align organizational effort and achieve higher levels of organizational performance. Measurement is a critical leadership function. As a means of organizing and using measurement to drive change, dashboards and scorecards are useful tools; when used properly, they can lead to accelerated rates of improvement and better alignment of effort across and down an organization.

Background and Terminology

Many healthcare organizations utilize some form of cross-functional or multidimensional measurement tools. The specific term *balanced scorecard* was first used by Robert S. Kaplan and David P. Norton in their 1992 *Harvard Business Review* article, "The Balanced Scorecard—Measures that Drive Performance." Based on a multicompany study, the article examines approaches to organizational performance management beyond the use of standard financial and accounting measures. Kaplan and Norton's theory was that reliance on traditional financial measures alone to drive performance limits the ability of a company to increase shareholder value. This investigational premise is consistent with the idea, advanced by quality guru W. Edwards Deming, that companies cannot be run by the visible numbers alone. To overcome this limitation, successful companies utilize a broader index of performance metrics to create a balance between financial and other important dimensions of organizational performance.

Kaplan and Norton's 1996 follow-up book, *The Balanced Scorecard— Translating Strategy into Action*, further examines the development of performance measures linked to organizational strategy. Rather than function simply as a balanced set of outcome measures for the organization, Kaplan and Norton observe that the balanced scorecard should be central to the leadership system deployed to get results. The above-referenced work is the original text on the development and use of balanced sets of measures at the organizational level to drive performance and the deployment of strategy.

Kaplan and Norton (1996) observe that most organizations collect nonfinancial performance measures that reflect important dimensions such as customers, service, and product quality. However, these measures are generally reviewed independently from financial results and with decreased leadership emphasis. Kaplan and Norton also observe that increased organizational alignment can be created by leaders simultaneously reviewing and monitoring the critical measures across multiple dimensions of performance, not just financial dimensions. And, rather than simply monitoring a broader set of outcome or process measures, Kaplan and Norton see a balanced scorecard as the key leadership tool central to deploying organizational strategy. Students are encouraged to read both the 1992 *Harvard Business Review* article and the 1996 book on the subject as background material for this chapter.

Dashboards

While in practice the terms dashboard and scorecard[1] are often used interchangeably, the words connote two different concepts. The term *dashboard* brings to mind the indicator panel on an automobile, which is most useful when the car is moving as a way for the driver to monitor key performance metrics such as speed, fuel level, engine temperature, and perhaps direction from digital display units. The driver could of course monitor many other metrics, such as tire pressure, manifold temperature, oil viscosity, or transmission efficiency; these might be useful information to a NASCAR driver in a high-performance race car but are not critical to the average driver's immediate mission to go from point A to point B. Instead, drivers rely on a core set of important high-level measures to inform the real-time process of driving the car.

The cockpit of an airplane is simply a more complex example of a collection of instruments that report important information critical to successful air travel. What is important to consider is that the driver of a car or the pilot of an airplane monitors multiple indicators of performance simultaneously to successfully arrive at the intended destination. At any given point in the journey, one indicator may receive greater focus for some period of time, yet overall success depends on the collective performance of all systems represented by the monitored indicators. Dashboards bring to mind a tool that reports the ongoing performance of the critical processes that lead to organizational success, rather than reporting on the success itself. Dashboards of critical process indicators are useful tools in healthcare organizations and have multiple applications discussed later in this chapter.

Scorecards

The term *scorecard* brings to mind a different image. Scorecards are used to record and report prior-period or past performance rather than real-time performance. Generally, these are outcome measures rather than process measures. School report cards, for example, report how an individual student fared against a specific grading standard, reported at some point after all work is completed and the "books are closed." Although there is a lag time in reporting, changes might be made to influence future outcomes by making changes in study habits and class attendance, devoting additional study time to specific subject matter, receiving outside tutoring, or making changes in homework preparation. However, these possible changes are the result of investigation of the current process rather than information available on the report card.

Golf scorecards are another example. They reflect the outcome of the previous holes played, compare the score for each hole to a target score (par), and are used to compare performance against other players or an overall stroke target for the game. In a competitive match, a player might use this report of past performance to influence the level of aggressive play required on future holes. Or he or she might monitor the cumulative score during play to judge the likelihood of achieving a desired overall score for the round. However, the scores from past holes generally do not tell a player much about what changes need to be made to improve success on future holes. Instead, the focus is on results. For many of us, golf might be more fun if we did not keep score. But if we never keep score, we will never know how our play compares to the target (par) or other players' performance, or how our play varies from round to round.

While the above distinctions between scorecards as outcome or results measures and dashboards as process measures may be logical, in practical application within healthcare, a bright line between the two rarely exists. Healthcare organizations are complex, and often a metric may be both a process measure and an outcome measure at the same time. As a result, many organizational scorecards contain a mix of outcome-, strategic-, and process-related measures. The key issue is how the measures and measurement sets are used by leadership to align priorities and achieve desired organizational results.

Scope and Use of Dashboards and Scorecards in Healthcare

Common Uses of Dashboards and Scorecards

Most healthcare organizations are awash in measures. One large organization in Florida routinely collects and reports more than 1,000 measures. While most healthcare organizations utilize some form of a dashboard/

scorecard at the senior leadership level, there is often a wide gap between the existence of a measurement set that an organization calls an organizational scorecard/dashboard and the actual use of the tool to create organizational alignment.

Commonly Used Measurement Sets

There is no lack of data collection in healthcare organizations. Hospitals routinely collect and review patient satisfaction and financial indicators and generally monitor a large, diverse set of quality indicators. As a condition of accreditation, the Joint Commission on Accreditation of Healthcare Organizations (Joint Commission) requires a specific set of quality indicators to be collected and monitored by the organization and provided to survey teams. The Joint Commission–required set of indicators track closely with quality indicators for specific clinical conditions (e.g., pneumonia and heart failure) promulgated by the Centers for Medicare & Medicaid Services (CMS) and collected on hospitals by CMS-contracted professional review organizations (PROs) in the late 1990s. In 2003, the American Hospital Association organized an effort to publicly report a set of common quality indicators in response to growing concern that CMS will at some point require public disclosure of a broad set of quality indicators. Currently, CMS requires long-term care facilities to collect a core set of quality and clinical indicators that are made publicly available through the CMS web site. While these activities are intended to spur healthcare organizations to pay attention to important quality indicators, in many organizations these types of clinical data reports are viewed as a functional form of compliance rather than true performance indicators that leadership actively seeks to improve.

Other healthcare organizations also collect a variety of performance measures that are used to both judge organizational performance and manage operations. Managed care organizations generally participate in a national data set known as the Health Employer Data and Information Set (HEDIS), which compares a variety of outpatient clinical performance indicators at the physician practice level, such as immunization rates and breast cancer screening rates in the covered population. Organized medical groups may also collect some form of patient satisfaction as well as the HEDIS clinical data set. Other nonclinical indicators that may be used by both health plans and physicians include waiting time to next appointment and medical cost per member, per month.

Quality Scorecards and Dashboards

Most commonly, healthcare organizations utilize some form of an organizational quality scorecard/dashboard both at the senior leadership level and to support the governance function. These scorecards tend to be reports of past achievement or quality control measures rather than drivers of future efforts, and they are not routinely used in the strategic manner contemplated by Kaplan and Norton. They are often populated with available or traditional measures, both outcome and process based. For example, it is not unusual to see a quality control measure such as the nosocomial infection rate on a governance dashboard, even absent an active improvement effort or link to organizational strategy. A classic quality control measure, healthcare organizations have monitored infection rates for years, generally only reacting when an outbreak occurs. Perhaps because of the absence of more important clinical outcome measures, some organizations include the infection rate on the organizational scorecard by default. "We need a clinical measure—what do we have? Stick the infection rate on there. . ."

Organizing by Categories of Measures

Measures collected by healthcare organizations traditionally fall into the categories of financial, volume, satisfaction, and clinical quality. These categories are often viewed by leadership as independent sets, useful in the day-to-day management of specific aspects of the organization. In some organizations, summary dashboards of key indicators have been developed and organized by category to facilitate review. For instance, leaders may routinely receive and review a financial report. At a different time, leadership may receive a customer/patient satisfaction or workforce report and then through some committee review process receive a report on clinical quality indicators. Quality scorecards or dashboards have become popular ways of reporting on clinical quality through medical staff committees and to the board. All of these reports may be organized into scorecard or dashboard formats that highlight the key indicators. While these may be useful approaches for review, format alone does not impart usefulness. Scorecards and dashboards should drive leadership behavior.

Financial and volume measures have traditionally driven management behavior in healthcare. One vestige of the drive to bring a business focus to healthcare in the late 1970s and the 1980s is that healthcare governing boards today tend to spend considerably more time discussing financial reports and indicators than quality or satisfaction reports. This is beginning to change at both the board and senior leadership levels, and boards are devoting more time to reviewing quality, workplace culture, and patient satisfaction data. While satisfaction measures have achieved new levels of importance and attention by leadership in many healthcare organizations, clinical quality metrics remain a challenge. Despite the increasing transparency of quality and safety problems in healthcare, clinical quality metrics for the most part remain underrepresented on organizational performance scorecards and isolated from day-to-day operations.

Dashboards and scorecards may be organized in a variety of formats ranging from simple tables to web-based graphical reports embedded in computerized decision support systems. Formats for reporting data include tables, radar charts, bar graphs, run or control charts, and color-coded indicator reports designed to highlight metrics that are out of line with targets or expectations.[2] In some organizations, each operating unit has a scorecard of key indicators that mirrors the organizational or corporate scorecard.

Simply taking available measures and deciding to format them into a summary dashboard (either department/category specific or cross-dimensional) is a start. However, the real power of using measurement comes from senior leaders organizing their leadership systems to get results. Figure 10.1 is one way of depicting the leadership system in a healthcare organization. The leadership system drives both organizational culture and alignment in daily work to achieve a desired level of organizational performance. One of the key elements of the leadership system is the measurement process, which includes the tools of dashboards and scorecards.

The challenge for healthcare leaders is to make sense of the multitude of measures and metrics that exist and are routinely available in most organizations. Scorecards and dashboards are useful tools for organizing important metrics. However, healthcare leaders struggle with the question, "What should we measure?" The answer is tied to the answer to another question, "For what purpose?" Form should follow function.

Applications of Scorecards and Dashboards
Governance and Leadership Measures

In healthcare organizations, three basic sets of measures should be considered for use in a scorecard or dashboard format. Figure 10.2 summarizes the three basic types of performance metrics and the interrelationship between the different types. At the governance level, a set of organizational performance measures should be defined and monitored. These measures should be linked to how the organization defines performance within the context of its mission, vision, and values. A governance-level scorecard of organizational performance measures should be a basic tool for all healthcare governing boards.

At the senior leadership level, a different set of measures should be used to align priorities and lead the organization and embody the concept of a balanced scorecard. The measures should be linked to the critical strategies, or *vital few* initiatives, of the organization and be used to drive desired results. As Kaplan and Norton (1996) suggest, strategic measures should be at the center of the organization's leadership system. While leadership's

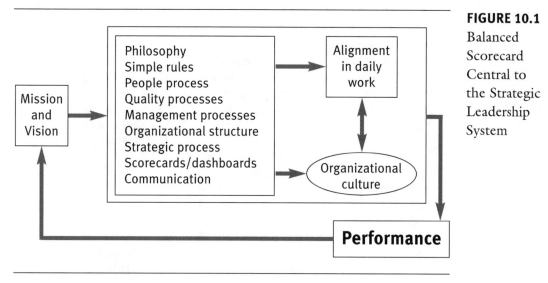

FIGURE 10.1
Balanced
Scorecard
Central to
the Strategic
Leadership
System

Source: Pugh Ettinger McCarthy Associates, LLC. Used with permission.

role is to deploy strategy, monitoring deployment is also a governance responsibility. A dashboard of strategic measures is a useful tool for leaders to set priorities and drive change. The same dashboard may serve as a scorecard for the board to monitor the deployment of strategy and be used to assess leadership effectiveness. An important relationship exists between the overall organizational performance measures and the strategic measures. Strategy should be about what drives desired organizational results. The test of good strategy and strategic measures is whether successful deployment of the strategies results in improved organizational performance as measured by the organizational scorecard.

Process and Management Measures

The third set of measures are process/operational measures. These measures are common in healthcare, and dashboards of critical operating measures are common tools in many healthcare organizations. Typical metrics found on these dashboards include quality control metrics, efficiency metrics, traditional quality/performance improvement measures, labor statistics, customer satisfaction indexes, and other routine operating statistics used in the day-to-day operation of the organization. The operational/ process measures monitored should be linked to the strategic measures. Organizational alignment is enhanced when, at the day-to-day work level, key processes that have a direct link to a specific organizational strategy are monitored and when the successful deployment of strategy improves one or more organizational performance metrics.

FIGURE 10.2

Different Sets of Measures for Different Purposes

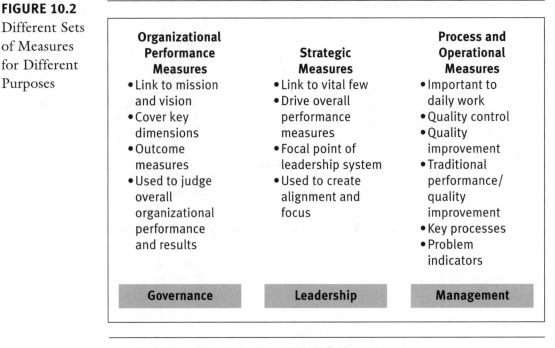

Organizational Performance Measures	Strategic Measures	Process and Operational Measures
• Link to mission and vision • Cover key dimensions • Outcome measures • Used to judge overall organizational performance and results	• Link to vital few • Drive overall performance measures • Focal point of leadership system • Used to create alignment and focus	• Important to daily work • Quality control • Quality improvement • Traditional performance/ quality improvement • Key processes • Problem indicators
Governance	**Leadership**	**Management**

Source: Pugh Ettinger McCarthy Associates, LLC. Used with permission.

Dimensions of Performance in Healthcare

So, what is good performance in healthcare? How do we know whether we are doing a good job? How should we organize our important measures to have the greatest effect? What should be on our organizational scorecard?

These are critical questions for healthcare leaders. Figure 10.2 makes clear that organizational performance is an outcome of the leadership process and should ultimately be measured by the effectiveness of the organization in meeting its mission and vision. Another way to think about performance is by important dimensions. Healthcare is clearly about more than a financial bottom line. The word *performance* is deliberately chosen here rather than the term *quality* because it is easier to argue that performance is a broader term that encompasses quality, although some advocates of quality improvement theory may legitimately argue otherwise. The point is that performance and/or quality in healthcare should be considered broadly; therefore, it is important to identify the multiple dimensions that might define performance.

Using a framework of the traditional financial, satisfaction, human resources, and clinical dimensions is one method. However, many organ-

FIGURE 10.3

Critical
Dimensions of
Healthcare
Organizational
Performance

- Patient and customer
  (satisfaction)
- Effectiveness (clinical outcomes)
- Appropriateness (evidence and
  process)
- Safety (patient and staff)
- Equity

- Employee and staff satisfaction
  (culture)
- Efficiency (cost)
- Financial
- Flow (wait times, cycle times,
  and throughput)
- Community/population health

Source: Pugh Ettinger McCarthy Associates, LLC. Used with permission.

izations have found it beneficial to think more broadly about what constitutes the important dimensions of performance in healthcare. Figure 10.3
lists some of the critical dimensions that can be used to define healthcare
organizational performance.

In *Crossing the Quality Chasm*, the Institute of Medicine (IOM 2001)
suggests a different framework for thinking about performance in healthcare. IOM recommends that patient care be reorganized and redesigned
to achieve six specific aims:

1. Safety
2. Effectiveness
3. Patient centeredness
4. Timeliness
5. Efficiency
6. Equity

Some organizations have found these six aims to be a useful framework for defining organizational performance and the type of metrics that
should be on the organizational scorecard.

A third approach to organizing performance results is to use the
Baldrige National Quality Program (BNQP) criteria. The criteria for Category
7, Organizational Performance, define specific classes of performance results
that applicants are expected to track and report on. Figure 10.4 shows the
relationships between the various results required by BNQP.

Aside from the three examples discussed here, other frameworks can
be used to develop and define the important dimensions of organizational
performance. Almost all frameworks are built on the traditional financial,
human resources, satisfaction, and clinical foundations. Religiously affiliated healthcare organizations often include dimensions of performance
related to the mission of the sponsoring organization in addition to the
other possible dimensions described.

FIGURE 10.4

2003 Baldrige
National
Quality
Program
Category 7
Results

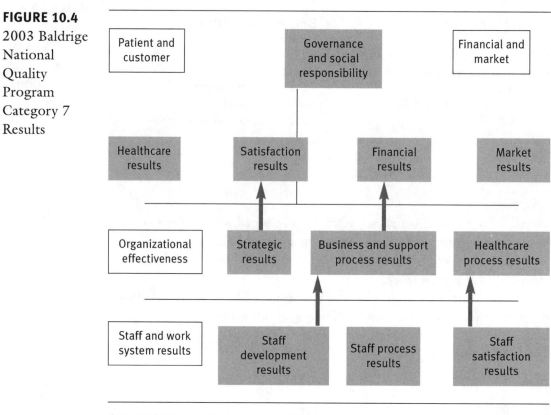

Source: Pugh Ettinger McCarthy Associates, LLC. Used with permission.

Clinical and Operational Issues

Creating an Organizational Scorecard

The approach to developing an organizational scorecard should go beyond simply organizing existing measures into a new format or framework. Deciding on an appropriate framework for the organizational scorecard is a first step. Once the framework is chosen, the next step is to define the important dimensions of performance relevant to the mission of the organization. Senior leadership and the governing body should engage in a constructive dialog to identify and define the important dimensions of performance and the required results for the organization. Once the dimensions are agreed to, leaders and governing boards should attempt to answer the question, "How will we know?" for each of the chosen dimensions and select appropriate outcome measures.

At the organizational level, the ideal cycle time for performance is quarterly. However, some important metrics may be difficult or too expensive to obtain on a quarterly basis, and the organization may be forced to default to one or more annual measures. Sometimes, the appropriate outcome measure for a dimension will not exist; either a proxy measure must be used or an investment must be made to develop new metrics.

"How many measures should be on an organizational scorecard?" is a question often asked by healthcare leaders and trustees. The answer is, "Enough to define the required results in each of the important dimensions." Initially, most organizations nominate far more measures than is practical and tend to include multiple process measures rather than outcome measures. Usually, this is the result of enthusiasm for the process and desire to include more detail. While additional measures may be interesting, the question should remain focused on results. Discipline in the measure selection process can be achieved if focus is maintained on answering the question, "What result do we want?" rather than, "What are good measures for . . .?" In the for-profit corporate world, the answer to the question of results is fairly straightforward—increased shareholder value (defined as more than temporary stock price). In the not-for-profit healthcare provider world, the results may be more multifaceted, but they are just as measurable.

The organizational scorecard should be used by the governing body and senior leadership to monitor overall organizational performance in a balanced manner. It should also be used to assess CEO and leadership performance. While it is likely that boards and senior leadership will continue to look at supporting reports such as financial and clinical quality reports and other sources of additional performance detail, the organization should be guided by the required results defined by the set of organizational performance measures.

Organizational performance measures should be benchmarked when possible against other similar types of organizations and specific targets noted on the scorecard. This statement is made with the caveat that benchmarking does not mean comparing to the average. Instead, benchmarking should identify great or best levels of performance reported, and strategies are deployed designed to close the gap between current performance and the benchmark. Benchmarking in healthcare is a challenge, but it is becoming easier in some areas. Information on patient and employee satisfaction benchmark performance is available through the proprietary databases maintained by survey companies. Comparative financial and workforce information is also available through multiple sources, some free and some available by subscription. Comparative clinical outcome metrics are becoming more widely available. However, it should be noted that for some clinical and safety issues, the target should be 100 percent. What level of medication error is acceptable to patients? How do you choose which qualified cardiac patient should not get evidence-based clinical care? Increasing reliability in healthcare around key results is supported by setting best-in-class targets and high expectations on performance scorecards.

Using the six IOM aims, one could begin to create an organizational scorecard by crafting potential measures for each, examples of which may include the following:

1. Adverse drug events per 1,000 doses (safety)
2. Functional outcomes as defined by hospital mortality rates, compliance to best practices guidelines, disease-specific measures, readmission rates (effectiveness)
3. Patient satisfaction (patient centeredness)
4. Number of days until the third next available appointment (timeliness)
5. Hospital costs per discharge (efficiency)
6. Effectiveness indicators by race/ethnicity and gender (equity)

One of the ironies in healthcare is that although we measure many things, little agreement exists as to the important outcome measures for an organization. The key is to understand the critical dimensions of performance and utilize the emerging national areas (e.g., the IOM aims) to guide development.

Creating Alignment

Creating alignment in organizations is a critical leadership function. Leadership has been a hot topic for many years, especially discussion of how to create and communicate a compelling vision. Innumerable works have been written about managing people, executing change, and managing organizations. However, not as much ink has been devoted to the leadership function of creating alignment between the compelling vision and the day-to-day work of organizations. Figure 10.5 identifies the important leadership actions that create alignment. Scorecards and dashboards can be useful tools supporting the measurement, executive review, and strategy processes used to link overall direction to the day-to-day work of the organization. Different measurement sets organized into scorecards or dashboards support the three different core leadership functions (see Figure 10.6).

One approach to creating alignment is to use the identified organizational performance dimensions as a framework for measurement throughout the organization. Metrics may be different in every department or division, but they are linked by consistent focus at every level of the organization. For example, many healthcare organizations have identified patient satisfaction as a key dimension of organizational performance. In a competitive market, the organization may also determine that one of its critical strategies is to improve patient satisfaction to build market share. The

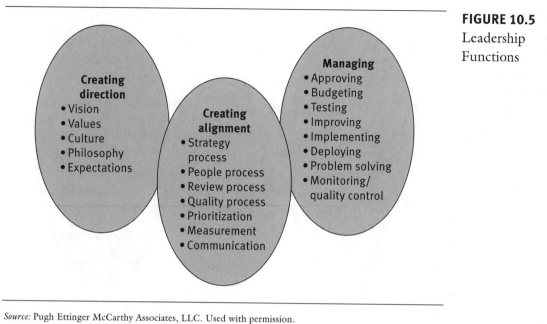

Source: Pugh Ettinger McCarthy Associates, LLC. Used with permission.

FIGURE 10.5

Leadership Functions

strategic dashboard would feature a set of metrics that validate that improvement in satisfaction is taking place. To link this strategy to daily work, every operating unit would monitor some metric that relates to patient satisfaction with the services the department provides as well as monitoring and improving key processes that are known to positively affect satisfaction. An emergency room might monitor patient satisfaction information for its service, and the appropriate metric would be on the departmental operating dashboard. The emergency room might also have an improvement project to improve flow that results in reduced waiting time, a key process that affects the satisfaction of emergency patients. In this example, clear links exist among the organizational performance dimension of satisfaction, strategic measures, and day-to-day improvement efforts and operation of the emergency department.

Figure 10.7 depicts a second method of creating alignment in an organization around a critical strategy or project. This fictitious organization has determined that reducing mortality among heart attack patients is an important effort for the population served. At the governance level, overall cardiac mortality might be monitored as an organizational performance measure. In this example, the hospital has determined that the two key leverage points, or critical strategies, for reducing cardiac mortality in its organization are to (1) ensure that all cardiac care is delivered per

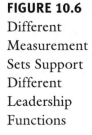

FIGURE 10.6
Different
Measurement
Sets Support
Different
Leadership
Functions

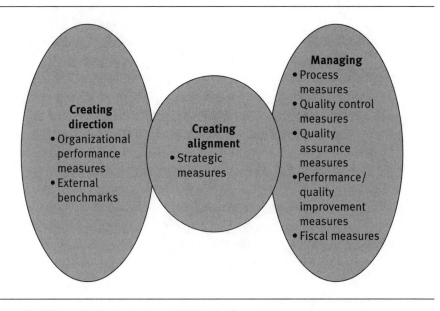

Source: Pugh Ettinger McCarthy Associates, LLC. Used with permission.

evidence-based care plans and (2) reduce the time from presentation in the emergency department to initiation of interventional therapy.

Successful deployment of the two critical strategies is defined by the percentage of patients who received 100 percent of the required care elements and the percentage of patients with door-to-catheterization lab times of less than 90 minutes. These metrics are included on a strategic dashboard and regularly reviewed by senior management and the board. By the function of review and including these metrics on a strategic dashboard, senior leaders signal the importance of the project, have a method of monitoring the deployment progress, and have a method to link desired results (lower mortality) to specific actions (strategies and tactics).

The targets associated with the two strategies are important because they signal to management the significance of the change and the results that are required. Informed by the required results, departmental management and clinical leadership can then organize efforts to understand the key processes and the levels of reliability at which these processes must operate to achieve the desired results. Once identified, key process measures are added to the appropriate management dashboards and used on a real-time basis for further improvement or process control. For purposes of this example, the processes on the far right of Figure 10.7 are identified as the critical supporting processes. The theory is that improvement and

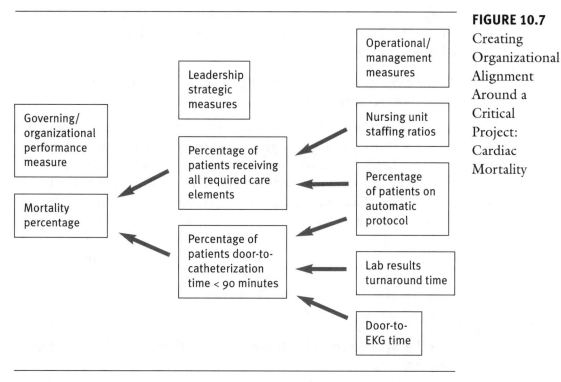

FIGURE 10.7

Creating Organizational Alignment Around a Critical Project: Cardiac Mortality

Source: Pugh Ettinger McCarthy Associates, LLC. Used with permission.

control of these process will lead to the required results in the strategic measures, ultimately affecting overall cardiac mortality.

Keys to Successful Implementation and Lessons Learned

Successful development of performance scorecards and dashboards is dependent on many factors. This section describes some of the critical issues and problems often faced by organizations in the development and use of performance measures.

Develop a Clear Understanding of the Intended Use

Healthcare management tends to be faddish. In some organizations, creation of the first scorecard is assigned to a member of the management team after a senior leader or board member has read or heard at a conference that healthcare organizations should have a performance scorecard. These efforts are doomed to failure. It is critical that the CEO, senior leadership team, and board have a clear understanding of why a scorecard is being created and how the board and senior leaders intend to use it. Many scorecards developed by organizations are sitting on shelves gathering dust, right next to the strategic plans.

Engage the Governing Board Early in Development of Performance Measures

A mistake that occasionally has been repeated is to have senior leadership present a performance scorecard to the board as an item of new business without adequate predevelopment discussion or involvement by the board. Ultimately, the governing body is responsible for the performance of the organization. This responsibility goes beyond simple fiduciary responsibility and includes clinical and service performance. Performance scorecards should reflect desired organizational results. Governing bodies must be involved in defining the important dimensions and choosing the relevant measures. Much of the work of development may be assigned to the leadership and clinical team, but final determination of the important dimensions and measures is a board responsibility.

Use the Scorecard to Evaluate Organizational and Leadership Performance

Once developed, the organizational performance scorecard should be central to the governance system of the organization. The scorecard should reflect the mission of the organization and be used by the board and leadership to evaluate progress toward achieving the mission and vision. Review of the scorecards by the governing board should occur at least quarterly. Since scorecards are about results, they can be useful in the CEO performance evaluation process and provide a balanced set of objective measures that can be tied to compensation plans and performance review criteria.

Be Prepared to Change the Measures

Developing a good organizational performance scorecard is a simple idea, but it is difficult to do. Any organization is unlikely to achieve a "perfect" set of measures the first time. Often, measures that reflect the real results desired for a performance dimension do not exist and have to be developed. Other times, it becomes clear after a couple of cycles of review that better measures than those being used might be desirable. Development of the scorecard is usually an iterative process rather than a single-shot approach. Organizations should continue to improve their scorecards as new understanding of the importance and desired results linked to each dimension surface and as better metrics are developed. To quote the philosopher Voltaire, "Perfect is the enemy of good"; organizations should work toward creating a good scorecard, not a perfect one.

Make the Data Useful, Not Pretty

Formats should first be useful and understandable. Many organizations struggle with fancy formats and attempts to create online versions. A good starting point is to construct simple run charts that display the measures over time and the desired target for each measure. Simple spreadsheet graphs can be dropped into a text document, four or six per page. The information conveyed, not the format, is important. Organizations have had mixed success with more sophisticated formats such as radar charts. Some boards find radar charts invaluable because all the metrics and targets can be displayed on a single page. Other boards have difficulty interpreting this type of graph. The admonition to start simple does not imply that other approaches will not work. One innovative computer-based display (see the Case Study section below) utilizes a radar chart backed by hot-linked run and control charts for each performance metric.

Integrate the Measures to Achieve a Balanced View

While some organizations may find it helpful to use scorecard and dashboard formats for financial and quality reports, the routine display of metrics in separate category-driven reports may be a reflection of a lack of integration. If an organization has developed a broader set of high-level measures and the category-based reports are supportive of the key measures, this characterization is likely invalid. However, if an organization chooses to use separate detailed scorecards of financial, quality, and service metrics that are independently reviewed, the tradition of placing more weight and emphasis on financial results will likely prevail, with clinical, satisfaction, and other dimension results receiving less intense and substantive attention, except when there is a crisis in any given area.

Develop Clear and Measurable Strategies

Kaplan and Norton (1996) contend that strategic measures should be central to the leadership system and focus of senior leadership. Strategic dashboards and balanced scorecards are key tools that leaders can use to create alignment of effort. Unfortunately, in healthcare, strategy and strategic planning are generally underdeveloped. Many organizations engage in an annual process that is superficial and results in a set of vague objectives that generally are task oriented rather than strategic. Often, the strategic plan sits on a shelf until it is time to dust it off in preparation for the next board retreat. It is difficult to develop a balanced scorecard as envisioned by Kaplan and Norton if strategies are not clear, measurable, and truly strategic. In most organizations, a simple set of critical, or vital few, strategies exist; if successfully deployed, these strategies will accelerate progress toward achieving organizational mission and vision. These critical strategies or strategic themes should be identified, and a set of specific measures should be developed for each strategy. Some organizations find it useful to track deployment progress on a specifically designed strategic dashboard. Choice of the measures is important because the measures help to define what the strategy is intended to accomplish. For most critical strategies, innumerable ideas and potential tactics exist. All tactics, initiatives, or projects proposed should directly affect one or more of the strategic measures. If not, leadership should look elsewhere to invest scare resources.

Use the Organizational Performance Dimensions to Create Alignment of Effort

One strategy for using scorecards and dashboards to create alignment is to build cascading sets of metrics consistent with the key dimensions of performance on the organizational scorecard. Each operating unit or department is required to develop a set of metrics for each of the key dimensions. For example, if patient safety is a key dimension, each nursing unit might track and seek to improve the fall rate or adverse drug event rate on its unit. Or, if employee well-being is a key performance dimension, voluntary turnover rates might be tracked at each departmental level. One important caveat is that measures should not be collected on departments, but rather a set of measures or dashboard consistent with the key performance dimensions should be developed and "owned" by each department or operating unit. Executive review of departmental performance should be across the entire set of measures, rather than conducting a financial review one month and a service or clinical quality review at another time.

Avoid Using Indicators Based on Averages

Averages mask variation, are misleading, and should be avoided when possible in developing scorecards and dashboards. For example, the average time from door to drug in the emergency room may be below a preset operating standard. However, on examination of the data one might find that a significant percentage of patients do not receive treatment within the prescribed standard. A better approach is to measure the percentage of patients who receive treatment within a specified standard. Average waiting times, average length of stay, average satisfaction scores, and average cost are all suspect indicators.

When Possible, Develop Composite Clinical Indicators for Processes and Outcome Indicators for Results

The whole issue of clinical indicators is difficult. Healthcare organizations are complex and generally provide care across a wide continuum of patient conditions and treatment regimens. It is often difficult to determine which clinical indicators are truly important and representative of the process of care provided. One approach is to develop composite indicators for high-volume, high-profile conditions. For example, the CMS/PRO review set contains six cardiac indicators. Most hospital organizations track their performance against each of the indicators, which is appropriate at the operational level. However, at the senior leadership level it may be more useful to track the percentage of cardiac patients who received all six required elements. This tracking accomplishes two things. First, it limits the number of metrics on a senior leadership or governing board scorecard. Second, it signals that it is important that all patients receive all required aspects of care, not just four or five out of six. The same approach can be used for tracking performance in chronic diseases such as diabetes. Organizations can establish the critical aspects of care that should always happen (e.g., timely hemoglobin testing, referral to the diabetic educator, eye and foot exams) and develop a composite measure that reflects the percentage of patients who receive "good" care.

Another approach to developing clinical performance metrics is to consider the results rather than the process. Mortality and readmission rates are obvious results. Some organizations are beginning to go beyond these types of measures and look at clinical results from the perspective of the patient. A number of experimental questionnaires and approaches to assessing patient function are being attempted (see Chapter 9). The type of patient-centered questions that might be asked include the following:

- Was pain controlled to my expectations?
- Am I better today as a result of the treatment I received?
- Am I able to function today at the level I expected?
- Is my function restored to the same level it was before I became ill or was injured?
- Did I receive the help I need to manage my ongoing condition?
- Am I aware of anything that "went wrong" in the course of my treatment that delayed my recovery or compromised my condition?

When Possible, Use Comparative Data and External Benchmarks

Whenever possible, utilize external benchmark data to establish standards and targets. Many organizations track mortality and readmission rates on their scorecards. Mortality is a much stronger performance measure when it is risk adjusted and compared to other organizations to establish a frame of reference. Without that frame of reference, mortality tracking provides little useful information except to note directional trends. However, beyond establishing a frame of reference, organizations should set targets based on best performance in class rather than peer-group averages. Comparison to a peer-group mean tends to reinforce mediocrity and deflects attention away from the importance of the desired result intended by the performance measure. One of the best examples of this is the use of peer averages and percentiles provided by most of the national patient satisfaction survey vendors. Just being above average or in the top quartile does not necessarily equate to high patient satisfaction. A significant percentage of patients may be lukewarm about the care received or dissatisfied. Rather than basing targets on ranking (percentile based), better targets might be the average raw score or the percentage of patients who express dissatisfaction.

Change Your Leadership System

There is a saying that goes something like, "If you always do what you have always done, you will always get what you always got." One mistake some organizations have made is to roll out an elaborate set of cascading dashboards and scorecards and then fail to change the way the leadership system functions. Scorecards and dashboards can quickly become another "thing we do for compliance or the Joint Commission," outside the perceived "real work" of the organization. Leadership must make the review of measurement sets an integral part of the leadership function. When departments or operating units are reviewed by senior leaders, the unit scorecard/dashboard should be the primary focus of the review. If a strategic dashboard is developed, review of progress should be at least monthly or coordinated with the measurement cycles of the indicators. Governing boards should review the organizational performance measures at least quarterly. Review should not be done just for the sake of review, but for the purposes of driving change and setting priorities.

Focus on Results, Not Activities

A well-developed system of dashboards and scorecards allows leadership to focus on results instead of activities. Many results-oriented, high-performing organizations work from a leadership philosophy of tight-loose-tight. Senior leaders are very clear and "tight" about the results to be achieved and can measure results through the use of strategic and operational dashboards. At the same time, they are "loose" in the direct control of those doing the work, creating a sense of empowerment for those charged with achieving the results. Absent clear measures, leaders may tend to be tight and controlling of activities, micromanaging, and disempowering as viewed by others in the organization. Finally, when required results are clear, senior leaders can be "tight" about holding individuals and teams accountable for achieving required results.

Cultivate Transparency

One characteristic of high-performing organizations such as BNQP winners is that every employee knows how his or her individual efforts fit into the bigger picture. Healthcare has a long tradition of secrecy about results, in part a reflection of the historical view that quality is about physician peer review and in part a reaction to the malpractice environment. It is a big step for some organizations, but the results posted on the organizational scorecard should be transparent and openly discussed and shared with employees and clinical staff. Ideally, the results are also shared with the community served. Employees and clinical staff need to know the important dimensions of performance for the organization and the results, as well as the important process and management indicators and dashboards related to their daily work. Scorecards and operational dashboards should be widely shared and discussed.

The same is true for strategic measures. Many organizations consider strategy confidential, which is for the most part a ludicrous idea—successful deployment of strategy generally depends on what an organization itself does, not what its competitors may do. Sometimes, a specific tactic such as building a new clinic in a competitive part of town might need to be closely held because of market issues, but the critical strategy relating to growth of the enterprise should be no secret to anyone. It is very difficult to create awareness and improvements of key processes that support a strategy if the strategy and strategic measures are secret.

Case Study: St. Joseph Hospital

St. Joseph Hospital (SJH) in Orange, California, is the flagship hospital of the St. Joseph Health System (SJHS), sponsored by the sisters of St. Joseph of Orange. The system consists of 11 hospitals, all located in California, with the exception of Covenant Health, which is located in Texas. SJH and the Covenant Health operation are the two largest healthcare organizations in the system.

SJHS was an early adopter and developer of a systemwide approach to collecting and reporting a set of common performance indicators. Utilizing the four dimensions of the quality compass framework (financial, human resources, clinical, and satisfaction), a common set of performance indicators is collected monthly from each hospital in the system by the corporate office. Known internally as the "web," individual hospital radar charts are developed; on a periodic basis, the information is shared with the corporate health system board. The charts are used by hospital leadership and the local governing boards of each hospital to track progress, and the results are used in the individual CEO performance review process. Each indicator on the radar chart is backed by a run or control chart. SJHS has been innovative in the development of its scorecard tool, utilizing the system information to post monthly updates and allow access through the system intranet. While the indicators are fairly traditional, SJHS continues to modify and change indicators as the state of their art advances. Figure 10.8 is a representation of the monthly performance web for SJH.

While useful for tracking performance across the system by both the corporate office and the governing boards of the hospitals, the web was viewed as helpful but insufficient as a tool for driving change at SJH. Larry Ainsworth, CEO, realized early in 2002 that a different set of measures tied to organizational strategy was required to continue to progress and remain competitive in the Orange County marketplace. Traditionally, SJH utilized an annual planning process that yielded a business plan of more than 20 pages of objectives and proposed actions. An enormous amount of management's time was spent developing and tracking activities and objectives and reporting monthly to the board.

Instead of starting over, the senior leadership examined the business plan and from it concluded that five strategic themes underpinned all of the proposed objectives. The five vital few strategies identified by the SJH leadership team are displayed in Figure 10.9.

For each strategy, a team of senior leaders and clinicians was formed to develop specific proposed strategic measures and identify the required tactics for deployment. Many of the tactics developed were modifications of previously identified objectives and actions, but many were also new as the team considered tactics that would directly affect the strategic measures. Development of the visual strategy maps and associated measures for each tactic helped the hospital accomplish its aim of integrating previously separate quality, business, and strategic plans into a single approach. The visual strategy maps are viewed by hospital leadership as a critical tool for creating alignment and focus.

For each strategy, a dashboard of the key strategic measures was developed. This dashboard is reviewed monthly by the senior leadership team, and the results are shared with the governing board on a quarterly basis. Figure 10.10 is a sample of the strategic dashboard used to drive progress on their oncology strategy. In addition to the strategies being measurable, each proposed tactic is required to have a set of associated measures to guide deployment.

Mr. Ainsworth and his leadership team have made changes in the leadership system and begun routine, scheduled, in-depth review of each strategy by senior leadership. The review starts with the results of each of

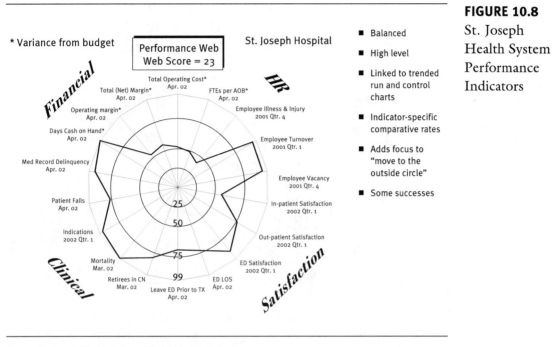

Source: St. Joseph Health System. Used with permission.

the strategic dashboard measures and continues with discussions of specific tactics and review of associated tactical measures. The identification of the five critical strategies and development of the strategy maps has also changed the review process by which the hospital board monitors progress.

Clarifying the key organizational strategies, developing key strategic measures for each, using the strategic measures to prioritize proposed tactics, and implementing changes in the leadership system to focus on strategy have resulted in increased organizational alignment around the improvement of important processes and increased organizational effectiveness. Importantly, positive effects are beginning to be noted on the system-required web of performance indicators.

Conclusion

Measurement is a critical element of the system of leadership in an organization. While most healthcare organizations gather hundreds of measures, the key is to organize the critical measures in such a way that they collectively tell a story about what needs to be achieved. Scorecards and dashboards are useful tools for organizing measures to drive and accelerate

FIGURE 10.9
St. Joseph
Hospital
Strategy Map:
Vital Few

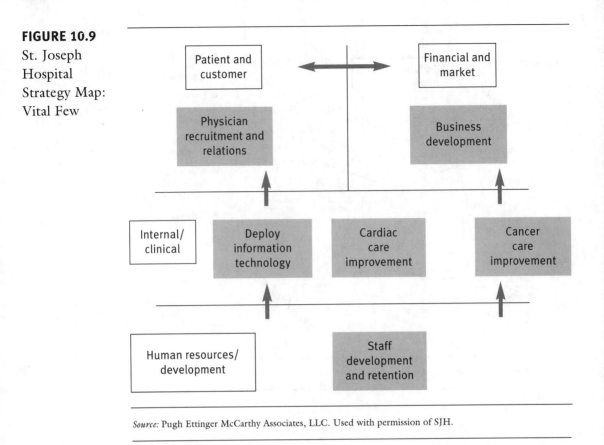

Source: Pugh Ettinger McCarthy Associates, LLC. Used with permission of SJH.

change. When used properly, they can create focus and alignment around the important dimensions of organizational performance as defined by the board and/or the core strategies that the organization seeks to employ.

Study Questions

1. In your experience with healthcare, what are the important dimensions of performance? How would you know whether or not an organization is performing well? What indicators do you think might be important to track for a hospital? A physician practice? A home care agency? A long-term care facility? A managed care organization?

2. What might be good indicators that reflect patient centeredness as recommended by IOM?

3. What are some of the pitfalls of overmeasurement? How do you determine what is important to measure in an organization?

4. Why is creating alignment an important leadership function? What are other methods of creating alignment, and how can the use of measurement support their deployment?

What are we trying to accomplish:
To be recognized for clinical excellence with increased market share in the provision of coordinated cancer care (oncology) services for Orange County and surrounding communities

Promise:
You will receive timely, comprehensive, current knowledge-based, and compassionate care at St. Joseph Hospital

FIGURE 10.10
Strategic Dashboard Used to Drive Progress on Oncology Strategy at St. Joseph Hospital

Volume, Profitability, and Market Share

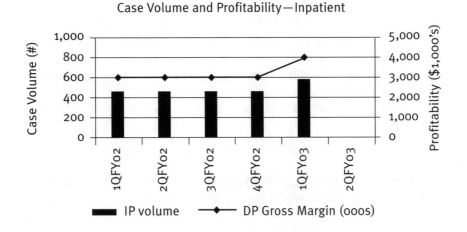

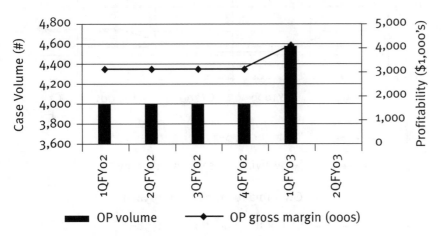

FIGURE 10.10
(continued)

Outcomes and Safety

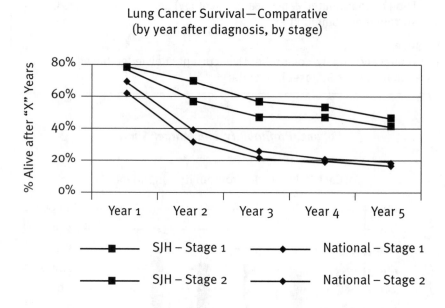

Lung Cancer Survival—Comparative
(by year after diagnosis, by stage)

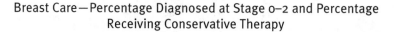

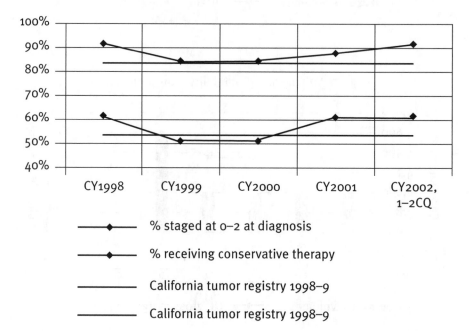

Breast Care—Percentage Diagnosed at Stage 0–2 and Percentage
Receiving Conservative Therapy

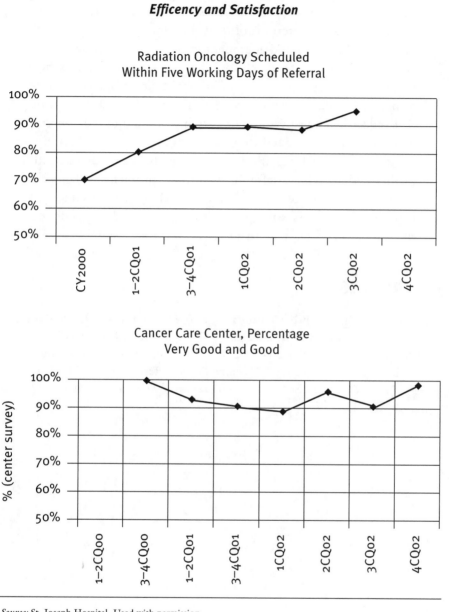

FIGURE 10.10
(*continued*)

Efficency and Satisfaction

Radiation Oncology Scheduled
Within Five Working Days of Referral

Cancer Care Center, Percentage
Very Good and Good

Source: St. Joseph Hospital. Used with permission.

Notes

1. In deference to the work of Kaplan and Norton (1992, 1996) and
    the specific concept in which leaders use a balanced scorecard of
    strategic measures, this chapter does not use the term *balanced*

scorecard except in direct reference to Kaplan and Norton's concept. Instead, the use of dashboards and scorecards is discussed in broader and generic terms in the exploration of a variety of applications to create focus and alignment in healthcare organizations.

2. A popular approach has been to utilize the stoplight color scheme of red, yellow, and green coding to highlight indicators where performance is judged against a predetermined standard. Indicators that reflect negative performance are highlighted in red, whereas indicators that are judged to be satisfactory or above expectations are given a green designation. Yellow can mean caution or need for further review. While useful for identifying problems or failure to meet a target, this format does not generally provide trended information useful for assessing progress or decline and, depending on the standard chosen, may reinforce poor actual results.

REFERENCES

Institute of Medicine. 2001. *Crossing the Quality Chasm: A New Health System for the 21st Century.* Washington, DC: National Academy Press.

Kaplan, R. S., and D. P. Norton. 1992. "The Balanced Scorecard—Measures that Drive Performance." *Harvard Business Review* 70 (1): 71–79.

———. 1996. *The Balanced Scorecard—Translating Strategy into Action.* Boston: HBS Press.

PATIENT SAFETY AND MEDICAL ERRORS

Frances A. Griffin and Carol Haraden

Patient safety has become one of the key issues facing healthcare leaders and managers today. Most hospital boards and chief executive officers currently cite patient safety as one of their top ten priority issues. Standards from regulatory and accrediting organizations contain a heavy focus on patients and continue to increase in scope, along with public demand for disclosure. Voluntary reporting systems for errors have been established with proposed legislation for mandatory systems. In the current environment, anyone working in healthcare management or leadership needs to understand the complexities of the patient safety issue and the underlying concepts of how errors and adverse events occur. This chapter provides an introductory framework to these areas and references to strategies that managers can use to improve patient safety in their own organization.

Background and Terminology

This chapter presents the contemporary challenge of improving patient safety and reducing medical errors. Harm is never the intention in healthcare delivery, but unfortunately it is sometimes the outcome. In addition to fears of a terminal diagnosis, debilitating disease, and pain, one of the greatest fears of patients is that a mistake will occur and the mistake will harm them. Horror stories of patients waking up in the middle of surgical procedures or having the wrong limb amputated, while rare, instill anxiety in those accessing the healthcare system. Fear of such events also hovers over the minds of healthcare practitioners, who worry about malpractice claims, loss of licensure, and, worst of all, the guilt of having caused harm rather than providing care and healing.

In 2000, the Institute of Medicine (IOM) published a landmark study on patient safety, *To Err Is Human*. Media attention to the report was swift and widespread, resulting in a sudden public awareness of the existence of a problem. Shock was expressed by the public at the estimate of up to 98,000 annual deaths in U.S. hospitals resulting from medical errors. Reaction among healthcare providers ranged from those who argued, and continue to, that the numbers were grossly overestimated (Hayward and Hofer 2001) to those who were unsurprised and even relieved that the information had been made public, in hopes that action now would be taken.

Published studies regarding medical errors, medication errors, and adverse events have been appearing in the literature for decades, providing the basis for the estimates in the IOM report. Lucian Leape, M.D., a leading expert on medical errors, has authored many studies. In 1991, he was one of the principal authors of the Harvard Medical Practice Study, which retrospectively reviewed hospital records for evidence of errors and adverse events (Brennan et al. 1991). The findings indicated that medical errors and adverse events were occurring far more often than reported and contributing to unnecessary deaths. Further studies have demonstrated that errors and adverse events commonly occur in healthcare settings other than hospitals. In 2003, Gandhi et al. reported that 25 percent of patients in ambulatory care practices had experienced adverse drug events. Other studies, in both the United States and Australia, have reported how adverse drug events result in additional visits to physician offices and emergency departments and increase hospital admissions (IOM 2000). The Commonwealth Fund found that 25 percent of patients in four countries reported experiencing some form of medical error in the previous two years (Blendon et al. 2003).

Patient Safety Defined

IOM (2000) defines *patient safety* as "freedom from accidental injury." At the core is the experience of the patient, with the goal that no patient will experience any unnecessary harm, pain, or other suffering. When a patient experiences harm or injury from a medical intervention, this is an adverse event (i.e., one not caused by an underlying medical condition) (IOM 2000). Adverse events sometimes are the result of an error, in which case they would be considered preventable. However, not all adverse events are the result of error; some medical interventions can cause harm (Shojania et al. 2002), even when planned and executed correctly. Some argue that such events are not really "adverse" and should not be considered as harm; instead, they would argue that such events are "known complications" or "associated risks" of certain procedures and interventions. However, the patient who experiences the adverse event receives little comfort from such an explanation.

Errors do not always reach patients, such as when the wrong dose of a medication is dispensed but detected prior to administration and corrected. Even when errors do reach the patient, they may not cause any harm or injury; for example, if an incorrect medication dose is administered, it may not differ enough from the intended dose to adversely affect the patient.

Beginning in the 1970s, much research has been conducted on human factors and the cognitive processes associated with errors. James Reason (1990), a renowned expert in human factors and error, defines error as an occasion on which a planned sequence of events fails to achieve its intended outcome. Errors originate from two basic types of failures according to Reason: a planning failure or an execution failure. An example in healthcare is the use of antibiotics to treat an infection. When an antibiotic is prescribed, it should be one effective against the bacteria causing the patient's infection; however, sometimes an antibiotic must be selected based on the physician's assessment of the most likely type of bacteria involved, as results of laboratory cultures may not yet be available. The antibiotic selected may be dispensed and administered in accordance with the physician's order but later turn out not to be the best choice. A planning error has occurred because the wrong plan was initiated, although the plan was carried out as intended. An execution error occurs when the plan is correct but not carried out as intended, for example, if the physician selects the correct antibiotic but it is either not dispensed or administered according to the order (e.g., wrong drug, wrong dose, wrong frequency). In either case, an error has occurred and the patient is at risk of harm.

Etiology of Patient Errors

Addressing patient safety and medical errors first requires an understanding of the underlying causes that contribute to errors and adverse events. Healthcare processes have become enormously complex over time, and the volume of information and knowledge currently available to practitioners is overwhelming, especially with the explosive growth of the Internet. New and rapidly advancing technologies have led to new treatments that offer many benefits but require training and expertise to be used effectively and safely. Thousands of new medications are introduced each year, far more than any one person could recall accurately from memory. Working conditions play an important role as well. Shortages of clinical personnel, high patient ratios, and long work hours all contribute to the risk that complex processes may not be executed as intended; that is, an error may occur.

It is important to recognize that when an error occurs, whether in planning or execution, it represents a systems problem (Leape, Berwick, and Bates 2002). This recognition has not often occurred with healthcare, and this is only beginning to change. Traditional response has been to blame an individual, usually the person at the end of a process that went wrong in many places and often many times previously. When an error leads to an adverse event or harm, emotions contribute to the situation: anger from patients and families, fear of lawsuits from practitioners, and guilt from those involved. The common response has been to identify a person at fault and take punitive action against that person, such as licensure removal, fines, suspension, or termination from employment. Punishment for being involved in an error discourages people from reporting (Findlay 2000).

Punitive action is only appropriate if an individual has knowingly and intentionally taken action to cause harm, which would be criminal or negligent behavior. An example is the case of a practitioner who injects a patient with a paralytic medication so that he or she can be the one to "save" the patient from the pulmonary arrest that would subsequently occur. Cases such as this are fortunately the exception and do warrant disciplinary action. However, most adverse events do not fit into this category, but rather are the result of a process breakdown. Blaming and punishing an individual and failing to change the process does not reverse the harm that has occurred and does nothing to decrease the likelihood of the same adverse event occurring again elsewhere in the organization.

Reporting of errors and adverse events is essential to know where changes and improvements can be made. Unfortunately, reporting of healthcare errors and events has been and remains low, within individual organizations as well as at state and national levels. This low level of reporting is largely due to the structure and response of the existing reporting systems, the majority of which are voluntary.

Some state regulatory agencies, such as state departments of health, have mandatory reporting for certain types of adverse events. The Joint Commission on Accreditation of Healthcare Organizations (Joint Commission) has attempted to gain further information from accredited organizations through its Sentinel Event standards. Excessive jury awards and high settlements in malpractice cases have contributed to the disincentive for reporting. When an error that causes no harm occurs, little incentive to report it may exist. As a result, the process remains unchanged and the same error continues to recur and may ultimately cause harm.

The Agency for Healthcare Research and Quality (AHRQ) released a report in response to the IOM report, providing information on evidence-based safety practices (Shojania et al. 2002). AHRQ defines a patient safety practice as "a type of process or structure whose application reduces the probability of adverse events resulting from exposure to the healthcare system." It is noteworthy that this definition does not reference "error" at all. Errors will always exist in healthcare. Processes will always have the potential to fail, and human factors will always contribute. However, adverse events and harm need not always occur (Nolan 2000). A system designed for patient safety is one in which errors are expected to occur, processes are designed and improved with human factors and safety in mind, and reporting is encouraged and rewarded. When safety is part of everyone's daily routine, the result is that while errors exist, adverse events do not.

Scope and Use of Patient Safety Considerations in Healthcare

Healthcare is not the only industry to have struggled with a poor safety record and public image problem. There was a period when aviation had nowhere near the safety record it has today. During the mid-twentieth century, as commercial air travel increased in popularity, accidents and deaths occurred at significantly higher rates than those seen today. This industry had to make significant changes to survive. This was accomplished by focusing on how to make systems safer and developing a different culture. The results are obvious when one considers how many planes are flown every day, the volume of passengers transported, and the number of those passengers who are injured or killed in airplane accidents. In just the first half of the 1990s, the number of deaths was one-third what it had been in the mid-twentieth century (IOM 2000). Sadly, we cannot say the same for healthcare and must even wonder if the opposite may be true.

While healthcare and aviation do have some distinct differences and the analogy is not perfect, much that the aviation industry learned is applicable. In fact, this application has already occurred in anesthesiology, the specialty now considered the benchmark for safe delivery of medical care. This was not always the case. In the 1950s, patients receiving general anesthesia were at a much greater risk of dying from the anesthesia than they are today. From the 1950s to the 1970s, changes decreased the rate of anesthesia-related deaths from 1 in 3,500 to 1 in 10,000 (Findlay 2000), a significant improvement. One key to the changes was that the initiative was led by anesthesiologists themselves, who developed standards of practice and guidelines not imposed on them by any outside regulatory agency. Much was taken from the practices developed in aviation, such as use of standardized procedures and safety checklists. More recent data show that anesthesia-related deaths have decreased to one in 300,000, a staggering difference from 40 years earlier (Findlay 2000). No breakthrough technology or newly discovered drug contributed to this improvement. Rather, a focus on the system of care and making many small changes that led to safer practices have all combined for an enormous difference in outcome (Leape, Berwick, and Bates 2002).

Teamwork and Patient Safety

The interaction of a team, in any setting, greatly affects the success of that team. Unsurprisingly, when the members of a team do not function well together or are not perceived by one another as having equally important roles, they do not handle unexpected situations well. Aviation learned this lesson the hard way. Reviews of the events in a cockpit prior to a plane accident or crash revealed that copilots and engineers were often unable to effectively communicate warnings to the pilot, the senior member of the team, or received negative responses when they did. Warnings that could have prevented the deaths of hundreds of passengers, plus the crew themselves, were frequently disregarded, poorly communicated, or not communicated at all. To change this environment, an initiative called cockpit resource management, later renamed *crew resource management* (CRM), was started. In CRM, crews learn how to interact as a team, with each member having equally important roles and responsibilities to ensure the safety of all on board. Appropriate assertion of concerns is more than encouraged; it is expected.

CRM has found its way into healthcare and is being used in a variety of settings. Operating room teams have many analogies to airline crews, and CRM training is being used to improve how surgeons, anesthesiologists, nurses, and technicians all work together to ensure the provision of safe care to the patient. Faculty at the University of Texas Center of Excellence in Patient Safety Research have studied airline crews and operating room teams to evaluate how they interact with one another and respond to errors and unexpected events. Using surveys to first assess team member perceptions of teamwork, hierarchy, and culture, the teams were then observed in their actual work environments to determine how many errors occurred, how many were serious, and how well the team resolved them. Teams that reported high levels of teamwork still had errors but experienced fewer serious ones compared to those who rated teamwork low. In addition, those rating teamwork high were more often able to effectively resolve conflict and prevent small errors from becoming adverse events; however, this appears to be true more often with airplane crews than operating room teams, as they have been receiving training in this area for much longer (Sexton, Thomas, and Helmreich 2000).

Attitudes about teamwork derive from the overall culture of an organization or unit. Enormous differences in culture can exist from one unit or department to another, even within the same organization. Individuals are most affected by the culture of the department in which they spend most of their time. Culture in a unit may not be obvious; on the surface, it may be deemed as fine if there are not frequent disputes and arguments among staff, physicians, and managers. Absence of such overt problems does not necessarily indicate a good underlying culture. Every department, unit, and organization should be constantly developing and enhancing its culture, regardless of how good it may appear or actually be, by focusing on and improving how all members of the healthcare team interact and communicate with one another. This certainly improves care to patients, but it has many other benefits as well.

When every member of the team feels valued and able to contribute, work satisfaction improves, thereby decreasing turnover, a costly issue in any organization. Improved communication among practitioners results in better coordination of care, early recognition of errors, and more rapid interventions, which contribute to operational benefits. At Johns Hopkins Hospital in Baltimore, a comprehensive program to improve teamwork and culture in the ICU resulted in a 50 percent decrease in length of stay, providing access for more than 650 additional admissions and $7 million in additional revenue (Pronovost et al. 2003). Other hospitals have used similar approaches to improve teamwork and communication among operating room teams. One technique is the adoption of preprocedural safety briefings prior to every operation, during which the entire team meets to review the case and potential safety issues. Following implementation of this and other changes, staff usually report less difficulty speaking up if they perceive a problem. Even more interesting, though, was that staff perception of high workloads being common actually decreased, even though no changes to workload or staffing levels were made (Sexton 2002).

Leading Improved Patient Safety

Leadership of an organization is the driving force behind the culture that exists and the perceptions it creates. For staff in any healthcare organization to believe that patient safety is a priority, that message must come from the top levels, including the CEO and board. Furthermore, that message must be visible and consistent. A visible approach to patient safety is not constituted by memos sent out by the CEO emphasizing its importance or by a periodic column in a staff newsletter. The only way frontline staff will know and believe that safety is important to the senior leaders in their organization is if the senior leaders visit the departments and units where the work occurs and talk directly with the staff about safety. Through the use of rounds and by soliciting input from staff, senior leaders can gain tremendous knowledge about what is happening in their organizations and take steps to make improvements (Frankel et al. 2003). To be convincing, the effort must also be consistent and sustained. When rounding is first started, it is not uncommon for staff to expect that it is the "idea of the month" and will be of short duration, especially if that has been the path of previous initiatives in the organization. Setting aside just one hour every week for senior leaders to round and talk with staff can have a powerful effect, as long as it occurs routinely and feedback is provided. In fact, some senior leaders have found the practice to be so beneficial that they have increased the amount of time spent on this activity.

Changing the culture and perceptions can take a long time and require tremendous effort and attention. Leadership presence on the front line is essential, but it represents only one piece of the package. The response to any event that occurs, whether an error, adverse event, or both, also significantly affects staff beliefs. Acknowledging that errors and adverse events are systems problems, not people problems, is a crucial first step. Following through on this idea with appropriate responses when something happens is critical. Many organizations have created nonpunitive reporting policies to encourage staff reporting of errors and adverse events without fear of reprisal, even if the reporter was involved in the event. These policies have met with limited success, especially at middle-management levels. Many managers, trained in the old pattern of find and blame the individual, struggle with the concept of nonpunitive policies as they mistakenly conclude that they imply that no employee, especially their "problem employees," will ever be disciplined. A true problem employee will usually accumulate enough offenses against other policies for the manager to take appropriate action. Even these individuals are as likely as all other employees to find themselves at the end of a systems failure. Such an instance is not the opportunity to be rid of the problem employee. In a nonpunitive environment, *every* error or adverse event is analyzed as a systems problem, and punitive action is not taken against anyone unless it is discovered that policy was deliberately violated with the intent to cause harm. Punitive action taken against anyone, even a problem employee, is recalled in the memory of the staff only as an example of how someone was punished for being involved in an error or adverse event. This will be remembered far longer than a senior leadership round that occurred during the same week.

It is important to consider what feels punitive from an employee's perspective, not just from management's. Managers sometimes consider formal disciplinary action, such as official written warnings, as the only type of punitive action. However, staff members certainly feel penalized when they are verbally criticized in front of others, when errors or adverse events in which they were involved are discussed at a staff meeting with emphasis on how "someone" made a mistake (even if names are left out), or when details of reported errors or events are attached to their performance appraisals. Any time a staff member walks away from an event feeling that he or she may have been at fault, or is viewed by management in that way, it perpetuates a punitive environment and decreases the likelihood that staff members will voluntarily report anything in the future.

Dealing with Adverse Events

Handling an adverse event in a healthcare organization can be enormously complicated. Emotions add further complexity, particularly when a patient has been harmed. External pressures can escalate the intensity of the situation when media and regulatory agencies become involved. All of these contributing factors increase our natural tendency to blame someone. Leaders are pressured at such times to identify the responsible parties and report what action has been taken. This is a critical time for leaders and managers to work together with everyone involved and prevent a blame-focused or punitive response. Human factors expert James Reason (1990) provides wonderful resources on this subject in *Managing the Risks of Organizational Accidents*. These resources include algorithms to analyze the sequence of events; with this tool, managers are prompted to consider key questions to determine whether a systems failure occurred. Rather than assuming that an employee simply did not follow a policy, Reason suggests that an investigator evaluate aspects such as whether the policy was readily available, easily understandable, and workable. One should also apply a substitution test, that is, how likely it is that the same event would occur with three other employees with similar experience and training under similar circumstances (e.g., hours on duty, fatigue, workload) (Reason 1990). If the event is quite likely, a systems problem exists.

Disclosure to patients and families is another difficult aspect for hospital leaders and physicians to manage when an adverse event occurs. Traditionally, this has not always been handled well, resulting in public perception that those in healthcare "cover up for each other." Punitive responses from regulatory agencies, accreditation bodies, and licensing boards discourage healthcare organizations and practitioners from reporting events unless mandated by law. Lawyers dissuade practitioners from apologizing to patients when an adverse event occurs by telling them that doing so would be considered an admission of guilt. Fearful of lawsuits, practitioners and representatives of healthcare organizations stay silent or say little and speak vaguely. This leads to incredible frustration and distrust on the part of patients and families, who often know that something has gone wrong but find themselves unable to obtain a straight answer. All this silence does is increase the likelihood of a lawsuit being filed. Many who have filed malpractice lawsuits report that they were not motivated by the desire for a large financial settlement, but rather because they felt it was the only way to discover the truth about what happened and because no one ever said that they were sorry. Public concern about disclosure of events led to the Joint Commission adding standards that now require accredited organizations to inform patients or their legal guardians of any unanticipated outcome.

Involving patients and families in discussions about their care throughout the entire process is an essential element in changing culture. In the IOM report *Crossing the Quality Chasm*, patient centeredness is one of the key aspects of the recommended changes (IOM 2001). Every part of a patient's care should be centered around *the patient's needs first*, not the needs of physicians, nurses, other clinical personnel, hospitals, or other healthcare agencies. Care should be approached in an open fashion; patients and families actively participating in rounds and goal setting, verifying iden-tification before procedures, and verifying medications before administra-tion are just a few examples of how patients should be integrated into the process. A safety-focused culture must include patients, and open discus-sion in one area will encourage openness in other areas.

Reporting Adverse Events

Focusing on reporting will increase reporting, but often not substantially or for very long. Organizations need to know more about the errors and adverse events that are occurring to improve their systems. Most rely on voluntary reporting systems to gain this information, but, as previously mentioned, these are not the best sources and underreporting is a signifi-cant problem. To increase reporting, well-intentioned individuals in health-care organizations try a variety of initiatives. These often include strategies such as education fairs, posters, safety hotlines, shorter reporting forms, raffles, prizes for departments with the most reports, and other incentives. While implementing these strategies, heavy emphasis is placed on the guar-anteed anonymity of the various reporting mechanisms and assurances of nonpunitive approaches. For a short period, reporting increases, resulting in celebration and excitement about all of the new knowledge that will be gained. But over time, reporting starts to decline and usually ends up back where it was before, if not worse, leaving those who led the initiative feel-ing discouraged and disheartened. They may rally and try again, only to have the same cycle repeated.

This cycle occurs mainly because the focus has not addressed the core issue: the underlying culture. The heavy focus on reporting causes a temporary increase simply because of focus on the issue, but reporting does not become integrated into the daily routine; eventually it is talked about less often unless someone takes on the role of cheerleader and attempts to keep the momentum going. Incentives may also help, but their attraction is highest when they are new; over time, people either forget about incen-tives or are no longer motivated by them. The focus on guaranteed anonymity may cause the opposite of the effect desired. In a truly just cul-ture, one need not remain anonymous when reporting, for no fear of reprisal exists. Reinforcing guaranteed anonymity may leave staff with the impres-sion that the potential for punitive action still exists.

Hospitals that have seen dramatic and sustained increases in volun-tary reporting have not achieved them by concentrating efforts on report-ing mechanisms. Rather, they have focused on their culture and creating a safety-conscious environment. Leadership commitment to safety and strate-gies to improve teamwork among all levels are fundamental first steps. Once the dialog begins, feedback then becomes critical. As frontline staff begin to alert management to safety issues and opportunities for improvement, their belief in the new system will only be established when feedback is provided about their suggestions. As all of these changes take root in the organization, the culture changes and voluntary reporting increases, likely to levels not previously seen.

Even in a safety-conscious culture, errors will continue to occur, as will adverse events. Reason (1990) describes two distinct types of errors: active and latent. In an *active error*, the effects or consequences occur immediately; an example is placing one's foot on the gas pedal in a car, rather than on the brake, when engaging the shift out of park and thus crashing through the garage wall. *Latent errors*, though, exist within the system for a long time, not causing any harm until a situation arises where, in combination with other factors, the error becomes part of a chain of events resulting in disaster. The loss of the Challenger space shuttle was later found to be the catastrophic result of latent errors, as have many other well-known disasters (Reason 1990). When an adverse event occurs in healthcare, retrospective review frequently reveals latent errors as contributing factors.

Each occurrence represents an opportunity for learning and for sharing the lessons both internally and externally. In creating a safety-oriented culture, an organization must ensure that information about errors and action taken to reduce them is shared openly. Frontline staff can learn a great deal by hearing about the experiences of others, and organizations should provide mechanisms that encourage them to do so. Incorporating patient safety issues into change-of-shift reports or setting aside a regular time for staff to have safety briefings are just two of the ways in which communication and teamwork can be enhanced. It is also important to find ways for this information to transcend departments, units, and divisions. If an important patient safety lesson is learned in one area, sharing it across the entire organization is the only way to move the same issue in another area from a latent error to an identified issue that can be changed.

Learning from the external environment is also important. The most serious adverse events, such as removal of the wrong limb, are usually, and fortunately, rare. Most hospitals may have not had such an event occur for years, but that should not mean that complacency is allowed to develop. Every time a serious adverse event occurs at *any* hospital *anywhere*, the lessons learned from that event should be available to all hospitals so that all can analyze their own processes for improvement opportunities. Unfortunately, this is not easy to do, as legal issues from lawsuits and concerns about privacy prevent or hinder many organizations from sharing details. Organizations such as the Joint Commission and Institute for Safe Medication Processes have disseminated newsletters with information they have obtained about serious adverse events, without including identifying information about the organization or people involved, as a way to facilitate learning and improvement. Despite such worthwhile initiatives, the same events continue to occur.

Looking to Other Industries

Healthcare can also look to other industries for ideas about how to implement safer practices; in fact, we should do so far more often than we do. A common argument against looking at industry is that in medicine, "We are not making widgets." This is certainly true, and those of us working in healthcare professions carry a special and unique responsibility when rendering care to our fellow human beings. However, that does not necessarily mean we cannot learn from other industries. There are other industries in which an error can result in the loss of life, even hundreds or thousands at once; examples include aviation, air traffic control systems, nuclear power plants, and aircraft carriers. Despite enormous risks and extremely complex processes, these industries all have safety records well beyond healthcare's. So what can be learned from these types of organizations? In *Managing the Unexpected*, Weick and Sutcliffe (2001) describe these successes as *high-reliability organizations*. The approach to daily work is an expectation and preoccupation with failure rather than success. This results in constant, early identification of errors and error-producing processes, with continuous improvement to processes and routines. The safety records of such organizations alone are such that healthcare leaders would be foolish not to learn more about how they have been achieved and which aspects are applicable in their own organizations.

One tool developed in the industrial setting that has found application in healthcare is failure modes and effects analysis (FMEA). FMEA is a systematic, proactive method for evaluating a process to identify where and how it might fail and to assess the relative effect of different failures to identify the parts of the process most in need of change. FMEA includes review of the following:

- Steps in the process
- Failure modes (What could go wrong?)
- Failure causes (Why would the failure happen?)
- Failure effects (What would be the consequences of each failure?)

An advantage to using this approach is the evaluation of processes for possible failures and to prevent them by correcting the processes *proactively*, rather than reacting to adverse events after failures have occurred. This is a very different approach from root-cause analysis (RCA), which is conducted only after an event has occurred. Another significant difference is that RCA by definition suggests that an adverse event has only one cause; that rarely is the case. FMEA, in contrast, looks at the entire process and every potential for failure, so the perspective is broader. FMEA is particularly useful in evaluating a new process prior to its implementation and in assessing the effect of a proposed change to an existing process. Using this approach, organizations can consider many options and assess potential consequences in a safe environment, prior to actual implementation in the patient care process.

The goal in FMEA is an emphasis on prevention to reduce risk of harm to both patients and staff. Use of forcing functions, such as oxygen flowmeters that are designed to only fit into oxygen outlets and not compressed air or vacuum outlets, is a prevention technique that works well for many processes. Although prevention is an important aspect in making practices safer, it is not possible to prevent all errors. When an error does occur, another important consideration is how visible the error will be. In conducting an FMEA, it is recommended that a numeric value of risk, called a *risk priority number* (RPN), be assigned to the process; this is used to assess for improvement, evident by reducing the RPN. To calculate an RPN, one asks three fundamental questions about each failure mode and assigns each question a value between one and ten (very unlikely to very likely):

1. *Likelihood of occurrence:* How likely is it that this failure mode will occur?
2. *Likelihood of detection:* If this failure mode occurs, how likely is it that the failure will be detected?
3. *Severity:* If this failure mode occurs, how likely is it that harm will occur?

The second question regarding detection relates directly to the issue of visibility. If an error is very likely to occur but likely to go undetected, then in addition to prevention strategies, one should look for methods to alert staff that an error has occurred. An example is the use of alert screens in computerized prescriber order entry (CPOE) systems; if a prescriber makes an error while ordering medications, an alert screen can provide immediate notification so that a change can be made.

The third, equally important, aspect to making practices safer is mitigation. Despite well-designed prevention and detection strategies, some errors will slip through and reach the patient. The ultimate goal in patient safety, of course, is to not cause harm. When an error does reach the patient, quick recognition and appropriate intervention can significantly reduce the level of harm to the patient. Training staff in response techniques, through the use of drills and simulations, and ensuring that resources needed for interventions are readily available in patient care areas are strategies that can help mitigate adverse events (Nolan 2000). A comprehensive patient safety approach requires that changes be made to improve all three areas: prevention, detection, and mitigation.

Using Technology to Improve Patient Safety

Technology is often seen as a solution to safer care, and while advances have offered many fabulous ways to improve systems and processes, it is important to remember that each new technology introduces new opportunities for error that did not exist previously. A good basic rule prior to implementing any technological solution is to never automate a bad process. If a process is not working well, as evidenced by frequent errors or process breakdowns, adding technology to the process usually will not solve the underlying problems; in fact, it usually makes the situation worse, and as even more process failures become evident, the technology is blamed and subsequently abandoned or not used.

CPOE has been an example of this in some cases. Almost every hospital in the United States has either implemented or planned for this technology, which offers many benefits, such as decision support and elimination of illegible orders. Some hospitals have learned the hard lesson that implementation of CPOE should not coincide with the implementation of standardized processes that have not been previously used, such as order sets or protocols. These standardized tools work best when tested and implemented using paper systems first if a hospital does not yet have computerized ordering. This provides physicians with an opportunity to learn and become accustomed to the new processes, integrate them into their routines, and make suggestions for any needed improvements. When a CPOE system is introduced later, physicians will only need to learn the technical use and how to adapt the standard processes they already know to that environment. Introducing standardized ordering processes and CPOE simultaneously has generally been a recipe for failure of both.

New opportunities for error and failure are introduced with any new technology. Since technological solutions are often employed in systems and processes that are already quite complex, one must remember that any change to one part of the system can produce unexpected effects in another (Shojania et al. 2002).

Here, FMEA can serve as a useful resource, providing a mechanism for staff to evaluate the potential failures of the equipment and consider processes to prevent, detect, and mitigate those failures. The extra features of any technology must be used in a balanced manner. Overuse of any feature will diminish its effectiveness over time. For example, in a CPOE system, alerts and pop-up screens can provide critical prescribing information to users, even requiring the use of an over-ride in certain high-risk situations. But if too many pop-ups are utilized, users will eventually begin to ignore them; as a routine, users will proceed to the next screen, without actually reading the alert information, leading to the risk of a serious error bypassing the system. Audible alarms are another example, so their parameters should be set to only alarm when attention is required. If equipment alarms frequently, and for reasons that do not require immediate intervention, staff will quickly become complacent about the alarms. Observing the activity on a patient care unit where many ventilators are in use will usually provide a good example of this if ventilators are alarming frequently and for long periods. Bypassing screens and not responding quickly to alarms are not failings of the people involved—they are the expected by-products of improperly designed systems. Human beings are so overloaded with the visual and auditory stimulation of technology, a natural defensive mechanism is to shut some of it out. Safety designs in other industries already consider this, and healthcare must also.

Designing Safe Processes

To decrease the harm that occurs to patients, healthcare organizations must design patient care systems for safety. The underlying foundation for success in this journey is the creation and development of a safety-conscious culture. Processes and systems must then be assessed for change using the following key elements:

1. Incorporate human factors knowledge into training and procedures. Expect and plan for error rather than reacting to it in surprise.
2. Design technology and procedures with end-users, planning for failures (Norman 1988). Until all medical device manufacturers adopt this process, the burden falls to healthcare organizations as purchasers to seek devices that incorporate safe designs and to develop procedures to support safe use within them.
3. Decrease complexity by reducing the number of steps in a process whenever possible (Nolan 2000). As the number of steps in a process increases, the likelihood that the process will be executed without error decreases. Periodically review all processes to determine if any steps no longer provide value, as all processes tend to change over time.
4. Ensure that safety initiatives address prevention, detection, and mitigation (Nolan 2000). A combination of all three is necessary to reduce harm. FMEA can be an effective tool for this.
5. Standardize processes, tools, technology, and equipment. Variation increases complexity and the risk of error. Technology can offer

great benefits, but it must be applied to processes that already function fairly well. Equipment may include features that decrease the need for reliance on memory, an important aspect of safety; however, if too many different types of equipment are in use, users will find it difficult to move from one item to another. Imagine how difficult it would be to drive a rental car if every car manufacturer placed gas pedals, brake pedals, and shifts in completely different locations with varying designs! Yet this is exactly what occurs with many medical devices.

6. Label medications and solutions clearly and for each individual dose, including both generic and trade names. Use extra alert measures for drugs that have similar-sounding names. Unfortunately, the burden for adding processes to address this safety issue also falls to healthcare organizations, as patient safety is generally not incorporated at all in the selection of drug names.

7. Use bar coding. The Food and Drug Administration has adopted requirements for all medications, a worthy but long overdue measure. As supermarkets have been using bar-code readers for years, healthcare is shamefully behind in this regard when one considers the difference in risk of administering the wrong blood product compared to charging the wrong price for a grocery item. This technology will become a standard part of healthcare delivery.

8. Use forcing functions to prevent certain types of errors from occurring, but be sure to maintain a balance and not overdo. Too many constraints will result in staff finding ways to work around them. Make things difficult that *should* be difficult (Norman 1988).

These elements are not new to quality improvement, industry, or in some cases even healthcare; yet they have not been widely adopted in healthcare. As we work toward decreasing and eliminating the unintended harm our systems cause, we must realize that our industry *can* learn from nonhealthcare industries. In fact, we must if we are to achieve any significant improvement in this area within our lifetime. The analogies are not perfect, and healthcare embodies some distinct and important differences. We are privileged to work in professions in which our interactions with our fellow human beings allow us the opportunity to care for them, hopefully curing them when possible, but when not, providing relief from their symptoms and ensuring dignified deaths. This privilege obligates us to use every possible resource and tool at our disposal, whether created in our own industry or not, to ensure that this care is delivered in the safest manner possible and never causes unintended harm. Every patient has that right.

Clinical and Operational Issues

Patient Safety Research

Many of the greatest breakthroughs in medicine that have led to improvements in patient care have come about through research. As clinicians continue to discover improved methods and interventions for treating and curing disease, new research will provide results that will alter the way in which care is delivered. Today, healthcare has known best practices for many clinical conditions, that is, multiple studies have demonstrated that these practices are reliable and general consensus exists among clinical experts. Practices include diagnostic tests identifying disease and assessing severity and the interventions that improve patient outcomes. Yet, despite the amount of knowledge that has been accumulated on these practices and the general acceptance that they are indeed best practices, huge variation in their adoption and use remains a problem (IOM 2000). One study found that most accepted best practices are documented as used in only 50 percent of appropriate patients at best (McGlynn et al. 2003). One could argue that failure to use a universally accepted treatment protocol, unless clinically contraindicated, is a planning error. The subject of optimizing physician performance is discussed in Chapter 9.

Physician Objections

The objection that many clinicians raise to using known best practices, or evidence-based medicine, usually centers on one of two interrelated issues. First is that the approach is "cookbook medicine" and an attempt to remove the clinician's expertise and judgment from the process. Evidence-based medicine, when used appropriately, does nothing of the kind. A clinician's training, skills, and expertise are essential in evaluating a patient, assessing the symptoms and results of diagnostic testing, and pulling all of this information together to make a clinical diagnosis. However, once the diagnosis has been made, why would clinicians want to be concerned with determining on their own what course of treatment should be utilized when they can select from those that have already proven to be the best through extensive research? Clinicians should welcome these best practices, feel confident in the evidence, and determine whether any contraindication exists.

This leads to the second issue, "My patients are different." Naturally, every patient is different in that all are unique individuals; many patients, though, do not have contraindications to the evidence-based practices but still do not receive them. It is time for physicians to accept that using evidence-based best practices takes nothing away from their value and expertise as clinicians, but rather provides them with the tools to assist them in providing patients with safe, high-quality care that may improve outcomes.

Limitations of Research

While research provides wonderful new knowledge, it has some limitations. Insistence that complete and thorough research must first be completed prior to any change being implemented hinders improvement and the adoption of safe practices. It is also an unrealistic expectation, as complete evidence for everything will never exist (Leape, Berwick, and Bates 2002). Some practices to improve patient safety just make sense and do not need a research study to prove their effectiveness—they should simply be implemented (Shojania et al. 2002). For example, how could anyone who has ever seen an illegible medication order claim that we need to first conduct studies as to the effectiveness of computerized systems that reduce or eliminate the need for handwritten orders before implementing them? Or, why would research need to be conducted on the need for verification of patient identification prior to any medical intervention? Research provides wonderful information, but we cannot research everything and should not allow research to become an obstacle that prevents adoption of safer practices.

Effects of Fatigue

An area that has been researched in healthcare and other industries is the effect of fatigue on errors and safety. Studies have shown that an individual who is sleep deprived demonstrates cognitive function at the ninth percentile of the overall population (Shojania et al. 2002); a person who has been awake for 24 straight hours often demonstrates actions and errors similar to a person who is legally under the influence of alcohol. Despite this knowledge, healthcare remains one of the only high-risk professions that does not mandate restrictions of hours (Leape, Berwick, and Bates 2002). Recent rules regarding the work hours of resident physicians have only begun to scratch the surface. No requirements exist for physicians who are not in training or other clinical personnel within the healthcare setting. Since many personnel work at more than one organization, no one is watching the overall perspective. The situation is not an easy one to address, since with current shortages in most clinical professions and increasing numbers of hospitalized patients, most organizations rely on staff overtime to meet staffing levels, especially in states where staffing ratios have been mandated. All of this contributes to high workloads, increased work hours, and greater fatigue for all staff, circumstances known to factor in the commission of errors.

Economics and Patient Safety

Healthcare is experiencing turbulent times, and financial pressures weigh heavily on every healthcare leader. In addition to staffing shortages, there are concerns regarding reimbursement, malpractice coverage, regulatory requirements, and access for the uninsured. Any healthcare CEO would agree that patient safety is important, but in actual practice it becomes a low priority at most organizations (Shojania et al. 2002). Distractions from all of the other aforementioned issues consume so much time that safety is easily lost.

Many factors affect healthcare, and economics is one—an important one, but not the only one (IOM 2000). Unsafe practices contribute to cost in many ways, including, but not limited to, efficiency, increased length of stay, turnover, absorbed costs when an error or adverse event occurs, malpractice settlements, and increased premiums. The dollars lost to lack of safety every year are staggering, to say nothing of the consequences to the patients who are harmed, which cannot always be measured in financial terms.

Patient safety must become a priority for healthcare leaders in action as well as word. The current system is broken, and changing it requires will (Nolan 2000). In a safety-oriented organization, everyone takes responsibility for safety (Findlay 2000). All organizations should strive to function that way, all employees and clinicians should want to work in that kind of environment, and all patients should demand to be treated in such a setting. Hopefully someday in the near future, we will be able to claim that all of healthcare has achieved the safety record anesthesia currently has. Hopefully someday, hospitals will be included in the list of high-reliability organizations. We must start working toward that end so that all patients can confidently access any part of the healthcare system without fear of harm.

Case Study: OSF Health System

The OSF Health System began its journey toward safer healthcare in earnest after release of IOM's *Crossing the Quality Chasm* report (IOM 2001). OSF Health System operates six hospital facilities, various physician office practices, urgent care centers, and extended care facilities in Illinois, Wisconsin, and Michigan. Like many organizations, OSF took the call to action contained in the report seriously. Unlike most organizations, it has actually created some of the safest systems of care in the United States. Following is the organization's story of transformation.

This important story begins with developing a culture of improvement and moves into testing cycles, implementation, spread, and hardwiring change. It is difficult to overstate the level of commitment and amount of work that have enabled OSF to achieve its successes.

True to all organizations that create transformative and lasting change, OSF employed a top-down and bottom-up improvement strategy. The corporate office and individual hospital leaders made safer care a top strategic priority. They added muscle to that declaration by tying the executive compensation package to adverse drug event (ADE) and mortality rates. OSF also began building the robust infrastructure needed to create and sustain change at the front line. It named physician change agents at the corporate office and several hospital sites. The change agents report directly to the CEO, and their role is designed to allow them to work at all levels of the organization and instigate improvement driven by strategic priorities.

To kick-start its safety project, OSF enrolled St. Joseph Medical Center into the Quantum Leaps in Patient Safety collaborative with the Institute for Healthcare Improvement (IHI). St. Joseph Medical Center was one of 50 international teams that formed a learning community that would lead to unprecedented change over the next year. An OSF team of early adopters representing administration, medical staff, nursing, and pharmacy was established and given the explicit task of creating a strong and successful prototype. The team would then use those successful changes to spread improvements throughout the organization. Leadership provided both human and financial resources and removed barriers so that the team could do its best work. This combination of a fully engaged leadership and a creative and committed frontline team was responsible for creating the unprecedented level of safety that was to come.

Changes that needed to be made were improving the safety culture and maintaining a cultural survey score above 4, using the medication reconciliation process to ensure that patients were on the correct medications at every point in their care, employing FMEA to reduce the risk and improve the reliability of the dispensing system, and standardizing the dosing and management of high-risk medications. All of these changes were in the service of the grand aim: reduce ADEs by a factor of ten. At the start of the journey, medication events were occurring at rates that translated into the occurrence of adverse events for every 1,000 doses given. The group's goal was to decrease the number of adverse events to parts per 10,000; this would mean that it would take about a full year to realize the same number of adverse events that were then occurring in a month.

With culture defined as "the predominating attitudes and behavior that characterize the functioning of a group or organization," a comprehensive redesign of the culture and care systems was initiated at OSF St. Joseph Medical Center to reduce the potential rate of harm to patients. In evaluating areas for improvement, reducing adverse events involving medications was identified as the opportunity that affected the largest population of patients.

Reducing Adverse Drug Events

The drastic reduction in ADEs that OSF aimed to create required multifaceted changes in many processes. No single change or small combination of changes can take an organization to that level of safety. OSF began by measuring the current rate of harm caused by medication using a trigger tool developed during the Idealized Design of Medication Systems sponsored by IHI. Charts were sampled randomly and reviewed by trained clinicians to gain an accurate assessment of the number and type of ADEs occurring in the hospital. Twenty randomly selected medical records were initially reviewed using the ADE trigger tool. The review indicated the hospital's ADE rate to be 5.8 per 1,000 doses dispensed; the goal was to reduce this rate to 0.58 ADEs per 1,000 doses.

OSF learned a tremendous amount about the medication harm in its system. The organization was also concerned about the rate of reported actual and potential errors. These errors had not caused harm yet, but they represented a tremendous potential for learning and improvement. OSF came to believe that the incident-occurrence reporting system produced reports that revealed only the tip of the iceberg in identifying these events. To improve the rate and the organization's learning, an ADE hotline was established. Because the hotline is located in the pharmacy, a pharmacist is able to check it daily for reported events and proceed with an investigation into potential causes. This is a win-win situation, as the event is identified for evaluation and trending and the staff can report easily, quickly, and anonymously and save time by avoiding paperwork associated with completion of an occurrence report. The error reporting and potential error reporting rates improved markedly.

A key change in the reduction of ADEs is the use of a medication reconciliation process. Medication reconciliation is the act of comparing the medications the patient has been taking with the medications currently ordered. Because a patient's care is often fragmented and he or she is under the care of multiple physicians, medications prescribed by the cardiologist may be missed when the patient is admitted to the hospital by the orthopedist. The reconciliation process allows the caregiver to identify the correct medications and discover those that were missed and may need to be continued, discontinued, or require special dose or frequency adjustments based on the patient's changing condition.

The comparison between ongoing and currently ordered medications is conducted in three phases: admission, transfer, and discharge. On admission reconciliation, the home medications are compared to the initial physician orders; on transfer reconciliation, the medications the patient was taking, as indicated by the previous nursing unit, are compared to the orders on the current unit, and discharge reconciliation compares all current medications taken in the hospital to those the physician orders for the patient on discharge. Any variances between the lists should be "reconciled" by the nurse or pharmacist and the physician within 4 to 24 hours, depending on the type of medication. By adding a physician signature line, this tool can also save staff time and potential transcription errors by serving as the physician order sheet.

Standardization of orders based on best known practice reduces variability based on individual clinician practices and can dramatically reduce the number of ADEs. OSF used pharmacy-based services and order sets to accomplish standardization and saw a strong reduction of ADEs. For example, to address dosing high-risk medications such as anticoagulants, a single, weight-based heparin nomogram was developed for use throughout the medical center. Additionally, both inpatient and outpatient Coumadin dosing services are offered by the pharmacy. Renal dosing services are conducted on all patients with a creatinine clearance of less than 50 mL. Development of a perioperative beta-blocker protocol has resulted in a dramatic and sustained reduction of perioperative myocardial infarctions and realized an unexpected benefit of reduced narcotic usage in patients receiving a perioperative beta-blocker.

One of the most fundamental and important changes was the availability of pharmacists on the nursing units to review and enter medication orders. This allowed pharmacists a first-hand look at the orders to identify potential dosing errors and drug interactions.

Cultural Changes

The organization had to transform its culture while creating remedies for care processes and high-risk medications. This work, while less evident, was essential to create and maintain a culture of safety that could sustain and improve safety over time. This work involved embedding safety into the very fabric of the organization, inserting safety aims into the organization's mission and corporate strategic goals, job descriptions, and meeting agenda. The transformation involved regular communication and reminders through meetings, conference calls, visits, and learning sessions. It was ever present and unrelenting.

In addition, specific changes made the importance of safety visible to frontline employees. The first change was the introduction of unit safety briefings. The staff gathers at a specified time for a five- to ten-minute review of safety concerns on the unit that day. Staff identify concerns involving equipment, medications, and care processes that pose a safety issue. The patient safety officer assigns the reported issues to the appropriate personnel for investigation and resolution. To close the communication loop, identified issues and their resolution are summarized and presented to staff monthly.

The second change was the institution of executive walkthroughs. A senior leader visited a patient care area weekly for the purpose of demonstrating commitment to safety through gathering information about the safety concerns of staff. The walkthroughs also served to educate the senior executives about the type and extent of safety issues within their organizations. The issues were logged into a database, owners were assigned for resolution, and a feedback loop to staff was established.

To measure the effect of all changes on the safety culture, a survey was conducted every six months to measure the cultural climate of the staff surrounding patient safety initiatives. The survey is a modified version of the J. Bryan Sexton/Robert Helmreich survey used by the aviation industry and NASA. Respondents include 10 percent of each hospital and medical staff. The survey is used as a tool for measuring the extent of a nonpunitive culture of reporting safety concerns and the effectiveness of safety initiatives, communication among team members, and overall teamwork.

Results

The drug-dispensing FMEA risk score was reduced by 66 percent in two years as a result of multiple action steps. Medication lists for discharged patients are retrieved hourly as pharmacy technicians make their rounds to deliver medications. Nursing unit stock medications have been reduced by 45 percent, adult IV medications have been standardized, and all non-standard doses are prepared by the pharmacy. An IV drug administration reference matrix directs dosage, guidelines, and monitoring information for nursing staff, and the pharmacist compares lab values to orders to identify potentially inappropriate dosing. Anesthesia staff have contributed to reducing potential dispensing events by assisting in standardization of epidural-safe pumps with use of colored tubing.

All of OSF's hard work has led to the following results:

- Medication reconciliation was introduced in the summer of 2001; as of May 2003, admission reconciliation usage ranged from 85 percent to 95 percent, transfer reconciliation was at 70 percent, and discharge reconciliation was at 95 percent.

- The organization completed the ordering FMEA, worked on reducing the risk at every step, and reduced its hazard vulnerability score from 157 to 103, a 34 percent reduction.

- Changes aimed at improving medication safety as well as specific interventions designed to improve the culture of safety were instituted. Culture survey results in the first year improved from a baseline score of 3.96 to 4.28 (maximum score of 5).

- The organization continues to work extremely hard at making progress every day. The proof of ultimate success comes in the form of the most important outcome, the rate of ADEs that cause patient harm. In June 2001, that rate was 5.8 per 1,000 doses dispensed; by May 2003, the rate had been reduced to 0.72 per 1,000 doses, nearly a tenfold reduction in harm.

Conclusion

Healthcare should be safer than its current state, and we, as an industry, need to push for change at a faster rate. Every day, patients are harmed by healthcare processes and systems; we can do better and have a moral obligation to do so. Within healthcare organizations, leaders must visibly demonstrate their commitment to safety and set the example for establishing a safety-conscious culture. The expectation must be set for all members of the healthcare team to work together as a true team, incorporating safe practices and awareness into daily operations. Ultimately, the goal should be for every sector of healthcare to work together toward safety: manufacturers incorporating human factors into design of medical devices, educators of healthcare providers including safety in their curricula, reporting systems and legal processes that do not assign individual blame for systems problems, and reimbursement systems that promote safe, quality care. Errors will always occur, yet many changes can be made to reduce their frequency and severity so that harm is eliminated. Healthcare has many good people working very hard to provide excellent, safe care to the patients they serve, and we should design systems and processes that enable them to do just that.

Study Questions

1. Describe how current reporting systems for medical errors and adverse events contribute to the issue of underreporting.

2. List three elements for designing safer processes and systems and provide a real example of each (preferably healthcare examples).

3. Explain why the perspective of the patient is the most important determinant as to whether an adverse event has occurred.
4. Provide an example of an error that can occur in a healthcare process and lead to patient harm. Then, describe a strategy or several strategies that would accomplish each of the following:
    a. Prevent the error from resulting in patient harm
    b. Detect the error when it occurs and before the patient is harmed
    c. Mitigate the amount of harm to the patient

REFERENCES

Blendon, R. J., C. Schoen, C. DesRoches, R. Osborn, and K. Zapert. 2003. "Common Concerns amid Diverse Systems: Health Care Experiences in Five Countries." *Health Affairs (Millwood)* 22 (3): 106–21.

Brennan, T. A., L. L. Leape, N. M. Laird, L. Herbert, A. R. Localio, A. G. Lawthers, J. P. Newhouse, P. C. Weiler, and H. H. Hiatt. 1991. "Incidence of Adverse Events and Negligence in Hospitalized Patients: Results of the Harvard Medical Practice Study I." *New England Journal of Medicine* 324: 370–76.

Findlay, S. (ed.). 2000. *Accelerating Change Today for America's Health: Reducing Medical Errors and Improving Patient Safety.* Washington, DC: National Coalition on Health Care and Institute for Healthcare Improvement.

Frankel, A., E. Graydon-Baker, C. Neppl, T. Simmonds, M. Gustafson, and T. K. Gandhi. 2003. "Patient Safety Leadership WalkRounds." *Joint Commission Journal on Quality and Safety* 29 (1): 16–26.

Gandhi, T. K., S. N. Weingart, J. Borus, A. C. Seger, J. Peterson, E. Burdick, D. L. Seger, K. Shu, F. Federico, L. L. Leape, and D. W. Bates. 2003. "Adverse Drug Events in Ambulatory Care." *New England Journal of Medicine* 348: 1556–64.

Hayward, R. A., and T. P. Hofer. 2001. "Estimating Hospital Deaths Due to Medical Errors: Preventability Is in the Eye of the Reviewer." *Journal of the American Medical Association* 286 (4): 415–20.

Institute of Medicine. 2001. *Crossing the Quality Chasm: A New Health System for the 21st Century.* Washington, DC: National Academy Press.

———. 2000. *To Err Is Human: Building a Safer Health System.* Washington, DC: National Academy Press.

Leape, L. L., D. M. Berwick, and D. W. Bates. 2002. "What Practices Will Most Improve Safety? Evidence-Based Medicine Meets Patient Safety." *Journal of the American Medical Association* 288 (4): 501–507.

McGlynn, E. A., S. M. Asch, J. Adams, J. Keesey, J. Hicks, A. DeCristofaro, and E. A. Kerr. 2003. "The Quality of Health Care Delivered to Adults in the United States." *New England Journal of Medicine* 348 (26): 2635–45.

Nolan, T. W. 2000. "System Changes to Improve Patient Safety." *British Medical Journal* 320 (March 18): 771–73.

Norman, D. A. 1988. *The Design of Everyday Things.* New York: Doubleday.

Pronovost, P., S. Berenholtz, T. Dorman, P. A. Lipsett, T. Simmonds, and C. Haraden. 2003. "Improving Communication in the ICU Using Daily Goals." *Journal of Critical Care* 18 (2): 71–75.

Reason, J. 1990. *Human Error.* New York: Cambridge University Press.

Sexton, J. B. 2002. Presented at the Institute for Healthcare Improvement National Forum.

Sexton, J. B., E. J. Thomas, and R. L. Helmreich. 2000. "Error, Stress, and Teamwork in Medicine and Aviation: Cross Sectional Surveys." *British Medical Journal* 320: 745–49.

Shojania, K. G., B. W. Duncan, K. M. McDonald, and R. M. Wachter. 2002. "Safe but Sound: Patient Safety Meets Evidence-Based Medicine." *Journal of the American Medical Association* 288 (4): 508–13.

Weick, K. E., and K. M. Sutcliffe. 2001. *Managing the Unexpected: Assuring High Performance in an Age of Complexity.* San Francisco: Jossey-Bass Publishers.

INFORMATION TECHNOLOGY APPLICATIONS FOR IMPROVED QUALITY

Richard E. Ward

Background and Terminology

This chapter introduces information technology (IT) opportunities to enhance healthcare quality. The healthcare industry simultaneously faces increased complexity, escalating economic pressure, and heightened consumerism. These three trends drive an increased interest in finding ways to improve the quality and efficiency of healthcare processes and to apply IT to meet this challenge.

Complexity

Healthcare involves the coordinated effort of multiple professionals from multiple clinical disciplines and specialties, working in multiple settings over time. This is particularly true for patients with severe illnesses and chronic diseases. As life expectancy increases and the population ages, a greater proportion of patients face severe illnesses, often complicated by multiple comorbid conditions. New scientific discoveries and medical technologies lead to constantly changing clinical processes. Furthermore, as medical knowledge grows, it becomes ever more difficult for individual clinicians to keep up with it all. There is an increasing awareness that the knowledge base of medicine is essentially unmanageable by traditional paper-based methods (Shortliffe and Perreault 1990). As a result, healthcare has become more specialized, increasing the need for interdisciplinary coordination. Quality patient care is dependent on successful management of this complexity.

Yet healthcare organizations are poorly equipped to meet the challenge of complexity. Despite the inspiring dedication of talented, highly trained healthcare professionals on an individual level, the track record of the health system collectively is poor for many basic healthcare processes. The healthcare system can be confusing to patients and clinicians alike, leading to frequent errors and suboptimal care. The literature is full of studies exposing such problems; Table 12.1 provides just a few examples.

TABLE 12.1
Examples of
Problems in
Healthcare
Delivery

Medication Errors	As new medications are developed and prescribed to patients with multiple comorbid conditions, the chance for unintended side-effects grows. Because of poor processes and systems for managing this complexity, 106,000 fatal adverse drug reactions occur each year in the United States, equivalent to a Boeing 747 crashing every other day with no survivors (Lazarou, Pomeranz, and Corey 1998). The cost of fatal and nonfatal adverse drug events is estimated at $110 billion per year.
Failure to Receive Needed Interventions	A study assessed the quality of care provided to heart failure patients discharged from an Ivy League medical center (Nohria et al. 1999). Among those who were "ideal candidates" for ACE inhibitors, drugs proven to reduce mortality and rehospitalization rates, 28% were not prescribed the drug and another 28% were receiving doses lower than those recommended in large clinical trials. In the same study, 25% did not receive dietary counseling, 17% were not educated about exercise, 91% were not instructed to track their daily weight, and 90% of the smokers had no documented advice to quit.
Poor Follow-up	A study in a large Midwestern medical group found that 17% to 32% of physicians report having no reliable method, not even a paper-based method, to make sure that the results of all tests ordered are received (Boohaker et al. 1996). One-third of physicians do not always notify patients of abnormal results. Only 23% of physicians reported having a reliable method for identifying patients overdue for follow-up. Not unexpectedly, this lack of a follow-up process causes errors. Among women with an abnormal mammogram, which requires follow-up in 4 to 6 months, 36.8% had inadequate follow-up (McCarthy et al. 1996).
Unjustified Variation in Care	Numerous studies have shown that healthcare is delivered in a highly variable manner unjustified by differences among patients. Comparing different geographical areas, rates of coronary artery bypass grafting, transurethral prostatectomy, mastectomy, and total hip replacement varied three- to five-fold across regions (Birkmeyer et al. 1998). Rates of surgical procedures for lower extremity revascularization, carotid endarterectomy, back surgery, and radical prostatectomy varied six- to tenfold across regions. This level of variation does not represent appropriate consideration of different patient situations. Rather, it demonstrates a fundamental lack of reliability and consistency in the process of implementing evidence-based best practices across the United States.

The economic consequences of healthcare processes unable to meet the challenge of increasing complexity are severe. By the late 1990s, healthcare expenditures in the United States totaled $1.1 trillion annually, representing 13.5 percent of the gross national product (Braden et al. 1998). According to a report prepared for the Senate Labor Relations Committee by the Health Care Financing Administration (now the Centers for Medicare & Medicaid Services), one-third of that cost is attributable to adverse drug reactions or other "avoidable or inappropriate care"; that represents one of every three dollars wasted.

Economic Pressure on Physicians

The economic pressure from this $1.1 trillion market is being transmitted through payers and employers to physicians and other healthcare professionals. The U.S. Congress has repeatedly passed cuts in Medicare reimbursement and failed to reverse the cuts as they wreaked havoc on the financial health of hospitals and medical groups. Private payers have followed suit, applying pressure to healthcare providers to reduce utilization and accept lower reimbursement rates. This pressure has been increasing for a long time, but it has only recently reached a sufficient intensity to motivate fundamental change. Hospitals and medical groups have already picked almost all of the "low-hanging fruit" available for cost savings. Facilities have been closed, patient copayments have been increased, and inpatient length of stay has been reduced to the point of becoming a public relations problem. Simply to maintain income, clinicians are forced to see more patients with fewer resources and do so under externally imposed rules and regulations.

At the same time reimbursement rates are falling, payers and employers are demanding evidence of improving quality and outcomes. To maintain their position on preferred physician lists and referral panels, physicians are challenged to produce data on quality, outcomes, satisfaction, utilization, and cost to prove they are offering a good value for the healthcare dollar.

However, healthcare organizations are ill prepared to respond to this pressure for accountability and economic efficiency. A few entrepreneurial clinicians have attempted to regain control of their practices by taking on financial risk in their agreements with managed care organizations, only to suffer financial losses because they were poorly equipped to manage this risk. Medical groups in competitive markets are being forced to lay off physicians or close down entirely. The groups that remain are highly motivated to find a better way.

Consumerism

In recent years, healthcare consumers have rejected a paternalistic approach to medicine and triggered a backlash against managed care. Consumers' loyalty to their doctors has declined; if their needs are not met, they complain to their elected representatives or go straight to their lawyers to sue their healthcare providers. An increasing number of states are allowing such litigation against health plans. Consumers are demanding information, choice, control, and improved service from the healthcare industry.

A report commissioned by the Kellogg Foundation found that 65 percent of healthcare consumers feel that *they* should have the most control over healthcare decisions affecting them; 31 percent say that their physicians should have the largest say, and fewer than 1 percent report that insurance companies should control decisions. However, only 22 percent report that they actually do feel in control of healthcare decisions, and only 15 percent say their physicians have control. As a result, one of three respondents characterized the healthcare system as "in critical condition" or "terminally ill."

This gap between consumer expectations and current reality is widening as consumers experience precedent-setting improvements in customer service in other industries. They are exposed to 800-number call centers, web-based e-commerce, service guarantees, and higher levels of standardization and quality in products and services in general. Healthcare providers and administrators are themselves consumers and are beginning to shake their own heads at the lag in healthcare service quality. In larger healthcare organizations, members of boards of directors are often executives in companies involved in service quality improvements. As a result, healthcare organizations are coming to understand the need to make fundamental changes in the way in which their own "product" is delivered. Healthcare organizations are now ready to make the commitment to take care process improvement concepts pursued on a pilot or demonstration basis over the past two decades and implement them on a large scale throughout their practices.

Taking a Lesson from Other Industries

The challenges of complexity, economic pressure, and heightened consumerism are not unique to healthcare. Since the 1980s, many other industries have faced similar challenges. Banking, insurance, retail, transportation, and manufacturing have all faced increased complexity from technology advancement. Many of these industries were redefined as a result of deregulation. Many faced intense economic pressures from international competition. All faced increased consumer expectations and demands.

In response, many companies in these industries turned to IT to achieve fundamental transformation of key business processes for "enterprise materials management" and "customer relationship management," revolutionizing the way they get their work done and interact with customers. These new applications enable companies to offer their customers increased access to information and services, with a higher level of customization to meet their complex, individual needs. They also enable companies to improve retention of existing customers and attract new business. At the same time, the new IT applications increase companies' capacity to serve more customers and reduce the cost of providing each service.

Internet

A number of recent technology developments have led to an explosion of interest and investment in applications to redesign materials and customer relationship management processes in other industries. The most important of these technologies is the Internet itself. The Internet provides ubiquitous information access to service providers across geographical locations and traditional organizational boundaries. The Internet also provides access directly to customers. Internet technology permits applications to be provided as a service, like telephones and cable TV, rather than as a software product that requires substantial up-front capital.

Business Process Applications

Second, sophisticated, flexible business process applications have benefited from recent improvements in the underlying technologies of database management, application integration, and workflow automation. *Workflow automation* is defined by the Workflow Management Coalition as the "computerized facilitation or automation of a business process, in whole or in part" (Hollingsworth 1995). Workflow-enabled applications offer the flexibility to create and modify workflow process definitions that describe the sequence of tasks involved in managing production and providing customer service. These process definitions are then used by a *workflow engine* that tracks and manages the delivery of services to particular customers, routing tasks and information to the right person at the right time to get the work done smoothly, efficiently, and correctly. Workflow technology is being integrated with telephone devices, web application servers, and e-mail to establish "contact centers," bringing nonhealthcare business process applications to an exciting new level.

Connectivity and Messaging

Third, connectivity and messaging standards have matured, including the common object-request broker architecture (CORBA), extensible markup language (XML), and, more recently, "web services" standards. Using such standards, business process applications can incorporate other third-party components, reducing the cost of development and maintenance.

Remarkably, the kind of business process applications widely used in other industries has so far not penetrated into the healthcare sector. The time to adapt IT tools and approaches to meet the unique needs of clinicians and patients has arrived.

The Emerging Field of Medical Informatics

Medical informatics is the scientific field that deals with the storage, retrieval, and optimal use of biomedical information, data, and knowledge for problem solving and decision making (Shortliffe and Perreault 1990). Practitioners in this field include individuals with medical training who extend their knowledge of IT and individuals who start off as IT professionals and specialize in healthcare applications. As early as 1984, a report by the Association of American Medical Colleges identified medical informatics as an area for which new educational opportunities are required and recommended the formation of new academic units in medical informatics in medical schools. The National Library of Medicine (NLM) sponsors University Medical Informatics Research Training Programs in 18 institutions throughout the United States. NLM also holds week-long training courses and offers opportunities for advanced studies. With greater opportunities for training, the supply of qualified medical informatics professionals will increase, enabling more healthcare institutions to improve their capabilities for quality management by adding medical informatics skills to the mix.

Two Tiers of Clinical IT

Almost all healthcare organizations use IT for clinical processes, and most consider clinical information systems to be of strategic importance. But different organizations have different visions and different objectives for clinical IT investments. It is helpful to consider two tiers of clinical IT: information access and care management.

IT for Information Access

The information access tier centers on a vision of IT providing "fingertip access to the right information at the right place and time." Organizations with an information access vision speak of the ultimate goal of achieving a "paperless medical record." Such organizations are seeking primarily to solve information access problems, including the following:

- Paper chart at wrong location
- Paper chart can only be used by one person at a time
- Multiple paper charts, each incomplete
- Paper chart poorly organized
- Paper summary sheets not up to date
- Paper chart takes up too much space
- Cannot easily find clinical references, practice guidelines, and patient educational material
- Too much time spent on insurance eligibility, formulary, etc.

In general, organizations focused primarily on a vision of information access are seeking to achieve incremental benefits, with modest return on investment (ROI). They are not applying IT to achieve strategic imperatives. Such an information access vision is reasonable and perhaps prudent given the long history of slow progress in clinical applications. Most of the current clinical information systems market is designed to address information access problems and even products from the newer e-health companies. But an information access vision fails to address the need for the kind of fundamental transformation of business processes that characterizes the successful use of IT in other industries.

IT for Care Management

The second tier of clinical IT, which can be described as a care management vision, seeks to use IT to enable successful continual improvements in the process of caring for individual patients and a patient population. Understanding the vision of IT for care management requires a clear definition of care management itself. On the most general level, all of healthcare can be conceptualized as a system involving two fundamentally different core processes: decision-making processes and care-delivery processes (see Figure 12.1).

Decision-making processes involve a clinician working with a patient to determine which, if any, healthcare interventions should be pursued at a given point in the patient's care. In this context, the phrase *healthcare intervention* is used broadly, encompassing everything from deciding on the components of a physical examination to deciding whether diagnostic testing or pharmaceutical or surgical treatment is needed. The output of this decision-making process is the plan of care for the patient. The care delivery process, in contrast, involves the execution of the plan of care. The results of executed interventions, in turn, affect subsequent decision making. Even the most complex clinical processes can be broken down into cycles of deciding on a plan, executing the plan, and deciding on the next plan based on the results achieved.

FIGURE 12.1
Two Core
Processes
Involving
Patients and
Clinicians

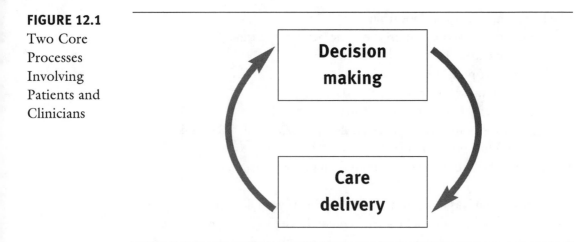

Quality is defined differently for decision-making and care-delivery processes. For decision-making processes, quality means "doing the right thing"—identifying the right alternatives and choosing the right one. For care-delivery processes, quality means "doing it right"—carrying out the plan of care without making mistakes or wasting resources. As illustrated in Figure 12.2, decision-making and care-delivery processes interact with four important care management subprocesses to form a general framework for care management.

The first important care management subprocess is *measurement*. Given organizational commitment to measurement and the appropriate set of clinical IT capabilities, data to support outcomes measurement and quality indicators can be collected as part of routine care-delivery processes. The data needed for measurement include characteristics of the patient, his or her risk factors, the medical interventions offered, and both immediate and long-term health and economic outcomes experienced by the population, including functional status, quality of life, satisfaction, and costs.

Measurements, in turn, support two other important care management subprocesses: *establishing best practices* and *performance reporting*. Best practices include practice guidelines, protocols, care maps, appropriateness criteria, credentialing requirements, and other forms of practice policies. The process of establishing best practices involves clinical policy analysis, which is supported by the scientific literature and by available outcomes information. In addition, when these two sources of information are incomplete (as they often are), expert opinion is utilized.

Recognizing that practice guidelines and other types of practice policies are meaningless unless they are used to affect clinician and patient decision making, the final important care management subprocess is *implementation*.

FIGURE 12.2
Care
Management
Process

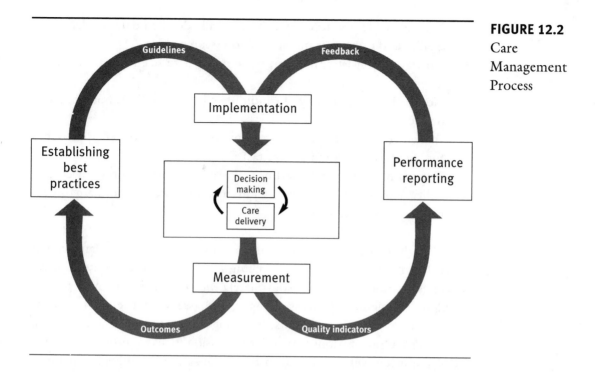

Implementation involves the use of a wide variety of methods, including clinician and patient education; various decision aids such as reminders, alerts, and prompts; and incremental improvements or more extensive reengineering of care delivery processes. A particularly important method of supporting implementation is the use of feedback of performance reporting data to clinicians, with or without associated incentives.

Since the 1980s, many healthcare organizations have attempted to implement many clinical practice improvements without the benefit of an IT infrastructure designed for that purpose. Many improvement efforts have achieved measurable success, at least on a small scale, during the time frame of the improvement project. But, in general, healthcare leaders have been disappointed at the success rate when improvements are rolled out to multiple settings. And they are disappointed in the durability of the changes. As attention turns to other processes and issues, the gains made from previous process improvements have tended to evaporate.

Organizations with a "tier two" vision seek to use IT to enable care management that is capable of large-scale, durable improvements in fundamental clinical processes, including decision-making and care-delivery processes. The care management vision involves the use of IT to solve problems such as the following:

- No affordable way to collect the clinically detailed data needed for quality and outcomes measures and research
- No way to consistently incorporate up-to-date scientific evidence into daily practice
- No feasible way to carry out multiple clinical practice improvement projects over time
- Inadequate tools to promote teamwork and "do it once" approaches for clinical and administrative tasks
- Too many intermediate parties and process steps required for care-delivery processes; documentation must be handled too many times, causing waste and errors

Healthcare organizations with a realistic vision of care management IT realize that the goal of such technology is not to directly improve processes. Instead, such technology merely *enables* efforts to identify process problems, implement process changes, and assess whether such process changes represent improvements. In other words, clinical IT is a tool, not a treatment. Organizations with a tier two vision focus on process improvement, not incentives. They focus not only on caring for individual patients presenting with medical problems but also on prevention and disease management on a population level. And they realize that different types of care processes involve different types of IT solutions.

Technologies for Different Types of Clinical Care Management Initiatives

Care management initiatives can be motivated by quality improvement, cost savings, or both (See Figure 12.3). Initiatives can be focused on simple clinical processes involving the delivery or avoidance of specific medical interventions to specific cohorts of patients. Or they can be focused on complex processes involving the coordination of many different clinicians from different disciplines to deliver a series of interventions over time. For simple processes, effective improvement methods include evidence-based guidelines, reminders, alerts, ticklers, and feedback of performance measures based on process variables (e.g., the percentage of two-year-olds who are up to date on all needed immunizations). The most important IT capabilities to support such process improvements include reminders integrated into medical records and physician order entry applications and access to an analytical data warehouse with comparative quality measures.

For more complex processes, such as managing diabetes or heart failure, typical methods include practice policies in the form of consensus-

FIGURE 12.3
Different Types of Care Management Initiatives Call for Different Methods and Technologies

	TYPES OF CARE MANAGEMENT INITIATIVES	
DRIVERS	**Simple Processes**	**Complex Processes**
Improve quality	Improve HEDIS rates • Mammography • Pap smears • Immunizations	• Improve survival rates for cancer or AIDS • Improve control of blood sugar for mild- to moderate-risk diabetics • Primary prevention of coronary artery disease events by reducing cardio-vascular risk profile
Improve quality and reduce cost	Improve HEDIS rates • Beta-blockers for patients who had heart attack	• Improve management of patients at high risk for hospital admission • High-risk asthmatics • Class III or IV heart failure • First six months after heart attack • Patients meeting "frail elderly" criteria • Discharge planning for hospitalized patients
Reduce cost	• Increase use of generic and in-formulary drugs • Avoid unneeded referrals and radiology studies • CT, MRI during first month of acute low back pain	• Attempts to attract only healthy members • Attempts to motivate physicians to order and refer less
Typical methods	• Evidence-based guidelines • Reminders, alerts, ticklers • Performance measurement with process variables	• Consensus-based algorithms and protocols • Continuing medical education • Patient education • Care managers
Enabling technologies	• Reminders integrated into medical records and ordering process • Analytical data warehouse with comparative quality measures	• Protocol-driven, team-based care supported by workflow automation technology • Outcomes data collection systems, including survey and structured documentation and access to comparative outcomes data

based algorithms, protocols, and care maps. Other methods applied to complex processes include improving the knowledge base of clinicians through continuing medical education; engaging patients in their own care through patient education; and using care managers, typically nurses, who aggressively track patient status and coordinate care for complex cases. The types of enabling technologies suitable for such complex processes include the use of workflow automation technology to support protocol-driven, team-based care (described more fully below). In addition, complex processes are best measured based on the overall outcomes achieved. Therefore, data collection systems that enable the administration of outcomes surveys to patients and structured documentation (template charting) tools that support the acquisition of data from clinicians are critical to providing the feedback loop needed to drive continual improvements in complex care processes.

Requirements and Architecture Framework for Clinical IT

According to the Institute of Medicine (IOM 2003), electronic records should support the following high-level functions:

- Physician access to patient information such as diagnoses, allergies, lab results, and medications;
- Access to new and past test results among providers in multiple care settings;
- Computerized order entry;
- Computerized decision support systems to prevent drug interactions and improve compliance with best practices;
- Secure electronic communication among providers and patients;
- Patient access to health records, disease management tools, and health information resources;
- Computerized administration processes such as scheduling systems; and
- Standards-based electronic data storage and reporting for patient safety and disease surveillance efforts.

As illustrated in Figure 12.4, most healthcare provider organizations have an existing portfolio of administrative and clinical information systems. Administrative systems include ambulatory practice management and inpatient admit/discharge/transfer systems and associated systems for appointment scheduling, registration, charge capture, patient accounting, and claims management. Additional administrative systems may include financial accounting, budgeting, cost accounting, materials management, and human resources management. Clinical systems include various applications used by clinical ancillary departments such as laboratory, radiology, and cardiology. Such systems include the capability of entering requisitions, tracking tests to completion, and capturing and communicating results.

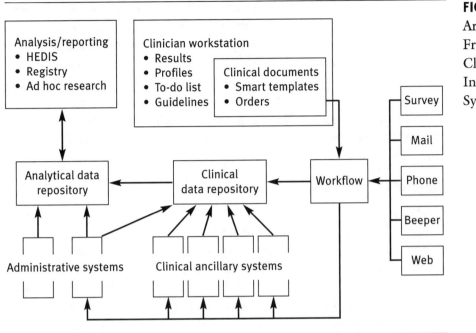

FIGURE 12.4
Architecture
Framework for
Clinical
Information
Systems

Data Repositories

Some healthcare organizations expand on this core of administrative and clinical systems by developing data repositories. *Analytical data repositories* and associated data analysis and reporting application take data primarily from administrative systems and make it available for routine and ad hoc reporting and research. Such systems go by many names, including decision support systems, data warehouses, data stores, executive information systems, and business intelligence systems. Such systems should include provisions for statistical analysis, including risk and severity adjustment, graphical analysis, and statistical modeling. Analytical data repositories are more useful if attention is paid to the quality of the data going into the repository, including the consistency of coding of procedures and diagnoses and the correct matching of all data for a single patient based on the use of an enterprisewide patient identifier or probabilistic matching algorithms.

A smaller percentage of healthcare organizations (fewer than half) have implemented *clinical data repositories* (CDRs), which take results data from various clinical ancillary systems, store the information in a database, and make the information accessible through some front-end application used by clinicians. Such systems are variously described as clinician workstations, electronic medical records, computerized patient records, and lifetime patient records. In addition to displaying results data, clinician workstation applications often enable the maintenance of patient profile information, including medical problem lists, medication lists, drug allergies, family and social history, and health risk factors such as smoking status, blood pressure, and body mass. Clinician workstations also may include a clinical to-do list, secure clinical messaging, and access to online medical reference materials such as internal practice guidelines, the hospital or health plan formulary, scientific articles indexed in MEDLINE, the *Physicians' Desk Reference*, and a collection of medical textbooks.

Template Charting

A small percentage of clinicians have access to an important feature of advanced clinician workstations, template charting. *Template charting* can be defined as the acquisition of unstructured and structured data as a single process carried out by a clinician during or immediately following a patient encounter to provide medical record documentation while simultaneously supporting other data needs such as billing, research and quality, and outcomes measurement. Template charting applications are also known as clinical documentation, note-writing, or charting applications. They permit a clinician to efficiently create clinical notes by incorporating material from previously prepared templates and then modifying the note as needed for a patient. Templates not only speed up the documentation process but also serve to remind the clinician of the data items that should be included, leading to more complete and standardized notes. Such notes are not only better for patient care but also produce as a by-product computer-readable, analyzable data that can be used for orders, requisitions, referrals, prescriptions, and billing.

More complete documentation can indirectly lead to increased revenue by supporting higher-level encounter and management (E&M) codes, leading to higher reimbursement for clinical visits. More complete structured documentation can provide the data inputs for clinical alerts, reminders, and order critique features. For example, by documenting drug history, drug allergies, and body mass, the system can analyze a new drug added to the plan of care for a clinic visit to determine whether it interacts with other drugs the patient is taking, whether the patient is allergic to the drug, whether the dose is inappropriate given the body mass, and whether there are other drugs that are more cost effective or in greater compliance with hospital or health plan formulary policy. Finally, more complete notes based on structured data can be used to support clinical research, quality assurance, and outcomes measurement, enabling evidence-based clinical process improvement.

As noted above, template charting applications are used to acquire both unstructured and structured data. Unstructured data include text from handwritten notes (incorporated into a computerized patient record through document imaging) or captured through voice dictation (followed by manual transcription or electronic voice recognition). Unstructured data can also take the form of clinical diagrams such as a diagram showing the anatomic location of a breast lump or distribution of low back pain. In contrast, structured data are captured as a number or code that is computer readable. Structured data include procedure codes, diagnosis codes, vital signs, and many physiologic parameters such as range of motion of a joint or visual acuity. Structured data also may include outcomes survey data collected from patients or clinicians.

A fundamental tradeoff must be made between the quantity and quality of structured data that can be collected (see Figure 12.5). This is true because of a limited tolerance by physicians to being "fenced in" by template charting systems that seem to keep them from expressing themselves as they wish. In practice, clinicians who use systems that attempt to capture the entire clinical note as structured data express frustration and demand that the structure of the data be loose. In this context, *loose* structure means that the system cannot demand that specific data elements be provided. Therefore, the resulting structured note represents a collection of computer-readable facts for aspects of the patient encounter the clinician thought to document, with no data on a large number of other aspects that were documented for other patients but not this one. Such a loose form of structured data is analogous to a database table with a large number of fields but mostly missing values.

On the other hand, more tightly structured data are characterized by rigorous, complete collection of data for a specified collection of data elements. In practice, clinicians using template charting applications that include tightly structured data tend to be unwilling to use the system unless the required data elements are kept to a small number for which the short-term utility is clear. Experts in medical vocabulary have traditionally advocated the use of standardized vocabulary for as much of the chart as possible, reasoning that whatever is collected using standardized codes can be pooled with data from a great number of patients and analyzed, and that the resulting large sample size will lead to conclusive results. But biostatisticians, epidemiologists, and health services researchers know that missing values severely limit the usefulness of data sets in ways not corrected by large sample sizes.

This insight applies not only to population research studies but also to the use of the data for more immediate purposes to drive reminders, alerts, and other decision aids. The logic rules used for such decision aids

FIGURE 12.5
Template
Charting
Tradeoff:
Quantity
Versus Quality
of Structured
Data

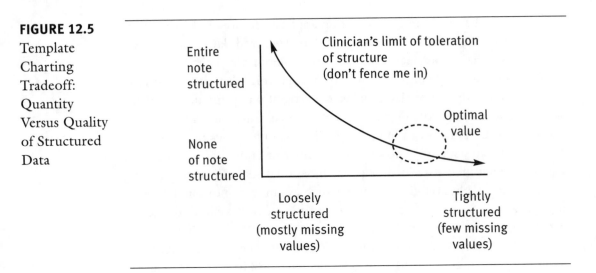

tend to require complete data for a small number of variables and often cannot be reliably applied when data inputs have missing values. Therefore, complete data are needed for both research and decision aids, two of the most important tools for clinical practice improvement. The philosophy should be to "start with the end in mind," defining the use of the data first, then characterizing the requirements of the data, and finally designing a data acquisition approach to meet those requirements. Therefore, when selecting a template charting approach, it is usually preferable to seek a solution that emphasizes the tight structuring of specified data elements rather than a loosely structured model.

Template charting applications also may include integrated decision support. By creating templates of orders that represent standing order sets, healthcare organizations can increase the standardization of testing and treatment. For example, a postoperative order set can help busy surgeons consistently remember all the services that should be at least considered for ordering after every surgical procedure. In addition, "smart templates" can incorporate clinical logic to conditionally include or exclude items within templates. For example, in a medical history template, gynecological history items may be automatically excluded from templates for men, and an order for a screening mammogram may be automatically offered in the template applied to a note for a woman who needs a mammogram. Finally, template charting applications are especially powerful if they are linked to reminders, alerts, and order critique rules that are processed immediately. For example, if a drug is included in the plan of care and the patient is allergic to the drug, the template charting application may alert the clinician by making that drug item display appear in red or displaying an appropriate alert message. In this manner, template charting can reduce medical errors.

Such examples also illustrate the importance of the functional integration of template charting applications and order entry applications. Many healthcare organizations fail to recognize this issue and implement separate applications with separate user interfaces for capturing unstructured clinical notes using dictation and for capturing orders. Many even implement separate devices for different kinds of orders. For example, many organizations use hand-held personal digital assistant devices for capturing prescriptions (drug orders) while using a full-sized computer for capturing laboratory or radiology orders. This approach offers important short-term benefits, including reductions in medication errors, but it may run the risk of being short sighted if the long-term goal is to completely integrate the process of developing a plan of care into the process of creating a clinical note.

Workflow Automation Technology Applied to Clinical Processes

As shown in Figure 12.4, a general framework for clinical IT to support clinical practice improvement includes a role for *workflow automation technology*. Workflow systems generally provide a capability for entering workflow specification data describing the sequence of tasks or activities in a work process, resources required to execute each task, and data needed to manage the flow of activities and execute each task. Workflow systems also generally include a component that manages the execution of individual workflows, such as a workflow to track the execution of a single medical order. This component is variously known as a workflow engine, workflow automation server, or workflow enactment service. This component tracks the status of each workflow, determines what task is needed next, determines what human or system resources to marshal to execute the task, and communicates with those resources to transport the needed data to and from the resources. In these systems, a workflow assessment is generally initiated by completing a computer-based form that provides the data needed to get the workflow started.

Improvements in Processes of Care

Workflow systems increase the efficiency of service delivery because they route the right task to the right person or machine at the right time. They increase the consistency and quality of service delivery because they track work according to workflow specifications that can define best practices.

They also increase the reliability of services because bottlenecks and errors can be identified and managed. Some workflow systems provide a generic framework that can be adapted to a wide variety of service-delivery processes.

In the context of healthcare, workflow automation provides the ability to encapsulate other ITs and services and make them available for incorporation into processes of care. Such services may include survey services; outbound recorded telephone messages; outbound e-mail messages; printing and mailing of generic or tailored educational materials; outbound fax; electronic pager or short-text messaging service; and requests for third-party services such as telemonitoring, care management, and disease management programs. Clinical workflow systems can also provide an interface to insurance eligibility and preauthorization transactions and to ancillary departmental systems for orders and order status checking.

Improvements in Change Management

Workflow automation technology offers the promise of improving teamwork and coordination across the continuum of care, including clinicians in different clinic locations, inpatient facilities, ancillary service providers, home health care, call centers, and other settings. It promises to coordinate care over time, ensuring the follow-up with each needed test or treatment and ensuring that a sequence of healthcare interventions happens consistent with a predetermined clinical protocol or care map. Workflow automation also enables clinicians to take charge of cycles of process improvement because it provides tools to permit changes to workflow specifications without always requiring changes to software. As a result, a team of clinicians can make a decision about a clinical process change and implement the change in the workflow system without having to go through a difficult process of writing proposals, obtaining capital funding, and waiting until the change makes it to the top of the priority list for overcommitted programmers.

When even small changes in care processes require navigating frustrating capital and IT development processes, clinicians leading such changes often resort to non-IT methods for implementing changes. They utilize racks of paper forms, rubber stamps, guidelines printed on pocket cards, signs taped to exam room walls, symbols marked on white-boards, decks of cards serving as tickler files, and various other low-tech alternatives. These approaches may prove effective in the short term at the local setting, but they tend to break down over time and at different locations, resulting in medical errors. By reducing the burden of making process changes that are scalable and durable, clinical workflow automation technology promises to be a powerful tool for reducing medical errors and improving the efficiency and quality of clinical processes.

Other Clinical IT Components

Telemedicine

In large, geographically distributed healthcare organizations, *telemedicine* capabilities allow clinicians to care for patients in remote locations. Such capabilities include a variety of technologies, such as multimedia telecommunications (e.g., video conferencing), to allow clinicians to interact with patients or other clinicians. Remote sensors allow physicians to extend their ability to observe patients. For example, in a home setting, remote sensors may include devices to capture and communicate body weight, blood glucose, peak expiratory flow, or pill count administered. In a clinic setting, a remote sensor can provide the capabilities of a stethoscope or ophthalmoscope. In the inpatient or intensive care setting, remote sensors allow the real-time viewing of vital signs, ECG tracings, ventilator outputs, and data from other devices. Finally, digital radiology allows radiographical images to be communicated remotely for interpretation by experts in another setting.

Rules Servers

Sophisticated clinical information systems include one or more *rules server* components used to apply clinical logic to healthcare data. These components are described using a variety of terms such as inference processors, expert systems, artificial intelligence, knowledge-based systems, smart systems, real-time decision support, and various combinations of these terms such as network-based real-time rule servers. In general, the role of such components is to increase the performance and decrease the maintenance cost of applying clinical logic as part of various features of a clinical information system. Such rules servers improve response-time performance by placing logic processing in close proximity to the clinical database and using high-powered processors optimized for such mathematical calculations. Rules servers decrease maintenance cost by avoiding the "hard coding" of clinical logic throughout many different applications and providing a single tool and a single syntax for creating, maintaining, and protecting clinical logic. By improving the standardization of the syntax used to represent clinical rules, such rules can be more easily shared across different parts of a healthcare organization or even across healthcare organizations. In this manner, centralized rule processors can help healthcare organizations treat their clinical logic as valuable intellectual property to be protected and leveraged.

Although inference processing may seem like an esoteric function, it is surprisingly ubiquitous within clinical information systems. For example, to load data into a CDR, an "integration engine" component is often employed that includes logic for routing data, reformatting and transforming data, and determining how data are to be inserted into database tables. In clinician workstation applications, clinical logic is applied to displaying abnormal values and intelligent summarization of clinical data for specific medical problems. In template charting, rules are applied to support "smart template" features that determine when specific parts of templates are to be included or activated.

Clinical Vocabulary Servers

Another important component of sophisticated clinical information systems is a *clinical vocabulary server*. Such a component, also known as a "lexical mediation" component, is responsible for translating codes, terms, and concepts to permit processing of rules. For example, in a centralized rules server, rules are best stated in terms of standard medical concepts, even though these rules may act on data collected using many different nonstandard codes. Vocabulary servers can be conceptualized as a special kind of rules server that applies rules that determine how nonstandard codes relate to standardized concepts and how standard concepts relate to each other. For example, the International Classification of Disease (ICD)-9 diagnosis code 864.12 corresponds to "Minor laceration of liver with open wound into abdominal cavity." A vocabulary server will help figure out that this same condition is represented in the Systematized Nomenclature of Medicine (SNOMED) vocabulary as DD-23522. In rule processing applications, it is also helpful to understand that this specific clinical concept is part of a more general concept of "laceration of liver," represented in ICD-9 as 864.05 and in SNOMED as DD-23502. Such logic is a prerequisite to a rule that might suggest an appropriate diagnostic algorithm for evaluating suspected laceration of the liver.

Vocabulary servers are included as part of the infrastructure of clinical software suites and also offered by some vendors as stand-alone components. A good vocabulary server includes up-to-date content regarding various standardized code sets for clinical use, such as the Logical Observation Identifiers Names and Codes and SNOMED. Such a vocabulary server will also offer standardized codes for administrative uses, such as ICD, Current Procedural Terminology, and National Drug Codes. A good clinical vocabulary offers concepts at a level of granularity that is specific enough to support clinical decision rules, but also practical for use by busy clinicians. A vocabulary server should provide a classification hierarchy to facilitate searching for terms and handling generalization, and it should be supported by routine maintenance and timely updates to keep current with continuously changing vocabulary.

Patient Surveys

A complete clinical information system designed to support clinical practice improvement should also include patient survey components to facilitate the acquisition of data directly from patients. A variety of technologies and methods are used for this purpose, including the following:

- Preprinted paper-based surveys or tailored surveys printed at the point of care (with subsequent data capture through manual data entry, scanning, or optical mark reading);
- Fax-based survey systems;
- Systems that allow a patient to directly enter information in a clinical facility using a touch screen or hand-held device;
- Web-based survey applications that allow a patient to enter data from home; and
- Telephone-based interactive voice response systems that utilize touch-tone entry or voice-recognition technology.

Evaluation of Systems

Important features to consider in evaluating such systems include the portability to deliver surveys to the patient at home, in a clinic waiting room, or in a hospital bed. Ideal systems reduce the risk of loss or breakage of valuable equipment. Survey systems should be suitable to deal with patient limitations, such as by offering larger type size for patients with poor eyesight, offering voice or pictures for patients who cannot read, and offering translations or pictures for patients who do not speak the predominant language. Patient survey systems should be adaptable to meet the changing needs of the healthcare organization, such as by permitting local customization of surveys to meet internal needs without requiring programming. They should ideally reduce the burden of patient data entry, such as by offering automated patient-level customization of surveys to avoid unneeded or duplicate questions and by offering branching logic for surveys with items that do not apply to all patients. Finally, good patient survey systems allow the flow of information to be bidirectional, permitting patient education to be combined with data acquisition. For example, "shared decision making" systems combine interactive video technology to educate patients about the pros and cons of alternative treatment options while simultaneously collecting data needed to assess the patient's comprehension of the information, document the patient's utilities and preferences, and collect additional data items needed to support patient care and research.

Study Management Capabilities

To support outcomes research and clinical research that are essential to implementing a care management vision of clinical information systems, such systems should also include study management capabilities. Study management systems handle the processes of identifying patients eligible for enrollment in a study, handle enrollment and disenrollment of patients into one or more study protocols, and determine which study subjects need which data collection forms at any given point in time. A good study management system should be able to handle multiple study protocols as a single process and track the status of data collection forms through the entire lifecycle to a final disposition. Such a process of administering data collection instruments should integrate with patient survey systems (described above) and facilitate the details of printing needed forms; cover letters and mailing labels for mailed surveys; reminder letters for overdue surveys; and referring physician letters, chart notes, and other reports based on completed surveys. Such systems should also facilitate the process of preparing the data to be analyzed or sent to an external research center for incorporation into a multi-institutional database. This type of data pooling process requires the ability to produce appropriately formatted data files for transmission to the data center, checking of data integrity, and acceptance of feedback regarding rejected records.

Such study management capabilities can take the form of a separate application dedicated to this purpose, leading to efficiencies in managing outcomes research and clinical studies. However, such an approach is inconsistent with the overall vision of tier two clinical information systems to support care management. The kinds of capabilities that are part of a study management system—identifying patients who need a service, tracking the delivery of the service to completion, collecting the structured data needed to support the goals of the process—are the same fundamental capabilities needed for clinical decision making and care delivery. The additional requirements of outcomes research and clinical studies should be seamlessly integrated into the routine clinical processes, enabling the healthcare organization to learn and innovate as a by-product of caring for patients. Such a vision has been clearly articulated and incorporated into the strategic plans of only a fraction of healthcare organizations, and it has been achieved in a frustratingly small number of settings.

Data Analysis and Reporting Capabilities

A complete clinical information system should also provide data analysis and reporting capabilities. Data analysis tools should not only support the needs of statisticians and data analysis professionals but should also provide "canned" graphical and tabular analysis of outcomes of populations of patients for healthcare leaders and other occasional users. Such tools may also provide predictions and formatted reports for individual patients to support informed medical decision making.

Case Examples

Flu Immunization Reminder Letters

One example of the use of IT to drive improvement in a simple care process involves a project to increase compliance with guidelines for adult influenza immunization at a large integrated delivery system in the Midwest. In the project, the team utilized IT along with other approaches to guide implementation, including staff training, patient education, and continuous quality improvement methods.

To increase the knowledge of the medical staff, the team created and disseminated a memorandum describing the flu guideline and included the guideline in a preventive services handbook printed as a soft-cover book designed to fit into labcoat pockets. The team also incorporated the flu guideline into a course on preventive services in its "managed care college" program, a continuing medical education program involving about 85 staff members in a series of lectures and mentored improvement projects. The team increased patients' knowledge by including an article about flu immunization in the magazine distributed by the organization's health maintenance organization and by commissioning a poster and tent cards featuring a cartoon character explaining the benefits of flu immunization to be deployed in clinic locations.

The team developed institution- and physician-level performance measures based on analysis of billing data present in the analytical data repository. The team conducted a small-scale study to validate the measures by calling a random sample of patients and asking them about flu immunizations that they received within the clinic and in other community locations such as churches, shopping malls, or senior centers. They found that 15 percent to 20 percent of all immunizations administered were through locations outside the scope of the billing data of the organization. Therefore, a decision was made to use the institutional performance measure as a way to measure improvement over time or compare performance of interventions to increase performance. But the team decided to forego dissemination of physician-level performance measures to avoid subjecting the overall performance measurement program to criticism because of inclusion of a measure known to be biased in the pessimistic direction.

The team then implemented Saturday Flu Shot Clinics during the flu season, placing the clinics close to lobby entrances to create the quickest possible visit for patients. To support these clinics, an analysis of the analytical data repository was done to prepare reports listing which patients were known to have received the immunization before, the date of service, and the patient's primary care physician. Finally, to encourage patients to seek out flu shots, computer-generated reminders were created. To evaluate the effectiveness and cost effectiveness of such reminders, a randomized trial was conducted; 24,743 patients were assigned to one of three interventions and a control group receiving only the benefit of other aspects of the flu shot improvement program described above. The intervention arms of the trial included (1) a generic, untailored postcard; (2) a postcard with a tailored message; and (3) an automatically generated tailored letter from the patient's primary care physician, mentioning risk factors present in the patient's records that put him or her in a risk category requiring a flu shot.

As shown in Figure 12.6, there was a dose-response relationship, with the expected increases in performance as additional features of the reminder were added. Overall, the tailored letter increased compliance with flu shots by about 5 percentage points. Although this may seem like a small increase, it represents an important improvement on a population level. The letters cost $0.42 to produce and send using an outside service with expertise in mass mailing. The vaccine itself cost $4.09. According to studies published elsewhere, the expected annual hospital cost for influenza is reduced from $355 to $215 when patients receive flu shots. Based on the size of the population for this institution and the prevalence of influenza, a cost-effectiveness model calculated the net savings to be $118,000 in a nonepidemic year and $268,000 in an epidemic year. Furthermore, the program was thought to have achieved additional noneconomic benefits to the organization in the form of satisfaction by patients with the attentiveness of their primary care provider and the organization in general to their personal health needs.

Diabetes Care Management

An example of IT applied to complex care processes is the use of a web-based population management tool to support the management of diabetes (Baker et al. 2001). As with the flu immunization project described above, the diabetes care management team used a multimodality approach to improving diabetes care. The team created a practice guideline for various diabetes-related interventions and made this available in paper form and through a link from an intranet diabetes care management application. This application was accessible through a web browser anywhere within the organization and could be reached through a link included as a pull-down menu within the main window of the clinician workstation application. In

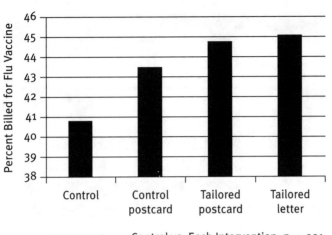

FIGURE 12.6
Results of
Randomized
Trial of
Alternative
Reminders
for Adult
Influenza
Immunization

addition to displaying the diabetes practice guideline, this care management application also offered the ability to view statistics describing the characteristics of the diabetes patient population for an individual care provider, a local clinic setting, or larger aggregations such as region and institutionwide (see Figure 12.7).

The care management application also offered a diabetes patient registry including the ability to generate lists of diabetes patients. These registry lists take the form of a grid with rows for each diabetes patient and columns displaying key variables related to diabetes care, including the date and value of the last glycated hemoglobin (HbA1c) test, whether the patient received two HbA1c tests during last year, whether the patient received a dilated eye exam during the last year, the date of the last eye exam, whether the patient received a microalbumin test during the last year, and the date and values of the last lipid profile test, including total cholesterol, LDL ("bad") cholesterol, and triglycerides. This care management application allowed the clinical staff to view a preliminary risk stratification, generating lists of patients who require diabetic services such as a primary care visit, HbA1c testing, and eye exams. These lists included patient contact information, making them more actionable.

The application also serves to provide practice feedback and comparative benchmarking. Feedback is presented in the form of graphs showing the percentage of patients who had good, intermediate, or poor control of blood glucose (as indicated by average HbA1c test results), comparing an individual care provider, the average for the local practice setting, and wider regional, institutional, or national averages. Other graphs show the trend line of the percentage of the diabetic patient panel that received needed diabetes services or is in good blood glucose control.

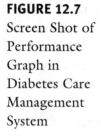

FIGURE 12.7

Screen Shot of
Performance
Graph in
Diabetes Care
Management
System

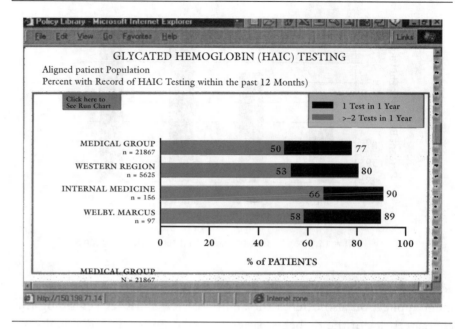

An evaluation of the diabetes care management application revealed
that the during the first year of use, 29 percent of primary care physicians
initiated a session; these physicians used the system an average of eight
times. More important, nonphysician staff from 94 percent of the primary
care clinics initiated at least one session, averaging 30 sessions per year. A
statistical model was developed to evaluate the effect of the system on
guideline performance related to 13,325 diabetes patients, controlling for
patient sociodemographic and clinical characteristics and the testing history of the patient, primary care physician, and primary care clinic. As a
result of using the system, compliance with diabetes practice guidelines
improved. Among physicians who used the system at least eight times, their
patients were 17 percent more likely to get two HbA1c tests, 12 percent
more likely to get a cholesterol test, and 4 percent more likely to get a reti-
nal exam. Among clinics that had staff use the system at least 30 times,
their patients were 34 percent more likely to get two HbA1c tests.

The diabetes care management team applied the knowledge gained
from evaluating the first-generation improvement program to drive the
next cycle of improvements. From the evaluation, the team learned that
10 percent of diabetes patients were not seen in the clinic during the prior
12 months. Therefore, the team concluded that an outreach intervention

was needed to engage patients in their care. Subsequently, the team implemented computer-generated, tailored letters from primary care physicians to the diabetes patients not seen in the clinic. The team also learned in the evaluation that 50 percent of the patients seen in the clinic during the prior 12 months did not receive needed tests and exams. Therefore, the team developed a system using workflow automation technology to track receipt of diabetes-related tests (along with a number of preventive services) and prompt the clinician for needed services. This reminder system was incorporated into the user interface for the clinician workstation and provided clinicians with a health maintenance report to track diabetes (and other) interventions and remind them of due dates.

Overall Return on Investment of Clinical Information Systems

To assess the effect of various clinical IT investments on cost savings and revenue enhancement, an ROI model was developed. The model includes assumptions based on a review of the literature for studies providing evidence of cost savings or revenue enhancement, including MEDLINE, vendor materials, and analyses published by IT consultants. Each of the identified benefits was categorized and associated with a functional area that corresponded to the type of IT investment (see Table 12.2).

Assumptions were made based on institution-specific input regarding such variables as personnel costs, costs of software and associated implementation, volume of activity, and payer mix. For each assumption, an unbiased best estimate was made, along with a range of uncertainty bounded by pessimistic and optimistic estimates. In addition, for each calculated cost or revenue effect, an assessment of the strength of evidence was assigned, judging both general and institution-specific assumptions underlying the estimated effect. This strength-of-evidence assessment was coded as strong evidence, medium evidence, poor evidence, and educated opinion.

The results of the model are highly dependent on institution-specific variables. For example, the bottom-line impact of using disease management to reduce the rate of hospitalization is to reduce revenue in fee-for-service patients and reduce cost in globally capitated patients. Therefore, the same effect has a dramatically different financial effect depending on payer mix. The model is highly sensitive to other institution-specific variables such as assumed speed of implementation, order in which functional areas are implemented, and compensation levels of different types of personnel. Nevertheless, the following model results for a hypothetical healthcare organization are included to illustrate the general struc-

TABLE 12.2
Clinical IT
Benefit
Categories
and
Associated
Functional
Areas

Benefit Category	Functional Area
Information access	Clinical data repository
Improve decision making	Physician ordering with alerts
Information capture	Clinical documentation
Improve process	Workflow automation and disease management
Improve market share*	Patient/community access

* No literature measuring market share outcomes of clinical systems offering patient/community access was identified, so this functional area was not included in this generation of the ROI analysis.

ture of such ROI calculations and provide a high-level prospective on the relative benefits of different clinical IT investments and the sensitivity of the estimates to the desired threshold for evidence.

The hypothetical healthcare organization has 300 physicians across all specialties, a teaching hospital, and a payer mix that includes 50 percent capitation. The model assumes a six-year implementation period, beginning with implementation of a CDR, followed by implementation of physician ordering, clinical documentation, and, finally, workflow automation and disease management (see Figure 12.8).

As shown in Figure 12.9, the "uptake" of the clinical information system components by clinicians and other personnel is assumed to take some time following the initial implementation of the component, such that full utilization of all components is expected to take a total of ten years.

Clinical information systems may have a large number of different effects on the net income of a healthcare organization (see Table 12.3). The largest-magnitude effects, based on the assumptions used for this hypothetical organization, are increased revenue from enabling clinicians to see more outpatients and having high-quality documentation capable of supporting higher E&M billing codes, and cost savings in the population of capitated patients resulting from disease management interventions and efforts to reduce unneeded utilization of pharmaceuticals and laboratory tests. Note that the different effects have different levels of evidence supporting them. One large category of benefit is the $7.5 million net income effect (net of revenue losses from fee-for-service inpatients) of reducing unnecessary inpatient utilization of lab and pharmacy services. The University of Indiana, Regenstreif, had similar-magnitude

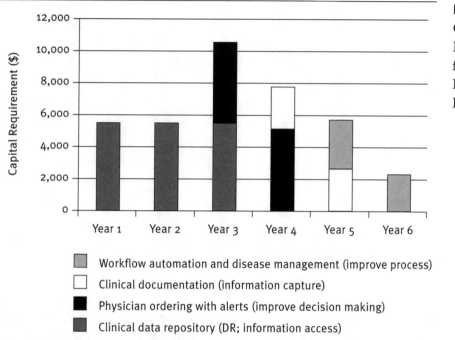

FIGURE 12.8

Capital Requirement for Hypothetical Institution

Legend:
- Workflow automation and disease management (improve process)
- Clinical documentation (information capture)
- Physician ordering with alerts (improve decision making)
- Clinical data repository (DR; information access)

effects across all categories of inpatient charges (not assumed for this model). If true, that would increase the effect from 2.3 percent to 13 percent of inpatient net revenue, creating an additional $29 million benefit for the hypothetical institution.

The overall annual effect on the healthcare organization's bottom line (net income) ranges from just over $20 million to almost $70 million, depending on whether the decision maker demands the best evidence before considering a specific cost or revenue effect to be trustworthy or whether less-certain effects are considered and counted (see Figure 12.10). The best evidence is available for certain categories of benefits, particularly related to order entry and clinical documentation. Intermediate quality of evidence is available for various categories of benefits related to the use of a CDR.

The literature includes many studies documenting dramatic benefits from disease management interventions, including many using supportive IT. Most such studies focus on common conditions such as asthma, congestive heart failure, and diabetes. But there is little evidence of the effect of implementation of disease management approaches more broadly across a larger number of clinical conditions. Furthermore, few studies directly assess the contribution of clinical information systems to disease manage-

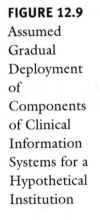

FIGURE 12.9
Assumed
Gradual
Deployment
of
Components
of Clinical
Information
Systems for a
Hypothetical
Institution

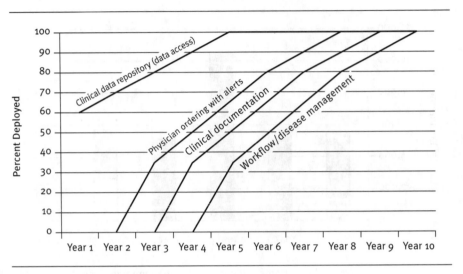

ment effectiveness. Such a study would attempt to compare the same disease management approach in settings with and without various supporting IT capabilities and track the effect over a long enough period to determine when the manual processes may begin to break down as the initial enthusiasm over a new disease management process wanes and staff turn their attention to other priorities. Over longer periods, disease management processes that are seamlessly incorporated into clinical information systems seem likely to suffer less breakdown. But such comparative studies have not been done, so this model rates evidence of disease management effects of clinical IT investments as being supported by educated opinion only. The magnitude of benefits from disease management capabilities also is highly dependent on the assumed proportion of patients for whom reimbursement is based on capitation or disease-specific subcapitation arrangements. In settings where reimbursement is predominantly fee-for-service, disease management interventions—usually uncompensated—have the effect of reducing the need for subsequent care. In such settings, disease management leads to increased cost and decreased revenue.

Figure 12.11 shows that the calculated ROI over a ten-year period ranges from extremely favorable (2,372 percent) to negative (–107 percent), depending on the range of uncertainty (from pessimistic to optimistic) and degree of evidence required to count a specific effect. This underscores the need for more rigorous clinical trials and effectiveness studies of clinical information system components and the importance of careful collection of institution-specific data to support ROI calculations needed for planning and investment decision making.

Source of Change in Net Income	Change in Net Income at Full Implementation (thousands)
Revenue from improved visit capacity	18,445
Disease management—all diseases other than CHF, asthma, diabetes	14,331
Decrease in down-coding behavior for E&M coding	12,726
CHF disease management in clinic	4,278
Reduced unnecessary inpatient lab utilization	4,050
Reduced unnecessary inpatient drug utilization	3,403
Diabetes disease management	2,373
Quicker prescription refill by clinic nurses	1,913
Increased claims acceptance from improved coding	1,818
Reduced need for transcription	1,521
Reduced preventable adverse drug events	1,511
More efficient NP/RN/clerical support task allocation	1,316
Decreased lost charges from improved coding	1,260
Quicker information access by clinic nurses	918
Reduced inpatient lab utilization for fee-for-service patients	668
Reduced need for chart pulls	600
Reduced inpatient drug utilization for fee-for-service patients	561
Asthma disease management in emergency room	515
Quicker visit prep (support staff)	426
Reduced need for lab result filing	108
Reduced need for medical record supplies	40
Reduced need for chart copies	0
Reduced outpatient drug utilization for capitated patients	?
Outsourcing enabled by workflow tools	?
Decreased encounter prep errors	?
Physician-to-RN/PA/NP task allocation	?
Savings from demand management of capitated patients	?
Revenue from new patients	?

TABLE 12.3
Net Income Effects of Clinical IT Investments in a Hypothetical Healthcare Organization, Assuming Lowest Threshold of Evidence

Note: CHF = congestive heart failure; ? = insufficient information to estimate.

FIGURE 12.10

Net Income Effect of Different Clinical Information System Investments for Different Thresholds for Required Strength of Evidence

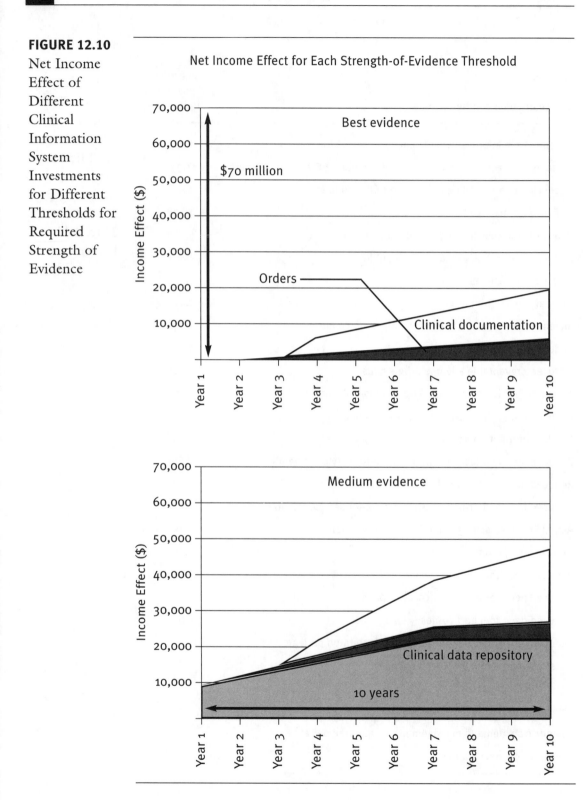

Net Income Effect for Each Strength-of-Evidence Threshold

FIGURE 12.10
(continued)

Net Income Effect for Each Strength-of-Evidence Threshold

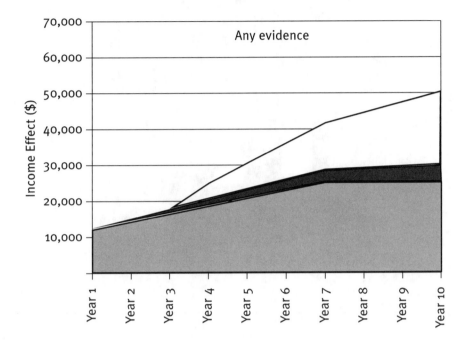

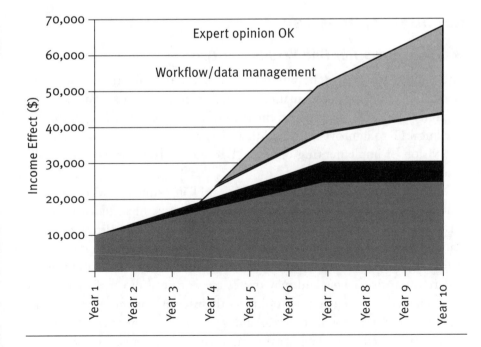

FIGURE 12.11
ROI for
Clinical
Information
Systems
Investments in
Hypothetical
Institution
Varies Based
on Standard of
Evidence and
Degree of
Optimism of
Estimating
Assumptions

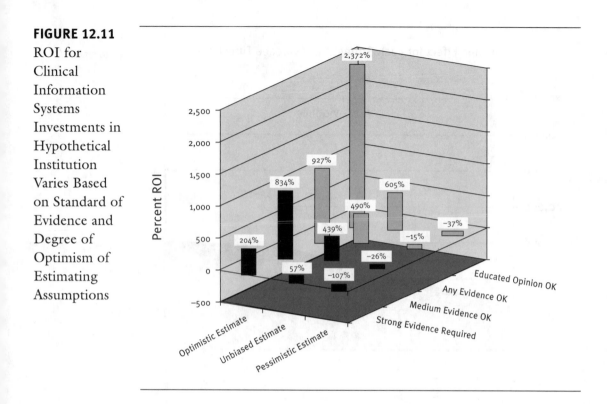

Key Strategy Debates

Waiting Versus Tier One Versus Tier Two

The biggest strategic debate within healthcare organizations regarding investments in clinical information systems is between those who want to minimize clinical IT investment, those who want to pursue a tier one vision of clinical IT to improve information access, and those who advocate a tier two vision of implementing clinical IT to enable transformation of care management processes.

The argument for minimizing clinical IT investment rests on the fact that such investments are not proven to be effective in sufficiently rigorous studies, and, more important, the low proportion of healthcare organizations that have already implemented clinical IT on a large scale is evidence that such investments are not yet sufficiently mainstream. Healthcare leaders are often risk averse and may prefer to wait until most of their peers have pursued a strategy before doing so themselves. Furthermore, declining revenue, poor capital reserves, and a long list of other priorities competing for limited funds support the argument to wait longer on large-scale clinical IT investments.

The argument for pursuing a tier one information access vision is largely based on a "walk before you run" philosophy and on the realization that the CDR components at the heart of the information access vision are also prerequisites to more ambitious tier two care management strategies. The arguments for information access are the easiest to articulate, require the least amount of potentially controversial process changes by clinicians, and can be implemented by IT staff who do not necessarily need to understand the details of clinical processes and methods of clinical practice improvement. Finally, the community of IT vendors has developed products with features that primarily focus on the information access vision, so the majority of peer references from institutions that have pursued clinical IT investments focus on a tier one vision.

The argument for pursuing a tier two care management vision is that the potential for gaining sustainable competitive advantage for the organization is greatest in this area. Rather than worrying that clinical IT might *require* process changes by clinicians, advocates of the care management vision describe a proactive goal of *enabling* process changes by clinicians. They point out that process improvement is the whole point of deployment of IT in other industries and that evidence-based improvement in clinical processes is consistent with the mission and vision of healthcare institutions and with the professionalism of clinicians. The vision for clinical IT investments to support care management is often best articulated by clinical leaders because it requires the ability to understand and describe clinical decision-making and care processes and the methods of biomedical research and quality improvement. Proponents of this tier two vision are most successful in competitive markets, especially those with active, vocal, and organized purchasers and consumers—including business coalitions, local payers, and patient/consumer advocates. In such markets, the need to make changes to create a noticeably different experience for patients and decrease waste and cost is top in the minds of leaders and a greater sense of urgency exists.

Balancing the Needs of Clinicians and the Organization

When making decisions about tier one or two clinical information systems investments, a balance must be struck between the goals of healthcare organizations making the financial investment and the goals of the individual clinician users making the investment in process change and learning to use new systems.

The organization balances between costs and benefits to the organization, whereas the clinician balances between the benefit to the user and burden of use (see Figure 12.12). Organizational costs include not only the cost of software and hardware but also other costs such as the disruption

FIGURE 12.12

Model for
Balancing
Organizational
and Clinician
Needs

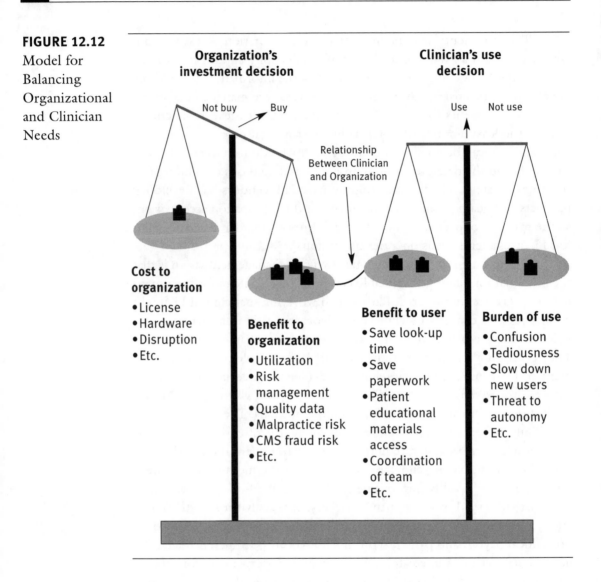

that implementing new systems and processes causes within facilities. The
organizational benefits include better management of utilization, cost, risk,
and quality. On the clinician side, user benefits include time savings and
improvements in coordination and effectiveness of care, whereas the burden of use includes confusion, tediousness, and decreased productivity during the learning process, as well as a more general concern that using systems
that structure documentation and integrate practice guidelines and protocols may erode the sense of autonomy and professionalism of clinicians.
The organizational and clinician decision making are inextricably linked
because the potential to make clinicians satisfied or angry is part of the cal-
culus of the organization, while the effect of improved care processes on

the financial health and competitive advantage of the organization is in the interests of individual clinicians as well.

Investment Pathways in Integrated Settings

Another strategy debate taking place in many healthcare organizations relates to defining the optimal pathway and sequence for making investments in clinical IT. In settings that have preexisting legacy clinical systems, often mainframe applications used in the inpatient environment, organizations must choose a pathway for migrating from such systems to using a CDR and associated inpatient clinician workstation applications (see Figure 12.13). Since the legacy applications include features that go beyond clinical processes, a key decision is to invest in a comprehensive, integrated suite of applications that cuts across clinical and administrative processes versus implementing clinical systems separately. Within the domain of clinical systems, a decision must be made to pursue a unified clinical system versus selecting separate best-of-breed applications for different clinical areas such as laboratory, radiology, and intensive care.

In settings with both inpatient and outpatient facilities, a decision must be made whether to purse an inpatient CDR separate from an ambulatory electronic medical record application or to pursue a single integrated clinical system that cuts across inpatient and outpatient settings. Although major clinical IT vendors promote their respective systems as fully capable across inpatient and outpatient settings, different products have distinct advantages in one setting over the other, making this strategy decision difficult.

The Role of Departmental Care Management Systems

Another debate going on within many healthcare organizations relates to the role of departmental solutions versus enterprise-level solutions. As illustrated in Figure 12.14, this debate can be characterized as an "ice versus spikes" problem. IT leaders with responsibility on the enterprise level, such as a chief information officer, typically place the highest priority on developing applications that offer benefits to the greatest number of users. Because they have limited financial and human resources to dedicate to clinical systems, they focus on deploying simple technologies that apply across the enterprise, analogous to a thin layer of ice across the entire pond. Such simple technologies include laboratory results retrieval, e-mail, clinical dictation, note writing (template charting), and workflow enhancements related to billing and other administrative processes that apply in all settings. IT leaders desire to make such investments in the context of a longer-term strategy to offer deeper, richer capabilities such as specialty-specific results reporting, clinical reminders and alerts, protocol-based care,

FIGURE 12.13
Debate About
Optimal
Pathway for
Clinical IT
Investments

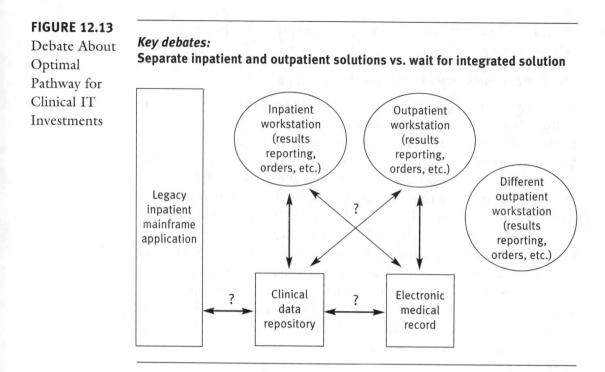

Key debates:
Separate inpatient and outpatient solutions vs. wait for integrated solution

population and disease registries, and tools to support quality and out-comes measurement and process improvement. But in the short term, they focus on the practical and "first things first"—and tend prioritize such deeper functions out of the current funding cycle.

In contrast, clinical leaders at the level of specialty departments or centers of excellence, such as cancer centers and heart and vascular centers, hold a different view. They believe themselves to have a mandate to transform clinical processes to dramatically improve care processes. They recognize that achieving large-scale, durable success in these efforts will require deeper clinical IT capabilities. They salute the long-term strategies for deploying such capabilities enterprisewide but express frustration with the slow pace of progress toward those goals. They would characterize the ice layer as one that is thickening at a glacial pace, and they do not want to wait that long. Therefore, they pursue deeper "spikes" of function within their own clinical domains, seeking to deploy systems that offer them the ability to transform their own clinical processes. Their clinical leadership position in a clinical domain of manageable size enables such leaders to drive the cultural change and attend to the details of the process changes to achieve success.

The ensuing debate about whether such spikes of departmental IT capabilities are desirable or undesirable can be fierce. The enterprise IT

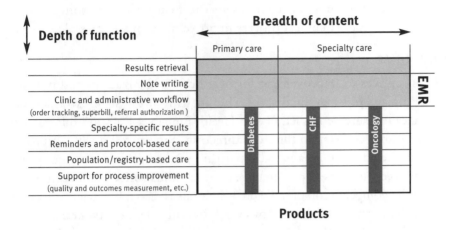

Key debates:
Ice vs. spikes: Enterprise Level vs. department Level

FIGURE 12.14
Ice Versus
Spikes Debate
Regarding
Enterprise
Versus
Departmental
Clinical IT
Solutions

leaders argue that the spikes are really "weeds" demanding support from IT, distracting them from making more rapid progress on enterprise-level goals. They actively resist proposals for such departmental capabilities. On the other hand, the departmental leaders argue that clinical process transformation is urgent and that the lessons learned in their departments will be important lessons that will generally apply across other departments. They argue that the technology investments for such changes are small compared to the investment in cultural and process change, and that even if the department-specific technology is eventually discarded as enterprise capabilities advance, the organization will be better off for having made progress on the cultural and process changes that take time to achieve.

The Challenge

Since the 1980s, some progress has been made in the healthcare field to establish a tradition for evidence-based medicine, quality improvement, and care management, and to develop clinical ITs that support these traditions. A number of important challenges remain, however. Overall healthcare quality is the sum of the quality of thousands of decision-making and care-delivery processes. The examples described in this chapter comprise a tiny slice of overall healthcare quality. It is unlikely that the level of resource intensity and leadership attentiveness that was applied to these examples could possibly be applied simultaneously to more than a few dozen processes within most organizations. Therefore, implementation of practice improvements must be an integral part of the overall practice of all clinicians. Only then will these methods scale up to the enormous task of improving thousands of healthcare processes.

Three fundamental changes in the healthcare environment are required to support clinical process improvement on a large scale.

Incentives

The incentives to improvement for healthcare organizations and individual clinicians must be increased. The growing interest in external performance measurement, such as with Health Employer Data and Information Set measures, is a step in the right direction. But overall quality improvement is likely to require a market structure where healthcare organizations face competition based on quality rather than just price competition and where the compensation of individual clinicians is driven by quality measures rather than just work effort. However, clinician-level quality measurement is a difficult proposition. Patient variation makes clinician-to-clinician comparisons difficult, even for the most common clinical practices. The subset of practices that can be measured represents a small fraction of all clinical practices. As a result, motivating clinicians to focus on improving measurable processes is like encouraging students to "study for the test," calling into question the generalizability of the measures to assess overall practice quality. Furthermore, some warn that the use of quality measurement to drive clinician incentives or as a basis to identify bad apples for remedial attention is counterproductive to the use of measurement for learning and improvement. (See Chapters 8 and 9 for further discussion of these issues.)

Clinician Education

The second fundamental change needed is the education of clinicians in the methods and tools of quality improvement and medical informatics. More substantial changes are needed in medical school curricula, residency training, board exams, and perhaps in the criteria used for medical school admissions.

IT

As described above, the third fundamental change needed is a substantial investment in IT to support clinical practice. Although information systems have been applied to administrative processes within healthcare organizations, the sophistication of systems to support patient care and quality improvement is lacking. Other industries, such as financial services and manufacturing, invest a substantially larger portion of their budgets in IT. Scalable, durable quality improvements will require systems that offer three important capabilities.

First, information systems must permit the acquisition of structured data on patients, healthcare interventions, and outcomes as part of the routine care-delivery process. Second, information systems must offer decision aids such as reminders, alerts, and prompts to clinicians at the moment clinical decisions are made. Third, information systems must facilitate the complex logistics of coordination of care involving many disciplines in many settings according to protocols and guidelines. The tide is beginning to change in this regard. When the Leapfrog Group promoted computerized physician order entry (CPOE) adoption as a patient safety initiative in 1999, survey data indicated that fewer than 2 percent of hospitals had already installed such a system. More recent surveys indicate that 25 percent of hospitals have implemented the technology and another 45 percent have begun planning for CPOE (Health Information and Management Systems Society 2003). Implementation is moving from academic medical centers and government facilities to community hospitals, and all major vendors are now emphasizing CPOE in their marketing strategies (Hobbs, Bauer, and Keillor 2003).

In addition to patient care (providing care to individuals) and evidence-based clinical practice improvement (working to improve the care of populations), clinicians and healthcare leaders have a responsibility to advocate and drive change in their environments to enable large-scale, durable improvement. In a world with incentives, education, and technology to support quality improvement, the public can expect dramatic, measurable improvements in the overall effectiveness of our healthcare system.

Study Questions

1. What different types of clinical IT capabilities are needed to support efforts to improve simple versus complex clinical processes?
2. What types of problems are addressed by clinical information systems?
3. What are the essential components of clinical information systems, and what types of benefits are associated with these components?
4. What are the common differences in the priorities and perspectives of enterprise-level IT leaders versus department-level clinical leaders?

REFERENCES

Baker, A. M., J. E. Lafata, R. E. Ward, F. Whitehouse, and G. Divine. 2001. "A Web-Based Diabetes Care Management Support System." *Joint Commission Journal on Quality Improvement* 27 (4): 179–90.

Birkmeyer, J. D., S. M. Sharp, S. R. Finlayson, E. S. Fisher, and J. E. Wennberg. 1998. "Variation Profiles of Common Surgical Procedures." *Surgery* 124 (5): 917–23.

Boohaker, E. A., R. E. Ward, J. E. Uman, and B. D. McCarthy. 1996. "Patient Notification and Follow-up of Abnormal Test Results, A Physician Survey." *Archives of Internal Medicine* 156 (Feb. 12): 327–31.

Braden, B. R., C. A. Cowan, H. C. Lazenby, A. B. Martin, P. A. McDonnell, A. L. Sensenig, J. M. Stiller, L. S. Whittle, C. S. Donham, A. M. Long, and M. W. Stewart. 1998. "National Health Expenditures, 1997." *Health Care Financing Review* 20 (1): 83–126.

Health Information and Management Systems Society. 2003. *2003 CIO Survey.* Southfield, MI: Superior Consultant Company.

Hobbs, G., J. Bauer, and A. Keillor. 2003. "New Perspectives on the Quality of Care: Reducing Medical Errors Through Cultural Change and Clinical Transformation." *Medscape Money & Medicine* 4 (2).

Hollingsworth, D. 1995. *The Workflow Reference Model.* Hampshire, UK: Workflow Management Coalition.

Institute of Medicine. 2003. National Academy of Sciences press release, July 31.

Lazarou, J., B. H. Pomeranz, and P. N. Corey. 1998. "Incidence of Adverse Drug Reactions in Hospitalized Patients: A Meta-Analysis of Prospective Studies." *Journal of the American Medical Association* 279 (15): 1200–1205.

McCarthy, B. D., M. U. Yood, E. A. Boohaker, R. E. Ward, M. Rebner, and C. C. Johnson. 1996. "Inadequate Follow-up of Abnormal Mammograms." *American Journal of Preventive Medicine* 12 (4): 282–88.

Nohria, A., Y. T. Chen, D. J. Morton, R. Walsh, P. H. Vlasses, and H. M. Krumholz. 1999. "Quality of Care for Patients Hospitalized with Heart Failure at Academic Medical Centers." *American Heart Journal* 137 (6): 1028–34.

Shortliffe, E. H., and L. E. Perreault (eds.). 1990. *Medical Informatics: Computer Applications in Health Care.* Redding, MA: Addison-Wesley Publishing.

LEADERSHIP FOR QUALITY

James L. Reinertsen

Background and Overview

A useful general definition of *leadership* is "working with people and systems to produce needed change" (Wessner 1998). Since every system is perfectly designed to produce the results it gets, it follows that if better results are to be expected, systems (and the people in them) must change. Leadership is therefore essential to quality improvement, whether at the level of a small team of clinicians working to improve care for a particular condition or at the level of an entire organization aiming to improve performance on system-level measures such as mortality rates or costs per capita.

Studies of leaders, and leadership, have produced many theories and models (Bass 1990) of what is required to "work with people and systems to produce needed change." This complex mix of theories can be thought of at two levels: individual leadership and organizational leadership systems.

Individual Leadership

This set of leadership ideas is about what people must *be*, and what they must know how to *do*, if they are to influence others to bring about needed changes. Examples of these two aspects of individual leadership are described in Table 13.1. It is important to understand that it is not enough to have strong personal leadership attributes without knowing how to use them. Similarly, knowing the leadership toolbox without authentically embodying the characteristics required of leaders is insufficient for successful leadership. Both being and doing are needed. This is especially true when the changes required for quality improvement involve reframing of core values (e.g., individual physician autonomy) or remaking of professional teams (e.g., the power relationships between doctors and nurses). Many improvements in healthcare will require these kinds of deep changes in values, sometimes labeled *transformational changes* to distinguish them from *transactional changes*, which do not require changes in values and patterns of behavior.

TABLE 13.1
Individual
Leadership:
Being and
Doing

What Leaders Must Be (examples)	What Leaders Must Know How to Do (examples)
• Authentic embodiment of core values • Trustworthy: consistent in thought, word, and deed • In love with the work, rather than the position, of leadership • Someone who adds energy to a team, rather than sucks it out • Humble, but not insecure; able to say, "I was wrong" • Focused on results, rather than popularity • Capable of building relationships • Passionately committed to the mission	• Understand the system context in which improvement work is being done • Explain how the work of the team fits into the aims of the whole system • Use and teach improvement methods • Develop new leaders • Explain and challenge the current reality • Inspire a shared vision • Enable others to act • Model the way • Encourage the heart (Kouzes and Posner 1987) • Manage complex projects

Organizational Leadership Systems

The ideas and theories at this second level of leadership are not about individual leaders and what they must be and do, but rather about creating a supportive organizational environment in which hundreds of capable individual leaders' work can thrive. This is the system-of-leadership level.

One way to view this level is as a complex set of interrelated activities in five broad categories:

1. *Set direction.* Every healthy organization has a sense of direction, a "future self-image." Leaders' job is to set that direction. The task can be thought of as something like the creation of magnetic lines of force running through the organization, by which people will feel both pulled toward a future they find attractive and pushed out of a status quo they find uncomfortable.

2. *Establish the foundation.* Leaders must prepare themselves, and their leadership teams, with the knowledge and skills necessary to improve systems and lead change. They must choose and develop future leaders wisely and build a broad base of capable improvers throughout the organization. Often, they must take the organization through a painful process of reframing values before they can set forth toward a better future.

3. *Build will.* The status quo is usually very comfortable. It takes will to initiate and sustain change, especially in healthcare organizations, which seem to be highly sensitive to any discord and often grind to a halt because of one loud negative voice. One way to build will for quality improvement is by making logical and quantitative links, including financial linkages, between improvement and key business goals. Will can also be greatly enhanced when boards of directors pay attention to quality and hold senior leadership accountable for performance improvement.

4. *Generate ideas.* Many healthcare quality challenges require innovation if they are to be successfully met. Excellent organizations have well-developed systems for finding and rapidly testing ideas from the best performers, other industries, and other cultures and nations. They also find and use the thousands of ideas latent within the organization itself. Encouraging and developing ideas is a key aspect of the leadership system. Ideas are particularly important for achieving depth of change.

5. *Execute change.* The best improvement ideas will fail to have much effect if they cannot be implemented across the organization. Good leadership systems adopt, teach, and use a good change leadership model and consistently execute both small- and large-scale changes. System-level measurement of performance is an important element in executing change, as is the assignment of responsibility for change to line managers rather than quality staff. This organizational system is particularly important for achieving breadth of change.

A visual representation of the leadership system, with additional examples, is provided in Figure 13.1.

The model outlined above is one general version of a leadership system for quality transformation. A number of excellent organizations have established leadership systems that fit their own business contexts and missions (Tichy 2002). It is important to understand that any individual leader's work is set into the context of the leadership system of a specific organization. Some aspects of that leadership system (e.g., compensation, performance measurement) might support the leader's improvement work, and other aspects (e.g., human resource, budgeting, information systems) might be barriers to that work. Leaders will not achieve large-scale performance changes by simply improving their own leadership skills; they also need to work on improvement of the system of leadership in their organizations. This is in part what Deming (1986) meant when he stated that "Workers work in the system. Leaders work on the system."

FIGURE 13.1
Leadership
System for
Transformation

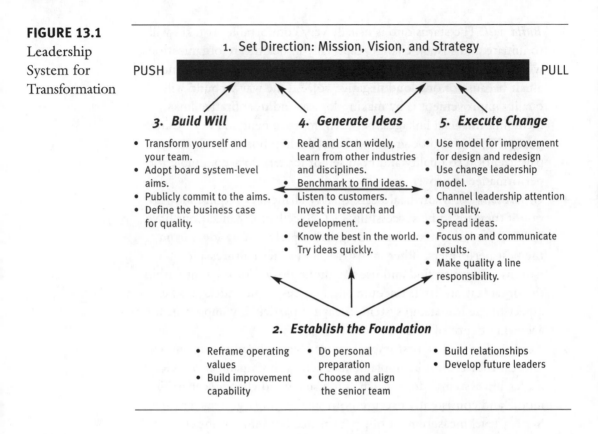

1. Set Direction: Mission, Vision, and Strategy

PUSH   PULL

3. Build Will

- Transform yourself and your team.
- Adopt board system-level aims.
- Publicly commit to the aims.
- Define the business case for quality.

4. Generate Ideas

- Read and scan widely, learn from other industries and disciplines.
- Benchmark to find ideas.
- Listen to customers.
- Invest in research and development.
- Know the best in the world.
- Try ideas quickly.

5. Execute Change

- Use model for improvement for design and redesign
- Use change leadership model.
- Channel leadership attention to quality.
- Spread ideas.
- Focus on and communicate results.
- Make quality a line responsibility.

2. Establish the Foundation

- Reframe operating values
- Build improvement capability
- Do personal preparation
- Choose and align the senior team
- Build relationships
- Develop future leaders

Important Leadership Concepts and Definitions

The following terms are helpful to understand when considering how to improve leadership:

- *Leadership:* working with people and systems to produce needed change.
- *Management:* working with people and systems to produce predictable results. (Note that management is not inferior to leadership; both are important for quality. Leadership, however, is somewhat more hazardous than management because it involves influencing people to change.)
- *Governance:* the process through which the representatives of the owners of an organization oversee the mission, strategy, executive leadership, quality performance, and financial stewardship of the institution. The owner's representatives are usually structured into a board of directors or board of trustees. (In the case of not-for-profit institutions, the "owner" is the community, usually through a state-chartered process monitored by the state's attorney general.)

- *Technical leadership challenges:* change situations in which there is a fairly high degree of agreement about the nature of goals as well as a fairly high level of certainty about how to achieve the goals (i.e., the problem has been faced before, and a method of solving it is known).

- *Adaptive leadership challenges:* change situations that require new learning, resolution of values conflicts, and resolution of deep differences in goals and methods of achieving the goals (very common in healthcare quality improvement work).

- *Boundaries of the system:* leaders must choose the boundaries of the system they wish to improve (e.g., their individual physician practice, the group of physicians in which they work, the entire medical staff of the hospital, the entire community of physicians, the entire profession). As Deming (1995) said, "The larger the boundary chosen, the greater the potential impact, and the greater the difficulty of achieving success."

- *Change leadership:* a framework or method for planning and executing major change (Kotter 1996).

- *Leadership development:* the processes by which an organization identifies, improves, evaluates, rewards, holds to account, and promotes leaders.

- *Transformation:* change that involves fundamental reframing of values, beliefs, and habits of behavior, along with radical redesign of care processes and systems, to achieve dramatic levels of improvement.

- *Vision:* a statement describing a future picture of the institution or care-delivery system. Good visions are usually specific enough that individual staff members can easily see themselves, and what their workday would be like, in that future picture. A quality vision for a hospital, framed in terms of the Institute of Medicine (IOM 2001) quality dimensions, might be a place with no needless deaths, no needless pain, no needless helplessness, no needless delays, no needless waste, and no inequities.

- *Mission:* a statement of the purpose of the institution, the reason it exists. This statement usually rests on the core needs of the institution's customers and on the core values of its people. In the case of hospitals, for example, a general statement of mission might be, "To cure when cure is possible; to heal, even when cure is not possible; and to do no harm in the process."

- *Strategic plan:* the organization's hypotheses about the causative relationship between a set of actions (e.g., capital investments, new structures, process redesigns, new staff capabilities) and achievement of system-level, mission-driven aims (e.g., reduced costs of care, improved levels of safety, lower mortality rates).

- *Budget:* the operational and financial expression of the strategic plan, usually for a defined period such as the next fiscal year.

Scope and Use of Leadership Concepts in Healthcare

From the introduction above, it should be obvious that effective leadership—at both the individual and system-of-leadership level—is essential to quality improvement. Look at it this way: if improvement did not require people and processes to change, leadership would not be needed. But change—often deep, transformative change—is a part of virtually every quality improvement activity, whether at the level of a small project within an office or department or a massive improvement effort involving entire communities. Leadership is therefore necessary.

It is tempting to think of leadership as the responsibility of those at or near the top of organizations, departments, and other structures. This hierarchical view of leadership is natural and, to a certain extent, useful. The CEO does have a larger system view and can accomplish some improvements that an individual nurse, administrator, or physician could not. The CEO's leadership opportunities to influence the system are greater, and so are his or her responsibilities for system-level results.

But it is incorrect, and often harmful, to think that the term *leadership* applies only to those in formally designated senior positions of authority. Healthcare organizations are large, complex systems and cannot be led effectively from a few senior executives' offices. These senior leaders cannot possibly have a deep understanding of the quality issues being faced every day by frontline staff serving patients. Facing, understanding, and improving performance at the critical interface between clinicians and patients is work that must be done by hundreds of capable individual leaders throughout the organization, supported by a well-aligned leadership system.

Finally, it should be emphasized that there exists no simple formula for successful healthcare leadership or for specific strategies that, if carried out, will result in organizational quality transformation. Care-delivery systems are "complex adaptive systems" (Zimmerman, Lindberg, and Plsek 1998), and therefore behave unpredictably, in large part because of the powerful influence of the professional, community, and macrosystem (regulation, policy, markets) context of each organization and care system.

For this reason, it would be presumptuous for leaders within organizations to believe that by working within their organizations alone they can transform those organizations to a dramatically higher level of quality performance. The example of vision given above ("a place with no needless deaths . . .") describes an organization so different from the ones in which we now work that getting there requires a fundamental state change, like going from water to steam. This sort of state change in healthcare will not be evolutionary, but revolutionary. Or, to put it into *Crossing the Quality Chasm* terms (IOM 2001), the gap between our current organizations and this vision is a chasm that cannot be crossed in two steps. All of these ideas—state change, revolution, crossing a chasm—suggest that when transformation does occur, it will be an emergent event, a surprise, something that comes about in the complex adaptive system that is healthcare not as a result of a detailed leadership plan but because of the convergence of multiple factors, some planned, others completely unplanned. The roads that lead to that convergence might come from multiple directions. Some of those roads can be built and traveled by leaders of hospitals and healthcare delivery systems, but these leaders by themselves can neither design nor build the other roads that might be required. The most robust plan to achieve transformation requires healthcare leaders to work on a plan to achieve those things that are within their control and simultaneously influence as much of their context as is possible, even though that context is out of their direct control. Healthcare organizational leaders should be aware of at least four routes to the transformational "surprise," only one of which (route 3) is more or less within their direct control.

Route 1: Revolution (Leadership from Below)

One critical factor in transformation of organizations will be a dramatic change in the culture of the professional workforce. The central themes of that cultural change are the following:

1. From individual physician autonomy to shared decision making
2. From professional hierarchies to teamwork
3. From professional disengagement in system aims to "system citizenship"

Why label this route to transformation *revolution*? If these changes were to occur in the health professions, particularly in medicine and nursing, and the organizations in which those nurses and doctors worked did not change responsively, the tensions between the workforce and their organizations would eventually kindle a "peasants at the gates with torches" sort of revolution, with the healthcare professionals demanding dramatic change from the leaders of healthcare organizations. For example, imagine 15 years of profound cultural changes taking place in newly trained physicians because of the new American Council on Graduate Medical Education requirements (Leach 2001), without any corresponding change in the way hospitals and group practices function. The new generation of physicians would likely revolt against the old systems and constitute a powerful force for dramatic change in all types of healthcare delivery.

Route 1 is particularly important for two of the three principal strategies of the *Crossing the Quality Chasm* report: use all the science we know, and cooperate as a system. Health leaders cannot simply wait for this cultural change to move through medicine, but should be aware of it and take steps both within and outside of their organizational boundaries to support and accelerate that cultural change. When possible, hospital and physician leaders should harness the energy from this slow tidal shift in the culture of medicine and use it to drive needed changes inside their organizations. Route 1 is clearly one of the main highways to the emergent surprise called transformation.

Route 2: Friendly Takeover (Leadership from Outside)

The example mission statement depicts another sort of cultural change, the impetus for which could come from outside the healthcare organizational culture: a profound shift in power from the professional and organization to the patient and family. In many ways, healthcare is already well down the road on route 2. For example, patients and families have broken into the medical "holy of holies," the special knowledge that has defined our source of professional power. They watch open-heart surgery on TV and bring printouts of the latest scientific articles to office visits. Patients now can see various reports on the performance of nursing homes, hospitals, and physicians and will soon see many more such reports. The power of information is already in the hands of the public.

This shift in power is positive and needs to drive a broad range of changes, from how the aims of care plans are defined to radical redesign of how care is delivered, paid for, measured, and reported. Ultimately, this power shift to patients and families will result in them having as much control of their care as they wish to have. They will lead the design of their own care and make important decisions about resources. It is necessary to go down route 2 to implement the patient-centeredness strategy of the *Crossing the Quality Chasm* report.

As in route 1, healthcare leaders cannot make travel down route 2 happen by themselves. But they can be aware of its importance, its necessity for the transformation of their own organizations, and its power to help leaders drive needed change. A lot of patients are driving down route 2 right now, and the job of healthcare leaders is to find them and use their energy, and their leadership, to invite a friendly takeover of their hospitals and clinics.

Route 3: Intentional Organizational Transformation (Leadership from Above)

This route to transformation should be the one most familiar to CEOs and other senior executives. This set of leadership strategies, implemented with constancy of purpose over some years, would be likely to drive organizational transformation. It is important to reiterate that, because transformation is an emergent property of a complex adaptive system, it would be an error for leaders to assume that a well-built, well-traveled route 3 will get them to the vision without some convergence from the other routes, which are not entirely within the control of leadership.

Why *leadership from above*? Route 3 contrasts with route 1 in that route 1 sees the principal drive for change coming from those working at the front lines, whereas route 3 envisions the push coming from visionary leaders who want to place their organizational change agendas at the leading, rather than trailing, edge of transformation. From a traditional hierarchical organization perspective, this is leadership from above.

Route 4: Intentional Macrosystem Transformation (Leadership from High Above)

A fourth route that might be described does not begin with diffused, perhaps even unorganized, cultural changes in professions and patients as in routes 1 and 2, nor does it arise from within healthcare delivery organizations as an intentional act of leadership. Route 4 is a way to transformation that arises out of intentional acts of policymakers, regulators, and others in positions of authority outside the healthcare delivery system itself. Many of the characteristics of the example mission would be accelerated by, and perhaps even dependent on, such macrosystem changes.

For example, it is not a natural act of organizations to publicly disclose data on their performance, especially when the performance is suboptimal. Without public policy that requires it, widespread transparency would likely not be the norm in healthcare, aside from a few brave pioneers. In general, measurement, payment, and accountability regulations that would encourage and reward those who demonstrate evidence-based practices, patient centeredness, and cooperation would be a powerful driver of deep organizational change. This policy/regulation highway, route 4, cannot be directly designed or traveled by healthcare delivery system leaders, but it might be influenced, and its power harnessed, to accelerate the changes leaders want to bring about inside their organizations. The role of delivery system leaders in route 4 might be analogous to the military situation of "calling in fire on your own position." If such regulatory fire could be sensibly guided by what healthcare executives are learning and trying to accomplish, it might be exceptionally powerful in getting their organizations through some difficult spots on their own routes to transformation.

This, then, is the large arena for the application of leadership principles in healthcare: at the individual and system-of-leadership levels within care-delivery organizations, and in the professions, communities, and macrosystems that make up the broad context for our work. The best leaders will be able to work effectively across this arena.

Clinical and Operational Issues

Within healthcare delivery systems, some unusual quality improvement leadership challenges present themselves. These challenges are briefly described below.

Professional Silos, Power Gradients, and Teamwork

Physicians, nurses, pharmacists, and other clinicians all come through separate and distinct training processes. This separation often persists in the way work is organized, information is exchanged, and improvement work is done. This *professional silo* problem is compounded by a power gradient issue, namely that all other professionals' actions are ultimately derivative of physicians' orders. The net effect is to diminish teamwork and reduce free flow of information, both of which are vital for safety and quality. Quality improvement leaders must be capable of establishing effective multidisciplinary teams despite these long-standing challenges.

Physician Autonomy

Physicians are taught to take personal responsibility for quality and have a highly developed attachment to individual professional autonomy. This cultural attribute has an enormous negative effect on the speed and reliability with which physicians adopt and implement evidence-based practices. As a general rule, physicians discuss evidence in groups but implement it as individuals. The resulting variation causes great complexity in the work of nurses, pharmacists, and others in the system, and it is a major source of errors and harm. Quality improvement leaders will need to be able to bring about a reframing of this professional value. Perhaps the best way to frame it might be, "Practice the science of medicine as teams, and the art of medicine as individuals" (Reinertsen 2003).

Leaders and Role Conflict in Organizations

The clinicians who work in healthcare organizations tend to see the organization as a platform for their individual work and seldom feel a corresponding sense of responsibility for the performance of the organization as a whole. As a result, they expect their leaders (e.g., department chairs, vice presidents of nursing) to protect them from the predations of the organization rather than help them contribute to the accomplishment of the organization's goals. This puts many middle-management leaders in a quandary. Are they to represent the interests of their department or unit to the organization, or are they to represent the interests of the organization to their department? The answer to these two questions—yes—is not comforting. Both roles are necessary, and it is important for leaders to be able to play both roles and still maintain the respect and trust of their followers. This sense of role conflict is especially acute among, but not unique to, physician leaders (Reinertsen 1998).

Keys to Successful Quality Leadership and Lessons Learned

Transform Yourself

A leader cannot lead others through the quality transformation unless he or she is transformed and has made an authentic, public, and permanent commitment to achieving the aims of improvement. Transformation is not an accident. One can design experiences that will both transform and sustain the transformed state. Examples include the following:

- Personally interview staff at the sharp end of an error that caused serious harm.
- Listen to a patient *every day*.
- Read and reread both of the Institute of Medicine reports: *To Err Is Human* (1999) and *Crossing the Quality Chasm* (2001).
- Learn and use quality improvement methods.
- View the video *First, Do No Harm*[1] with your team and discuss it.
- Perform regular safety rounds with your care team.

Adopt and Use a Leadership Model

The leadership literature is replete with useful models and frameworks for leadership. Heifetz's model (1994) is particularly valuable when you are facing adaptive leadership challenges, which tend to be marked by conflict, tension, and emotion and by the absence of clear agreement about goals and methods. Many other models are available; as leaders learn them, they often reframe the models into ones that work well for their specific situations (Joiner 1994; Kouzes and Posner 1987; Northouse 2001).

Grow and Develop Your Leadership Skills

Good leaders in healthcare engage in the following three activities that help them continually grow and develop as leaders:

1. *Learn new ideas and information.* This is done by reading about, talking to, and observing leaders; going to courses (including courses outside the healthcare context); and other means of importing information.
2. *Try out the ideas.* Growing leaders take what they learn and use it in the laboratory of their practices, departments, and institutions. They use the results to decide which ideas to keep and which to discard.
3. *Reflect.* Truly great leaders tend to have maintained a lifelong habit of regular reflection on their leadership work. The method of reflection (e.g., private journaling, private meditation, written reports to peers, dialog with mentors and coaches) is not as important as that the reflection is regular, purposeful, and serious.

Avoid the Seven Deadly Sins of Leadership

Following is a list of behaviors and habits that are not predictive of success as a leader.

1. *Indulging in victimhood.* Leaders initiate, act, take responsibility, and approach problems with a positive attitude. They do not lapse into victimhood, a set of behaviors typified by "if only" whining about what might be accomplished if only someone else would improve the information technology system, produce a new boss, or remove querulous members of the team. Leaders do not say "tell me what to do, and I'll do it." They do not join in and encourage organization bashing. To paraphrase Gertrude Stein, "When one arrives at leadership, there is no 'them' there." Leaders face the realities in front of them and make the best of the situation they are in.
2. *Mismatching words and deeds.* The fastest way to lose followers is for leaders to talk about goals such as quality and safety and then falter when it comes time to put resources behind the rhetoric. Followers watch where their leaders' time, attention, and financial resources are deployed and are quick to pick up any mismatch between words and these indicators of the real priorities in the organization.
3. *Loving the job more than the work.* As leaders rise in organizations, some become enamored of the trappings of leadership rather than the work of improving and delivering high-quality health services. Their attention gets diverted to signs of power and status such as office size, reserved parking, salaries, and titles, and away from the needs of their customers and staff members. This is not a path to long-term leadership success. Leaders need to be focused on doing the job they are in, not on getting the next job.
4. *Confusing leadership with popularity.* Leadership is about accountability for results. Leaders often must take unpopular actions and

courageously stand up against fairly loud opposition to bring about positive change. When one is in a leadership role, it is better to be respected than to be liked.

5. *Choosing harmony rather than conflict.* In addition to popularity, leaders are also tempted to seek peace. Anger and tension, however, are often the markers of the key values conflicts through which leaders must help followers learn their way. Avoiding the pain of meetings and interactions laden with conflict, or soothing it with artificial nostrums, is a good way for leaders to miss the opportunity for real creativity and renewal that lies beneath many conflicts.

6. *Inconstancy of purpose.* Nothing irritates a team more than when its leader flits from one hot idea to the next, without any apparent long-term constancy of aim and method. An important variant of this is when the leader's priorities and actions bounce around like the ball in a pinball arcade game because the leader is always responding to the last loud voice he or she has heard.

7. *Unwillingness to say "I don't know," or "I made a mistake."* The best leaders are always learning, and learning cannot occur without recognizing what is not known or admitting mistakes. Good leaders are secure enough to admit when they do not have the answer and are willing to bring the questions to their teams.

Case Study of Leadership: Interview with William Rupp, M.D.

Luther Midelfort-Mayo Health System (LM), in Eau Claire, Wisconsin, although small in size, has gained a reputation as a successful innovator and implementer of quality and safety ideas. This fully integrated healthcare system includes a 190-physician multispecialty group practice, three hospitals, two nursing homes, a retail pharmacy system, ambulance services, a home care agency, and a partnership with a regional health plan. In a unified organizational structure with a single CEO and a single financial statement, LM provides 95 percent of all the healthcare services needed for the vast majority of the patients it serves.

The record of LM's quality accomplishments over the past decade is broad and deep and includes significant advances in medication safety, access to care, flow of care, nurse morale, and nurses' perception of quality. LM has been a highly visible participant in many of the Institute for Healthcare Improvement's (IHI) Breakthrough Series[2] and is now deeply involved in implementation of Six Sigma process management[3] (Nauman and Hoisington 2000) as well as the development of a culture to support quality and safety. William Rupp, M.D., a practicing medical oncologist, became chairman of the LM board in 1992 and CEO of LM in 1994. He has led the organization's drive to innovate in quality and safety. Dr. Rupp stepped down as CEO in December 2001. He was interviewed in February 2002 about the leadership challenges, and lessons learned, during his tenure.

JR: Under your leadership, LM has become known as a quality leader among organizations. Are you really that good?

WR: LM is making progress in quality, although we're clearly not as good as we'd like to be. What we *are* really good at is taking ideas from others and trying them out, quickly. For example, we heard about a red/green/yellow light system for managing hospital flow and nurse staffing at a meeting I attended. We tried it out within two weeks and refined it within three months. We believed that this traffic-light system was a tool for managing the flow of patients through the hospital and for directing resources to parts of the hospital that needed them. But when we tried it out, the traffic-light system turned out to have little to do with managing our flow. Rather, for us, it has been an extraordinary system for empowering nurses, communicating across nursing units, improving nurse morale, and avoiding unsafe staffing situations (Rozich and Resar 2002). Our nurse vacancy rate is now *very* low. It was a great idea, but not for the purpose we originally thought.[4]

JR: How did you get interested in safety?

WR: At an IHI meeting in 1998, our leadership team heard Don Berwick talk about medication errors. We had 20 LM people at the meeting, and our reaction was, "We can't be that bad, can we?" When we came home, we interviewed some frontline nurses and pharmacists about recent errors or near misses and were amazed at the sheer number of stories we heard. So we reviewed 20 charts a week on one unit for six weeks and found that the nurses and pharmacists were right—we were having the same number of errors as everyone else. We also identified the major cause of most of the errors in our system: poor communication between the outpatient and inpatient medication record systems.

We then took our findings from the interviews and the chart reviews and went over them with the physician and administrative leadership. The universal reaction was surprise and shock, but the data were very convincing, and everyone soon agreed we needed to do something about the problem. We put a simple paper-and-pencil reconciliation system in place for in/outpatient medications, and adverse drug events decreased fivefold.[5]

JR: What was your role as CEO in driving these sorts of specific improvements?

WR: I couldn't be personally responsible for guiding and directing specific projects like the traffic-light system, medication safety, and implementation of evidence-based care systems for specific diseases. But I could make sure the teams working on these problems knew that I was interested in them and that I wanted results. I met monthly individually with the project leaders, even if only for 15 minutes, to hear about progress. And I also made sure that my executive assistant scheduled me to "drop in" for a few minutes on the meeting of each team at least once a month so that all the members of the team knew that the organization was paying attention to their work. I know this sort of attention must be important because when specific projects didn't go well (and we had a few), they were projects to which I didn't pay this sort of attention.[6]

JR: Trying out new ideas and changes all the time must cause a lot of tension for your staff. How did you handle this?

WR: You're right—innovation and change is a source of tension. I found it exceptionally useful to have a small number of people working directly for me whose only role was to be change agents. Roger Resar, M.D., is a great example. His job was to find and try out new ideas, and when he did, I inevitably got calls from doctors, nurses, and administrators saying, "We can't get our work done with all these new ideas coming at us. Get Dr. Resar off our backs." At that point, my job was to support Roger, especially if the resistance was based simply on unwillingness to change. But I also listened carefully to the content and tone of the resistance. If I thought there really was a safety risk in trying out the idea, or if there was genuine meltdown under way, I would ask him to back down, or we might decide to try the idea on a much smaller scale.

For example, when we first tried open-access scheduling in one of our satellite offices, we didn't understand the principles well enough and the office exploded in an uproar. Rather than pushing ahead, I went to the office and said, "We really didn't do this very well. We should stop this trial. I still think open access is a good idea, but we just haven't figured out how to implement it yet." After we learned more about implementation, we tried it out elsewhere and are now successfully putting open-access in place across virtually the entire system (except for the office in which the uproar occurred). I shudder to think what would have happened if we had bulled ahead.

So, I'd say my change leadership role was to push for needed change, support the change agents, listen carefully to the pain they caused, and respond.

JR: That must be a hard judgment to make—when to back down on change and when to push ahead.

WR: The right answer isn't always obvious. In some cases the decision is easy, especially when the resistance conflicts directly with a broadly supported organizational value or is in opposition to a strategic approach that the organization has adopted after a lot of debate. For example, we are now well along in our adoption and implementation of Six Sigma process management. If an administrative vice president, or a prominent physician, or a key nurse manager were to come to me and say, "This process management stuff is baloney, I'm not going to do it," my response would be to say, "Well, process management is a major strategy of this organization, and if you can't help to lead it, then you'll have to leave."

JR: How do you deal with resistance to important initiatives, such as clinical practice guidelines, if the resistance is coming from doctors?

WR: We are fundamentally a group practice. Once we have made a group decision about a care process and have designed a system for implementing that process (e.g., our insulin sliding scale protocol, or our choice of a single hip or knee prosthesis), we expect our physicians to use the protocol. We monitor protocol usage and always ask those who aren't using the protocol to tell us what's wrong with the protocol. Sometimes they point out problems with the design. But most of the time, they simply change their behavior to match the protocol. One way or another, we don't back down on our commitment to evidence-based practice of medicine.

JR: During your tenure, did you ever have to face a financial crisis? Were you ever pressured to cut back on your investment in quality and safety?

WR: In 1998/99, we sustained financial losses for the first time in our history, due to the effects of the Balanced Budget Act. I received a lot of pressure from parts of the organization to reduce our investment in innovation and quality. They said, "Cut travel costs. Don't send the usual 20 people to the IHI National Forum." And the physicians said, "Put those physician change agents back into practice, where they can do real work and generate professional billings." I resisted both pressures. I felt that during rough times we needed more ideas, not fewer. So we sent 30 people to the IHI Forum. And we showed the doctors that for every dollar invested in change agents' salaries, we had generated ten dollars in return. The financial results have been good. Last year, we had a positive margin—3.5 percent.[7]

JR: I've heard of your work on culture change and "simple rules." What is all this about?

WR: In 1997, we realized that the rate of change in LM was not what it needed to be and that the biggest drag on our rate of improvement was our culture. We went through an organizationwide exercise in which we discussed our cultural "simple rules" with people from all levels of our organization. A leader cannot significantly change a culture until he or she can describe it and outline it on paper and the staff agrees with the description of the current culture. Only then can you begin to describe what you want a new culture to look and feel like, what you want it to accomplish for patients.

JR: What rules did you find were in place in your culture?
WR: We think the main characteristics of our old culture were embedded in the following rules:

1. Success is defined by quality.
2. Physicians give permission for leaders to lead (and they can withdraw it).
3. Physician leadership means "I'm in charge."
4. Results are achieved by working hard.
5. Compliance requires consensus.
6. Conflict is resolved by compromise.

We will keep the first rule, but the others are up for redefinition. We will not get to our long-term goals if these rules define our culture. How can we reach for exceptional levels of quality if we resolve all conflicts by compromise? How can we design and implement systems of quality and safety as our primary strategy if deep in our hearts we still believe that individual effort is what drives quality?

JR: How would you sum up the main lessons you have learned about the CEO's role in leadership for quality and safety?
WR: I don't think there's a prescription that works for every CEO, in every situation. This is what I have learned from my work at LM:

1. The CEO must always be strategically searching for the next good idea. On my own, I come up with maybe one good idea every two or three years. But I can recognize someone else's good idea in a flash, and my organization can get that idea implemented.
2. The CEO must push the quality agenda. He or she must be seen to be in charge of it and must make it happen. There are many forces lined up to preserve the status quo, and if the CEO doesn't visibly lead quality, the necessary changes won't happen.
3. The CEO doesn't make change happen single handedly. The leader does so through key change agents, and his or her job is to protect and support those change agents, while listening carefully to the pain they cause.

4. This whole experience has profoundly reinforced for me the concept of a system of quality. The professional culture that focuses responsibility for quality and safety solely on individuals is dead wrong. The vast majority of our staff is doing the best they can. Asking them to, "Think harder next time," or telling them, "Don't ever do that again," will not work.

Study Questions

1. What aspects of individual leadership (being and doing) does William Rupp demonstrate?
2. Examine Figure 13.1 and describe the elements of this organizational leadership model evident in the LM organization.

Notes

1. For more information, see the Partnership for Patient Safety's web site at www.p4ps.org.
2. See IHI's web site at www.ihi.org.
3. Six Sigma refers to an approach to performance improvement in which the organization's strategic goals are traced directly to certain key processes; those key processes are then managed toward a high standard of quality—3.4 defects per million opportunities, or "six sigma." For example, most hospitals' medication systems currently produce three or four medication errors per 1,000 doses, or three sigma. *Sigma* is a statistical term used to describe the amount of deviation from the norm, or average, in a population—the more sigmas, the greater the deviation (Kouzes and Posner 1987).
4. One of the most important tasks of leaders is to be on the lookout for good ideas. But leaders have more than an academic interest in ideas; they know that simply accumulating interesting ideas from other organizations, industries, and innovators is not sufficient. Good leaders apply ideas to their work environment and establish ways to test many ideas on a small scale, discarding those that fail.
5. Another task of leaders is to marshal the will to take action. Data about the problem, collected in a credible fashion, can create discomfort with the status quo, often a vital factor in developing organizational will.
6. The "currency" of leadership is attention. Choosing how and where to channel attention is one of the most important tasks of leadership.

7. Healthcare leaders often state that the business case for quality is weak, in that investments in quality and safety do not produce the same kinds of business returns as investments in expensive technologies and procedures. In the case of safety, however, the professional case overwhelms any concerns about the business issues; courageous healthcare leaders understand this. When Paul O'Neill was CEO of Alcoa, he refused to allow anyone to calculate Alcoa's business returns from improving workplace safety. He treated worker safety as a fundamental right of employment. If "first, do no harm" is a fundamental value of our profession, can healthcare leaders play dollars against patient harm?

REFERENCES

Bass, B. M. 1990. *Bass and Stogdill's Handbook of Leadership*. New York: The Free Press.

Deming, W. E. 1986. *Out of the Crisis*. Cambridge, MA: MIT Press.

———. 1995. *The New Economics for Industry, Government, and Education, 2nd ed*. Cambridge, MA: MIT Press.

Heifetz, R. 1994. *Leadership Without Easy Answers*. Cambridge, MA: Belknap Press.

Institute of Medicine. 1999. *To Err Is Human: Building a Safer Health System*. Washington, DC: National Academy Press.

———. 2001. *Crossing the Quality Chasm: A New Health System for the 21st Century*. Washington, DC: National Academy Press.

Joiner, B. 1994. *Fourth Generation Management, The New Business Consciousness*. New York: McGraw-Hill.

Kotter, J. 1996. *Leading Change*. Cambridge, MA: Harvard Business School Press.

Kouzes, J., and B. Posner. 1987. *The Leadership Challenge: How to Get Extraordinary Things Done in Organizations*. San Francisco: Jossey-Bass.

Leach, D. 2001. ACGME Outcomes Project. [Online document; retrieved 5/24/04.] http://www.acgme.org/outcome/comp/compFull.asp.

Nauman, E., and S. H. Hoisington. 2000. *Customer Centered Six Sigma: Linking Customers, Process Improvement, and Financial Results*. Milwaukee, WI: ASQ Quality Press.

Northouse, P. G. 2001. *Leadership Theory and Practice*. Thousand Oaks, CA: Sage Publications.

Reinertsen, J. L. 1998. "Physicians as Leaders in the Improvement of Health Care Systems." *Annals of Internal Medicine* 128 (10): 833–88.

———. 2003. "Zen and the Art of Physician Autonomy Maintenance." *Annals of Internal Medicine* 138 (12): 992–95.

Rozich, J., and R. Resar. 2002. "Using a Unit Assessment Tool to Optimize Flow and Staffing in a Community Hospital." *Joint Commission Journal of Quality Improvement* 28: 31–41.

Tichy, N. 2002. *The Leadership Engine*. New York: Harper Collins.

Wessner, D. 1998. Personal communication.

Zimmerman, B., C. Lindberg, and P. Plsek. 1998. *Edgeware: Insights from Complexity Science for Health Care Leaders*. Irving, TX: VHA Press.

ORGANIZATIONAL QUALITY INFRASTRUCTURE: HOW DOES AN ORGANIZATION STAFF QUALITY?

A. Al-Assaf

My favorite definition of *quality* is simple: incremental improvement. But to live up to this, a major task lies behind the definition. The term quality is being rapidly transformed to mean *performance improvement.* Therefore, for the above definition of quality, one must first know one's current performance so that if improvement does occur, a baseline for judgment exists. Still, one should also have in place a system to monitor progress toward improvement on a regular and continuous basis to verify whether improvement is actually happening. This system would require an adequate and effective infrastructure, process(es) for data gathering, process(es) for data analysis and reporting, and process(es) for identifying and instituting improvements, all of which require a strong management commitment and organizational intent to improve performance. Hence, the development of an efficient, appropriate, and effective system for sustaining incremental improvement is needed.

Now that quality has been defined, what is the difference between quality assurance (QA), quality improvement (QI), monitoring/quality control (QC), and total quality management (TQM)? According to the quality management cycle shown in Figure 14.1, each of these activities has certain steps to be followed to achieve the desired objectives.

- QA is the process of ensuring compliance to specifications, requirements, or standards and implementing methods for conformance. It includes setting and communicating standards and identifying indicators for performance monitoring and compliance to standards. These standards can come in different forms (e.g., protocols, guidelines, specifications). QA, however, is losing its earlier popularity, as it resorts to disciplinary means for standards compliance and therefore blames human error for noncompliance.

FIGURE 14.1
Quality
Management
Cycle

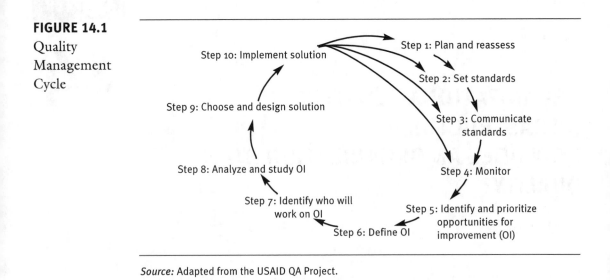

Source: Adapted from the USAID QA Project.

- QC, on the other hand, is defined by the National Association for Healthcare Quality (Brown 1994) as "a management process where actual performance is measured against expected performance, and actions are taken on the difference." QC was originally used in the laboratory, where accuracy of test results dictates certain norms and specific (and often) rigid procedures that do not allow for error and discrepancy. Thus, QC makes an effort to reduce variations as much as possible. QA and QC are complemented and sometimes overwhelmed by QI efforts and processes.
- QI is defined as an organized, structured process that selectively identifies improvement teams to achieve improvements in products or services.
- TQM or quality management in general involves all three of the above processes—QA, QC, and QI. TQM involves processes related to the coordination of activities related to all or any one of the above processes as well as the administration and resource allocation of these processes. Quality management becomes the umbrella under which all processes and activities related to quality fall. Quality management may also encompass such terms as continuous quality management and TQM/leadership/improvement.

Management Commitment

There are not enough words to describe how important management commitment is to the success of quality, at least in industries other than healthcare. Repeatedly, experts have demonstrated the value of management commitment to the quality process. Management can open doors, facilitate interventions freely, and coordinate resources easily. In most cases, management has the final say on activities. Therefore, implementation of quality in healthcare can be enhanced through management supporting QI activities and encouraging professional involvement.

According to Deming (1986), if top management's commitment is not there, the success of implementing quality in an organization is severely jeopardized. He further tells the prospective leader, "If you can't come, then send no one." Commitment to a cause means being involved, supportive, active, and participatory in that cause. Commitment also means leading the efforts, facilitating activities, participating in tasks, and providing the necessary and adequate resources to make QI a reality and a success. Commitment to a process or a program means taking pride and joy in supporting it. It includes enthusiastic initiatives to learn more about it. Commitment is certainly not just rhetoric and oral support, although even that is better than no support at all!

Commitment cannot be achieved without adequate understanding of what you want to commit to and why. Therefore, paramount in this step is increasing knowledge and awareness of the subject needing commitment. For healthcare quality, it is even more difficult to get unequivocal commitment from management without demonstrating results. Managers are usually quick to say, "Show me that it works or it has worked!" Healthcare quality must then be based on data and should always be driven by outcomes. With adequate planning and process design, commitment will be cultivated and positive results can be achieved.

The Role of the Coordinator of Healthcare Quality

Once commitment is achieved, the person in charge of the organization, usually the CEO, needs to identify a coordinator/director of healthcare quality (also known as the chief quality officer). This position is usually full time and may be filled by an experienced person in the organization with leadership skills and a clinical background; this person is given sufficient authority. A direct link is necessary between this individual and the CEO or the CEO's designee for maintaining credibility and authority. Actually, this position is so important that in some organizations the CEO assumes the role of chairing the quality council. This approach, however, has advantages and disadvantages. A prominent person like the CEO gives instant recognition and support to the quality department. He or she establishes commitment from day one, which sends a clear message to the rest of the organization that quality is important and everyone must follow. The disadvantage is that the CEO is not a permanent person, thus causing possible discontinuity of the process once he or she leaves. Regardless of whom the quality assurance/quality improvement coordinator or director is, once identified, this individual should be trained extensively in healthcare quality techniques and must prepare for the organization of the quality council.

Of course, the responsibilities of the quality coordinator are numerous; they include the following:

- Advocate and speak for healthcare quality.
- Facilitate the quality council.
- Serve as designated liaison with outside agencies related to quality activities.
- Coordinate strategic and operational planning for healthcare quality activities and allocation of resources.
- Develop and update the quality/performance improvement program and plan documents.
- Ensure compliance to accreditation standards.
- Initiate monitoring activities of performance measures.
- Serve on and coordinate most of the quality/performance improvement committees in the organization.
- Initiate process improvement teams.
- Coordinate selection of key personnel in quality.
- Coordinate the healthcare quality training plan.
- Facilitate intervention strategies for healthcare quality.

The Role of the Quality Council

The quality council or similar entity is formed to act as the steering body that will direct the healthcare quality process organizationally. It works as a coordinating committee of individuals representing the different aspects of healthcare and departments/units in the organization to formulate organizational policies toward healthcare quality. Experience shows that organizing the quality council is a necessity. Certainly, the membership of the council is important, and careful selection of these individuals should rest with the top official of the organization (CEO) with advice and assistance from the quality coordinator. Again, members should be prominent individuals in the organization representing different disciplines and units. Membership may be broadened to include other individuals from other units of the organization who should perhaps be in leadership positions to harness some of the voices of the workers. Once members are identified, a *charter*, or description document, needs to be developed, with roles and responsibilities delineated. The roles of the council are similar to the roles of the quality coordinator, giving it collective perspective and establishing itself as the central organizational resource in healthcare quality. Similarly, quality council members need to be prepared for their roles adequately and should be exposed to the concept of healthcare quality and its principles early on.

Mission and Vision

Once formed, the first agenda item for the quality council should be to ratify its charter. Each member should be aware of his or her roles and responsibilities as outlined in the charter. Members should get actively involved in the revision and redrafting of the charter to reflect actual involvement and ownership in the council. Another agenda item that needs to be addressed is the development of the mission and vision statements of the organization, which should reflect the desire for healthcare improvements. The council members should draft both statements with input from all key personnel in the organization. These statements are important in establishing the organization's constancy of purpose. They will serve as a constant reminder of the path on which the organization is moving and a map for its future.

Mission and vision statements should be concise, clear, realistic, and reflective of the true desire of the organization. For this reason, real input from other key individuals is necessary. A *mission statement* should answer questions like who we are, what our main purpose as an organization is, whom we are serving, what their needs are, and how to meet those needs. *Vision statements* are somewhat futuristic (visionary) and should answer the question of what the organization strives to be in the future (in three, five, or ten years). Once drafted, approved, and finalized, these statements should be communicated to the rest of the organization actively and consistently. Actually, some organizations post the mission and vision statements in prominent places and even print them on the back of personnel business cards. In this way, all improvement and other activities of the organization will be designed and targeted to achieve the vision and take place along the boundaries of the mission.

Allocation of Resources

Obviously, both physical and human resources are needed to initiate change. Resources are required for the necessary training and acquisition of knowledge. Resources are also needed for dissemination and increasing awareness of health professionals on the concept of healthcare quality. Additional resources will be required to monitor compliance to standards; draft, test, and enforce compliance to policies and procedures; identify opportunities for improvement and initiate and coordinate improvement projects; as well as disseminate the concept of quality and performance improvement at the grass-roots level and to the professional staff. Funds should also be set aside for potential structural changes and redesigns in processes or units to fit required improvements. In some organizations, funds are also used to acquire reference materials and establish a resource library on healthcare quality. Others may allocate certain funds to hire full- or part-time individuals as reviewers and quality coordinators to be disbursed throughout the different units and departments of the organization, whereas others use additional funds to publish a newsletter on quality or hold organizationwide seminars on the subject. Still additional funds may be allotted to provide incentives to the quality process by offering monetary and capital support to successful units or individuals that have demonstrated substantial improvements.

Another aspect of resource allocation in most organizations is establishment of a new central department/unit related to healthcare quality and performance improvement. This unit is organized with a number of health professionals from within (or recruited from outside) the organization, headed by the quality director, and linked directly to the CEO or the CEO's designee. The quality unit is given the mandate of setting the standards to be followed by the organization (e.g., in hospitals, standards usually come from the Joint Commission on Accreditation of Healthcare Organizations [Joint Commission]; in health maintenance organizations, the standards usually come from the National Committee for Quality Assurance). This unit is also charged with communicating these standards to the rest of the organization and its staff, disseminating information (QA/QI communication and training) related to healthcare quality, monitoring the quality of care delivered, and acting on opportunities for improvements in the system. The said unit receives financial and political support from the CEO and additional support from the organization's board, with broad authority for surveying and monitoring performance of any healthcare or service unit in the organization. The objective is to organize this quality unit so that it will take the responsibility of coordinating healthcare quality for the whole organization, with the direct input and participation of every other unit, to institutionalize and ensure sustainability of quality.

Organizational Structure

So what is the organizational structure of this unit on quality in a healthcare organization? To answer this question, one should outline the main and customary functions of this unit and decide what position the unit should occupy in the organization's hierarchy. Also to be considered is the support this unit should get through the committee structure of the organization. Therefore, the list of functions of this unit may include the following:

- Implement the organization's quality program.
- Initiate planning for quality initiatives.
- Set organizational standards for quality.
- Communicate standards to employees (organize seminars to increase awareness; disseminate information on standards; discuss mechanisms for compliance to standards; deliver workshops and lectures on standards; provide training on quality skills and methods).
- Monitor compliance to standards (identify measurable indicators for performance; collect data on indicators; analyze data on indicators; perform periodic audits; perform medical record reviews; perform retrospective reviews of care processes; perform outcomes measurement of patient care; measure satisfaction of customers, employees, patients, and providers; collect data on patient complaints and concerns; assist in meeting accreditation standards; review and update policies and procedures; identify and draft new policies and procedures).
- Identify opportunities for improvement in care and services.
- Initiate and coordinate improvement projects.
- Facilitate performance and productivity measurement and improvements.
- Coordinate all committees related to quality and performance improvement.
- Identify and acquire necessary resources for quality and performance improvement.
- Develop the organization's quality program document and annual plan.
- Evaluate the organization's quality program annually.
- Develop the annual quality report for the organization's board of directors.
- Coordinate all functions and activities related to the optimum utilization of resources.
- Coordinate all functions and activities related to prevention, control, and management of risks to the organization's internal and external customers.
- Take responsibility for coordination of an effective credentialing and recredentialing system for practitioners.
- Act as a liaison with all units to facilitate their performance improvement.

The quality unit will have access to the organization's data collected related to patient care and to all the services provided by the organization internally and externally. It will therefore work closely with the organization's information technology unit.

Considerable variation as to what constitutes a typical organizational structure of such a unit exists. In general, this unit has traditionally been under the medical staff affairs section of the organization, although the new trend is to move the unit to a higher level where it directly reports to the CEO. Considerable variation as to who reports to the unit also exists. Some organizations include both administrative and clinical functions under this unit, whereas others narrow the scope to include only the clinical functions. Other variations include adding utilization and case management activities or risk management and credentialing units.

The other functions of this quality unit are usually handled through the informal structure of the organization, that is, the committees. Again, there is considerable variation as to which committees belong to quality and which ones belong to medical staff affairs. In general, however, such committees as credentialing, peer review and clinical services management, utilization and case management, patient safety, risk management, infection control, and medical records review all usually report to the quality unit. In addition, although there is no reporting relationship, the organization's quality council (or similar entity) is aligned with the quality unit, and the unit's staff usually coordinates the council.

Increasing Awareness of Healthcare Quality

Healthcare quality as a concept has different facets, principles, skills, techniques, and tools. In addition, a vast amount of literature has been written about the subject. Therefore, an early activity of the quality council is for its members to participate in a seminar on healthcare quality. This seminar should be followed by intellectual discussions with a designated facilitator as to the application of this concept in the organization, taking into consideration the available resources, culture, and current health status and structure. A similar activity should be organized to present healthcare quality to other key personnel to gain further support and increase dissemination of the concept. Certainly, the facilitator's services could be used to present a number of short sessions with other key personnel and middle managers to discuss healthcare quality. These sessions, to be repeated at least annually, should be attended by at least the quality coordinator and some members of the quality council. They can serve as focus group sessions to get feedback on quality implementation and applications in healthcare as well as an avenue to increase awareness on the concept. Information and feedback gathered at these sessions can be used in the next planning phase at the operational level and in launching improvement projects and initiatives.

Mapping Quality Improvement Interventions

In collaboration with the quality council and using information collected during the planning phase, the quality coordinator may identify areas in the system with an opportunity for improvement. Identified areas should be selected carefully to include simple projects that require the least amount of resources and have the highest probability of success yet affect a large number of beneficiaries. Examples of such projects include the following:

- Improving the reception area of the organization;
- Improving the esthetics of the organization;
- Improving the timeliness of tests and services to patients;
- Identifying and improving patient safety areas such as infections, falls, complications, or medication errors;
- Initiating a campaign to improve reporting on sentinel events and their management efforts;
- Selecting a few areas that receive a high number of complaints from external customers and trying to improve them;
- Initiating a campaign of promoting health awareness to the public; or
- Leading an informational campaign on improvement initiatives, with participation of all units.

Other projects may involve the formal identification and selection of an improvement opportunity and the organization of an interdisciplinary team from the affected process to initiate improvements. Results are then organized and reported in a forum that maximizes sensitization to and awareness of improvements.

At the completion of improvement projects, the quality council should analyze the lessons learned and, based on certain criteria described below, prioritize services and organizational areas for further implementation of improvements in healthcare quality. Examples of such criteria used for the selection of services for intervention are as follows:

- High volume,
- Problem prone,
- High risk,

- High impact, and
- High cost

Other criteria used for selection of intervention venues and units may include the following:

- Availability and accessibility of necessary data;
- Relatively small, with a homogenous study population;
- Simple infrastructure;
- Well-defined and focused intervention proposed;
- Relatively stable and supportive leadership;
- High need for improvement;
- Additional resources not required for intervention;
- Health professionals willing to participate; and
- Feasibility of demonstrating improvements.

The quality council should decide whether to allocate certain resources for the proposed intervention area. Using the above criteria, the quality council will be able to choose the area or service specific to implementation of the intervention. The use of objectivity in selecting a system or area for intervention is crucial for successful outcomes.

Quality/Performance Improvement Program Document

One of the most important documents the quality unit must develop is the program description document. This document is considered one of the main pieces required for accreditation of the organization. In fact, an organization that lacks this document will never be accredited.

Figure 14.2 shows a suggested outline for the program. This document provides a description of the different activities of the quality unit and an outline of the scope of work in which this unit or the organization's quality program is engaged. It also describes the functions of the different individuals and committees associated with the quality program and serves as the basis for evaluating the progress of the organization toward quality.

This document should be reviewed, rereviewed, and approved at least once annually by the appropriate staff of the QA unit as well as the quality council and then forwarded to the organization's board of directors for final approval. These revisions and approvals should be documented, including approval signatures and dates.

Quality Plan

The second document that should be in place alongside the quality program document is the quality plan. This document should list all of the

FIGURE 14.2
Quality
Program
Document

- Purpose of document
- General program description and overview
- Statements of mission, vision, and values of the organization and the quality unit
- Goals and objectives of the quality program
- Strategies for performance improvement
- Organizational structure supporting performance improvement
  - Formal structure
  - Committee structure
- Roles and responsibilities of performance improvement program
  - Board of directors
  - CEO and executive team
  - Quality council
  - Quality/performance improvement unit
    - Quality director
    - Quality coordinators
    - Quality reviewers/specialists
  - Quality committees
  - Project teams
  - Departmental, section, and other unit leaders' responsibilities in quality
  - Staff responsibilities and involvement in performance improvement
- Scope of work and standards of care and service
- Authority, lines of communication, and accountability
- Delegation of services (if any)
- Reporting mechanisms
- Criteria for setting priorities on performance improvement projects
- List of indicators for monitoring performance improvement
- Methods of monitoring compliance to standards and measuring performance
- Procedures for tackling deficiencies
- Mechanism/model for improvement interventions
- Education and awareness activities on quality/performance improvement
- Rewarding results program
- Annual evaluation of quality/performance improvement
- Audits and reviews
- Confidentiality of information
- Credentialing and recredentialing
- Utilization management program documentation
- Case management program documentation
- Risk management and patient safety program documentation

activities/tasks related to quality that will be carried out the next year and their timelines. Actually, a better document is an action plan where the activities are listed in one column, followed by the name of the person responsible for each activity, timeline for completion, and indicator of when the activity is completed. In this way, both accountability and time expectations for completion of each activity are established. This document is useful for monitoring the performance of the quality unit and is important to allow follow-up on accomplishments.

Reassessment, Monitoring, and Continuous Quality Improvement

In today's healthcare arena, a number of issues have received increased attention from either healthcare consumers or the media. The 1990s can easily be dubbed the period of *performance measurement*. Providers, consumers, and purchasers all look for ways to satisfy one another through measuring and reporting on care outcomes. Accountability is at stake during this period. Several third-party organizations attempted to produce measures to report on these care outcomes. Nationally, a number of indicators have been developed and are being measured by healthcare organizations. Report cards are assembled, and benchmarking efforts are underway to identify and emulate excellence in care and services. All of these activities are being carried out in an effort to measure and improve performance in healthcare.[1]

Performance measurement includes such activities as the identification of indicators for performance. This is followed by collecting data to measure those indicators, then comparing current performance with a desired performance level. Several systems of measurements and indicators have already been developed.[2] The practice of measuring every project pre- and postimprovement initiative should be encouraged. In this way, reassessment will be much easier to accomplish. Reassessment and evaluation may use the same methods applied during the assessment and planning phases through different methods of data collection and analysis.

This discussion on performance measurement provides some highlights on assessing performance and improvement progress. *Monitoring*, on the other hand, is based on specific and measured indicators related to standards. It is a process of measuring variance from standards and initiating processes for action to reduce this variance. Monitoring is a necessary step for proper consideration and selection of QI projects and studies. It can also provide the organization an indication of the status of care and services provided at any point in time. In advanced systems of healthcare, elaborate and comprehensive systems of monitoring have been developed that utilize the patient's medical record for the abstraction of specific data elements. Data are then fed into a central database for analysis and monitoring. Each organization receives a periodic report showing aggregate data of national healthcare indicators compared to its specific set of data for the same indicators. Variance from the mean is then studied and acted on using the QA/QI process mentioned above.

A few words need to be said about the issue of continuous improvement. Improvements are not one-time activities. When a team has worked on a process and improvement is accomplished, this does not mean the team should abandon this process forever and move on to the next one. Improvement is a process, and a process is continuous. Monitoring should continue, and improvements should be initiated every time they are needed. The other principle involves incremental improvements in the standards once compliance is achieved. If high or even perfect compliance to a specific standard has been documented, upgrading this standard is the next prudent step to take; otherwise, the organization will stay in the status quo without further improvements taking place.

Quality Program Evaluation

The program, including its objectives, measures, and activities, should be assessed at least once every year to ensure its effectiveness and that its objectives are in line with the organization's mission and vision. This evaluation is also a mechanism to measure outcomes of the program and identify deficiencies, if any, in achieving the desired outcomes. New goals and objectives might be drafted and incorporated in the new annual plan, including any activities introduced for the next year. Some programs develop a list of specific and quantifiable outcomes to be achieved for the coming year. This list might include the number and type of improvement studies to be carried out, specific performance thresholds for identified outcome measures (e.g., HEDIS, ORYX), patient satisfaction rate goals, and compliance rate for accreditation and other standards.

Therefore, evaluation includes an annual review of all of the activities proposed by the program the year before and comparison with accomplished tasks. A summary of what has been accomplished should be developed and a justification of deficiencies included. A plan of action for the next year will then depend on the assessment of performance of the program and may include recommendations for process revisions or enhancement or modification in the program to ensure continuous progress in improvement.

One point should be emphasized: although evaluation of the program is a scheduled, once-a-year activity, that does not mean the program is not assessed more often. A difference exists between evaluation, which is a yearly retrospective activity, and monitoring, which is an ongoing and continuous activity where goals, progress, and accomplishments are assessed periodically, often throughout the year. This principle should always be emphasized to program staff.

Challenges, Opportunities, and Lessons Learned

A Quality Culture

After the full implementation of healthcare quality in an organization, community, or country, the next expected milestone is to establish a *quality culture*. Total healthcare quality coupled with a quality culture represents the *institutionalization* of healthcare quality. In a system where there is planning for quality, QA, monitoring, QI, and quality management, institutionalization is imminent. Therefore, institutionalization is achieved when appropriate healthcare quality activities are carried out effectively, efficiently, and on a routine basis throughout a system or organization (Brown 1995). Institutionalization is a state where quality is practiced and maintained routinely, without the need for additional outside resources. In such a state, expertise is available internally and commitment is fully integrated and maintained.

A quality environment or culture is achieved when quality activities become day-to-day activities. Such activities are not separate from the normal activities carried out daily by the system and its personnel. In such a state, each employee is aware of the quality concept, believes in it, practices its principles, and makes it part of his or her responsibility, not the responsibility of a department or another individual. Each individual is responsible for the quality structure, process, and outcome of his or her own task. Employees are making every effort at that level to make sure that the processes of QA (i.e., planning, standard setting, and monitoring) are maintained. In such a culture, employees are also practicing QI; that is, they identify variance from standards and select opportunities for improvements to set in motion individually or in collaboration with others to make improvements. In a quality culture, employees are empowered to achieve their goals. Individual goals are always in alignment with the organization's mission and vision statements.

Lessons in Institutionalization

- *Plan* for quality systematically and thoroughly. Delineation of responsibility, identification of scope of involvement, allocation of resources, and anticipation of changes should occur before activities in QA or QI begin.

- Secure *commitment* from management, and hopefully from the CEO. This can make the process of implementation of any new activity or project move rapidly. The involvement of the top manager in the early activities of planning is essential.

- Develop a *policy* for quality at the organizationwide level as early and as solidly as possible. A policy that is well prepared and developed in collaboration with senior staff will have a much better chance of survival, even with expectedly high turnover of managers and staff.

- Identify the *leader* or *champions* to lead the quality unit. A professional with authority, credibility, enthusiasm, and interest can be an asset to the acceleration and success of healthcare quality program implementation. This individual can act as facilitator and cheerleader for healthcare quality initiatives throughout the organization.

- Organize a steering committee or *council* of organizationwide representatives to give the healthcare quality process credibility, sustainability, and momentum.

- Form the *structure* for healthcare quality gradually and cautiously based on progress and understanding of the concept, scope, and practice. Organizing large structures of committees and councils early on may shift the focus to organizing issues and away from the actual mission of healthcare quality. The quality program should be synonymous with improvement of performance at all levels. At the beginning of implementation, staff should concentrate more on learning and understanding the concept and practice performance enhancements daily to achieve positive results. Too many committees with too many meetings and too many tasks distract from focusing on expected goals.

- Always have an *alternative plan* in case you are slowed down because of anticipated and frequent staff changes. Making a habit of not relying on one individual is helpful when trying to implement healthcare quality initiatives effectively. Train a number of individuals and prepare several qualified staff simultaneously. This practice will allow for wider selections of coordinators (representing and even being housed at different units) and enhance sustainability efforts.

- Keep quality activities closely related to the organization's main activities and its *mission* without unnecessary change in organizational structure and the allocation of additional resources. At least at the beginning of implementation, healthcare quality activities may be delegated to an existing staff or department as part of their normal responsibility and daily work.

- Prepare yourself to answer questions related to *incentives* for staff to participate. As long as healthcare quality activities are not required as integral parts of their job, employees will question their role in participation. A system of employee rewards and recognition based on healthcare quality achievements is necessary. A program for rewarding results is paramount for continuous improvement of performance.
- *Document improvements.* Measure performance of processes and programs before and after each improvement intervention. Always have quantitative data available for comparisons and measurements of effectiveness. It is also useful to calculate cost savings to measure efficiency. Providing measurable parameters gives credibility and sustainability to the process of healthcare quality.
- Actively *disseminate achievements* and healthcare quality awareness information to as many individuals in the system as possible. Make sure that participation is voluntary and open to everyone as opportunities for improvement are identified. Do not make it a private club; keep everybody informed and involved as much as possible.
- Build an effective process in one area/unit; this is more important than starting several incomplete processes in different locations and areas. Keep the improvement process *focused*.
- Always keep *adequate funding* available for the development of new projects and activities not originally planned. This will also give you the flexibility of shifting additional funds to areas where improvements are taking place more effectively. Adequate funds will increase the likelihood of sustainability.
- Finally, encourage and foster an environment of *learning*, not judgment. In particular, rely on data and facts in making judgments. Avoid the antiquated disciplinary method of management.

Remember, "Every system is perfectly designed to meet the objectives for which it is designed," according to Deming (1986). Therefore, making sure that the quality infrastructure is designed effectively is essential, and monitoring its performance regularly is even more important.

Case Example

It was only 8:00 p.m. as intern Jerry Garcia wheeled the new EKG machine into Ms. Smith's room, but Jerry could sense he was in for another sleepless night. Ms. Smith, who was 68 years old, had been admitted earlier in the day for an elective cholecystectomy. She now appeared acutely ill. She was pale and sweaty, her pulse was 120, her respirations were shallow and rapid, and her blood pressure was 90/60.

Jerry quickened his attempts to obtain the EKG. He momentarily considered asking a nurse for help, but reasoned that the night shift would not have received any more training on the use of these new EKG machines than he had.

The new EKG system was really great, he had heard. He had read an article in the hospital's weekly employee newspaper about it. It featured a computerized interpretation of the cardiogram, and this was supposedly tied into data banks containing previous EKGs on every patient. The effort to purchase the system was spearheaded by the chief of cardiology, who felt it provided sophisticated EKG interpretations during off hours and solved growing data storage problems. The EKG machines themselves were operated by technicians during the day, but they had long since gone home.

After affixing the EKG electrodes to the patient, Jerry looked at the control panel. He saw buttons labeled STD, AUTO, RUN, MEMORY, RS, and TIE. Other buttons, toggles, and symbols were attached, but Jerry had no clue as to what they meant. He could not find an instruction manual. "Hmmmm. . . . Totally different from my old favorite," Jerry thought as he began the process of trial and error. Unfortunately, he could not figure out how to use the new machine, and after 15 minutes he went to another floor to fetch his favorite machine.

"Admitted for an elective cholecystectomy," Jerry remarked to himself upon reading the EKG, "And this lady's having a massive heart attack! Geez. . . . She only came to the floor at 4:00; I hadn't planned to see her until 9:00!" He gave some orders and began looking through the chart to write a CCU transfer note.

Jerry's eyes widened when he came across the routine preoperative EKG, which had been obtained at 1:00 p.m. using the new computerized system. It had arrived on the floor four hours earlier, along with Ms. Smith. It showed the same abnormalities as Jerry's cardiogram, and the computer had interpreted the abnormalities appropriately.

Jerry returned to Ms. Smith's room. On direct questioning, she volunteered that her chest pain had in fact been present since late morning. However, she didn't want to bother nurses or physicians because they appeared so busy to her.

Jerry then discussed the case with the CCU team. They decided with some regret that Ms. Smith would not qualify for thrombolytic therapy (an effective treatment for myocardial infarction) because the duration of her symptoms precluded any hope that it would help her. Conservative therapy was initiated, but Ms. Smith's clinical condition steadily deteriorated overnight, and she died the next morning.

Jerry reflected about the case. Why had he not been notified about the first abnormal tracing? He called the EKG lab and found that a technician had noticed the abnormal cardiogram coming off the computer. However, he assumed the appropriate physicians knew about it and, in any event, did not feel it was his duty to notify physicians about such abnormalities.

For his part, Jerry assumed the new EKG system would notify him about marked abnormalities. In fact, when Jerry first read about the new system, he thought it would serve a useful backup role in the event he did not have time to review EKGs himself until late in the evening.

1. What is the main problem in this scenario?
2. What should be done about it?
3. How should this hospital organize for quality?

Study Questions

1. If you were assuming the chief executive position in a hospital and the chief quality officer position was vacant, what type of person would you seek to fill the position? Background? Experience?
2. How do accreditation and adherence to standards mix with the quality/performance improvement activities? Is there an optimal percentage of time a group should spend on one or the other?
3. What are the cultural barriers and enablers to achieving a successful quality improvement program?

Notes

1. In the international arena, the World Health Organization (WHO) organized and facilitated a number of activities related to quality assessment, performance improvement, and outcomes measurement (see work coordinated by the U.S. Agency for Healthcare Research and Quality at www.qualitymeasures.ahrq.gov/). A large number of countries and institutions participated in these activities and initiatives. All agreed that there has to be an organized mechanism to account for quality and continuous measures to improve performance in healthcare organizations (see WHO's report on health systems rankings at www.who.int/whr2001/2001/archives/2000/en/).
2. The Health Plan Employer Data and Information Set (HEDIS) is one example (www.ncqa.org/Programs/HEDIS/). This set contains more than 50 measures, primarily for preventive health services, against which organizations can compare their performance and therefore trend progress toward improvement. Other similar

systems include the U.S. Public Health Service Healthy People 2000 and 2010 list of indicators (www.healthypeople.gov/), the Joint Commission's ORYX clinical indicator system for hospitals (www.qiproject.org/ORYX/ORYX.pdf), the Canadian Council on Health Services Accreditation hospital indicators (www.cchsa.ca/), and the Centers for Medicare & Medicaid Services QISMC indicator system for managed care (www.cms.gov).

REFERENCES

Brown, J. A. 1994. *The Healthcare Quality Handbook*. Glenview, IL: National Association for Healthcare Quality.

Brown, L. D. 1995. "Lessons Learned in Institutionalization of Quality Assurance Programs: An International Perspective." *International Journal of Quality in Health Care* 7 (4): 419–25.

Deming, W. E. 1986. *Out of the Crisis*. Cambridge, MA: MIT Press.

Suggested Reading

Al-Assaf, A. 1997a. "Strategies for Introducing Quality Assurance in Health Care." In *Quality Assurance in Health Care: A Report of a WHO Intercountry Meeting*, 33–49. New Delhi: World Health Organization.

———. 1997b. "Institutionalization of Healthcare Quality." *Proceedings of the International Association of Management* 15 (1): 55–59.

Al-Assaf, A. F. 1998. *Managed Care Quality: A Practical Guide*. Boca Raton, FL: CRC Press.

———. 2001. *Health Care Quality: An International Perspective*. New Delhi: World Health Organization–SEARO.

Al-Assaf, A. F., and J. A. Schmele. 1993. *The Textbook of Total Quality in Healthcare*. Delray, FL: St. Lucie Press.

Juran, J., and K. F. Gryna. 1988. *Juran's Quality Control Handbook*. New York: McGraw-Hill.

Nicholas, D. D., J. R. Heiby, and T. A. Hatzell. 1991. "The Quality Assurance Project: Introducing Quality Improvement to Primary Health Care in Less Developed Countries." *Quality Assurance in Health Care* 3 (3): 147–65.

IMPLEMENTING QUALITY AS THE CORE ORGANIZATIONAL STRATEGY

Scott B. Ransom, Narendra Kini, Michael L. Jones, and

Elizabeth R. Ransom

Implementing change is a premier challenge in improving healthcare quality. While many of the initiatives described in this text are well supported in the literature and conceptually make logical sense, it is the rare leader who has successfully operationalized a significant improvement. How can it be that hundreds of manuscripts have been published and millions of dollars have been devoted to improving the healthcare system, yet few real improvements have been realized? Programs devoted to appropriately treating and screening for even the most common disorders have largely failed (see Table 15.1). Peer-review organizations across the country have spent countless hours and dollars to address these issues, yet, at best, only minimal improvements have been observed. A storm of efforts by leaders from such notable organizations as the Institute of Medicine (IOM),[1] the Leapfrog Group,[2] the Institute for Healthcare Improvement (IHI),[3] and the National Quality Forum (NQF)[4] have highlighted concerns about patient safety and medication errors; however, only minimal improvements have been experienced in hospitals. This chapter is devoted to optimizing change and improving quality. While conceptually easy, implementing change leading to improvement is the most difficult issue confronting contemporary healthcare leaders.

Incorporating quality as a core organizational strategy requires leadership from the board of trustees and the top executive team. Despite best intentions, developing a focus on improving quality is a challenge for most healthcare organizations because of their many competing agendas. Hospitals are confronted with nearly daily conflicts that can disrupt a quality focus; some of these include financial crises, union difficulties, Health Insurance Portability and Accountability Act requirements, review by the Joint Commission on Accreditation of Healthcare Organizations, malpractice concerns, employee morale, physician relations, and community advocacy. While every governing board wants a high-quality organization, it is the rare hospital that is able to maintain quality as its core strategy.

TABLE 15.1
Healthcare
Quality
Measures

Measure	1999	2000	2001	2002
Antidepressant Medication Management (acute phase)	58.8	na	56.9	59.8
Antidepressant Medication Management (continuation phase)	21.4	na	19.8	19.2
Breast Cancer Screening	73.4	74.5	75.5	74.9
Cervical Cancer Screening	71.8	78.1	80.0	80.5
Childhood Immunization Rates	63.6	66.8	68.1	68.5
Controlling Hypertension	39.0	51.5	55.4	58.4
Cholesterol Management After Heart Attack	45.2	53.4	59.3	61.4
Diabetes Care—Eye Exams	45.4	48.1	52.1	51.7
Diabetes Care—HbA1c Testing	75.0	78.4	81.4	82.6
Appropriate Asthma Medication Use	57.6	62.6	65.6	67.9

Source: National Committee for Quality Assurance (2003).

Leading organizations have expanded their view of quality to include important perspectives of patient, family, and employee satisfaction; clinical quality; and financial performance. A balanced tradeoff of these perspectives is important. What is the effect on patient satisfaction of the new food services vendor contract? What are the market share implications of purchasing a multimillion-dollar DaVinci robot to maintain the cutting edge of surgical innovation? What are the financial implications of adding a second MRI system? What are the quality, cost, and revenue effects of these new initiatives? These tradeoffs must be deliberately discussed and debated to make quality the core organizational strategy.

As quality takes center stage in the organization's thinking, a simple framework must be in place to ensure that improvement is possible. Langley et al. (1996) suggested a model for improvement based on three fundamental questions: What are we trying to accomplish? How will we know that a change is an improvement? and What changes can we make that will result in improvement? While these questions prompt an operational focus on improving the healthcare organization, the model requires a connection to the human dynamics of the organization for implementation. Expanding on the traditional model for improvement, the following six-step approach has been used to implement a quality strategy in the healthcare organization:

1. Develop an organizational vision for quality, with clearly outlined objectives, priorities, and expectations.
2. Recruit the best people possible to achieve results and provide necessary resources.
3. Hold individuals accountable for results.
4. Measure just enough to confirm improvement or stagnation.
5. Expect and encourage productive conflict in your organization.
6. Engage physicians and other key clinical staff in the process.

The approach places a strong emphasis on the organization's most important resource—people. People make decisions and set direction. People also will impede progress on improvement. This chapter provides a practical methodology for leaders to manage and implement change in the healthcare organization.

Implementing Quality in Healthcare Organizations

Develop an Organizational Vision for Quality

The essential trait of leadership is the courage to set a direction. The transition to a high-performance healthcare organization requires a leader to define quality and establish clear and specific priorities. While numerous conflicts occur in the typical healthcare organization, institutions that devote time to important strategic issues will succeed in achieving their goals. While most hospitals cite quality as an objective, few organizations actually define quality in any meaningful way. Given this reality, it cannot be a surprise that most organizations are stagnant in quality and have no real mechanism to move forward.

Top organizations spend time on what is important. If quality is the focus, time must be spent on quality. Leaders must set the key priorities for organizational focus and ensure that budgets and employee attention are focused on these areas. For most organizations, quality has been a difficult area on which to focus. Myriad daily activities present the organizational leadership with a challenge to provide this focus on quality. Top organizations develop clear and specific metrics of quality. This is highlighted in the budget and often used in the performance reward system for employees.

Leadership requires discipline to set the direction and remain fixed even during conflict. Leaders must remain focused on quality without being distracted by other issues. While these other issues need to be addressed, time and resources must be set aside for improvement to occur. For example, the Henry Ford Health System in Detroit, Michigan, has been proud of its attention to quality improvement. The CEO spends substantial time thinking about how to improve organizational performance. Many members of the management team go to national meetings and conferences devoted to quality. The organization annually commits resources to internal educational opportunities for younger leaders to learn about and operationalize quality improvement. Time and focus allow Henry Ford to improve.

Strategic planning is an exercise that allows the organization to decide its core business. Interestingly, for-profit organizations inherently focus on improving profits. Not-for-profit organizations have the opportunity to pursue a more mission-oriented existence. Nevertheless, not-for-profit groups must survive fiscally, which requires adhering to a budget. As organizations experience financial crisis, the focus is necessarily fiscal. Mazlow's theory of progressive needs indicates that survival requirements are a first priority; they can overshadow a quality focus until basic needs are met. Since a significant number of hospitals are experiencing financial hardship, a quality crisis has resulted. The organization in financial straits does not focus on quality and emphasizes a positive bottom line, which may compromise improvement and lead to a less-competitive organization. Hypothetically, then, only the financially successful one-third of hospitals have any chance at a quality focus. Rare exceptions to this rule exist, including that of Sutter Health.

Sutter Health in Northern California was in an organizational crisis because of poor financial performance and low employee morale. A new CEO led the organization to develop a competitive vision and goals. One goal was to inspire the staff to transcend the basic survival needs of their individual business units to achieve the vision. The CEO helped the management team, physicians, and employees deal with the crisis through a constant focus on the benefits of achievement of the vision. The focus on vision helped the staff go beyond the profit-only perspective by using the mission, values, and vision as the major decision rules. The road to profitability can be either the scorched-earth approach of layoffs and cost cutting, which is a short-term solution and destroys staff morale, or the leadership approach, which bonds staff together against a common enemy (i.e., the crisis to be overcome). The Sutter leadership emphasized the latter with a strong focus on quality, and they succeeded.

A key metric of Sutter's vision was to become a top 100 Solucient Hospital.[5] Sutter achieved this quality level through a disciplined focus on its core vision, with specific and measurable goals. The CEO emphasized that every decision must move the organization closer to the vision of the hospital. Collins and Porras (1997) researched the role of leadership during crisis and concluded that "Leadership is defined as top executive(s) who displayed high levels of persistence, overcame significant obstacles, attracted dedicated people, influenced groups of people toward the achievement of goals, and played key roles in guiding their companies through crucial episodes in their history."

Top healthcare leaders develop a vision for quality, with clearly outlined objectives, priorities, and expectations. This focus on vision is a mark of great leadership that can move the healthcare organization to optimal quality. While this focus may be uncommon, it does not take long to understand the dire consequences of our current clinical processes, which result in thousands of unexpected deaths, medication errors, and other mistakes. The focused organization budgets for improvement as the core business. Budget items that do not support the vision or core business should be eliminated. While this leadership focus will present challenges, it is the optimal way to achieve improvement.

Recruit the Best People Possible

"Leaders get the right people on the bus (and the wrong people off the bus) and set the direction," says Jim Collins, author of *Good to Great* (2001). The organization's strategy and focus should determine what is needed in a specific position. Prior to recruiting, top executives will set the expected outcomes for the position and only then find the best person to fill the role. All too frequently, organizations develop a position with no specific expectations. Unless the hiring executive can outline specific and measurable achievements expected for a position at 3, 12, and 36 months, the goals will likely not be achieved. The goals for the position may be specific or general depending on the position. The nursing manager's objectives may include reducing length of stay, improving patient or employee satisfaction, or implementing an improvement project to reduce medication errors. Meanwhile, the CEO may have objectives of driving the hospital to become the market leader in the community, maintaining a 4 percent margin, or developing a new cancer center. Only through clear expectations will the employee drive improvement. In addition, depending on the desired goals, the organization may need to recruit different types of people. An organization that hopes to build a new hospital may look for a CEO with this type of experience, whereas an organization going through a financial turnaround may require a different skill set for success.

Recruiting is an important skill. Top leaders recruit people with core values and priorities that fit the organization's vision. Understanding a potential recruit's values is difficult in a one-hour interview. Depending on the position, it may be important to gain insights by meeting the candidate in different settings with different people. Similarly, thoughtful reference checks are critical. The candidate should provide several references who are able to comment on the expertise and values of the potential recruit. Look to others familiar with the candidate for pertinent comments.

Associates from a different department can be a useful resource. The reference checks must probe for the candidate's core values, personality traits under pressure, goals, and qualifications. This process can be lengthy; however, to build a top organization, executives must develop an outstanding and cohesive team, which can only come from strong employees with appropriate values and priorities (see Table 15.2).

The effective leader must support the handpicked team for success (Thompson and Ware 2003). As Harry S. Truman indicated, "You can accomplish anything in life, provided you do not mind who gets the credit." The exceptional leader sets up his or her successor for success. If problems arise, the leader takes the blame. When success occurs, the employee gets the credit. Through a supportive environment, employees thrive and help achieve the organization's vision.

When employee changes need to be made, act immediately. General Electric has been known to have a rigorous evaluation system that requires executives to eliminate the bottom 10 percent of performers every year. By eliminating the lowest performers, the organization can pick new talent to help achieve the vision (Slater 1999). Top organizations look to put the best people on the biggest opportunities, not the biggest problems (Collins 2001). Rewarding top performers with outstanding projects allows the organization to move forward more quickly. In addition, rewarding top performers with the best projects will reduce the potential for the talented worker to look for alternative employment, as noted in *The War for Talent* (Michaels, Handfield-Jones, and Axelrod 2001).

Compensation is always a subject of controversy. Compensation should not be developed to motivate behaviors, but to keep the right people with the organization. Every compensation system has built-in corrupt incentives. Care must be taken in rewarding employees for performance (Ransom et al. 1996). As shown at Enron, executives and other employees will act in their best interests, at the risk of possible destruction of the organization. Compensation should be provided to recruit and retain the best and brightest. In addition, the organization should look to the recruit's real needs and desires. More money may not have the impact that an onsite childcare service may provide, for example. Look for ways to compensate employees who matter, and, if compensation is based on performance, carefully ensure that the compensation program is consistent with the organization's vision (Dye 2002).

Hold Individuals Accountable for Results

Providing good and valuable feedback is one of the most important, yet difficult, things a top employer can do to develop an optimal employee. Even top employees appreciate effective direction from a supervisor to

Recruitment Step	Time Required (weeks)	TABLE 15.2 Recruiting Process and Timetable
1. Interview key stakeholders for recruitment	1	
2. Develop a comprehensive position specification	1	
3. Ensure appropriate support for position specification	1	
4. Identify and screen appropriate candidates for position	8–12	
5. Conduct preliminary interviews with 4–6 top candidates	1	
6. Conduct two preliminary reference checks on top candidates	1	
7. Conduct second interviews with 2–3 top candidates	1	
8. Conduct 3–12 additional reference checks on top candidates	1	
9. Ensure support for top candidate with key stakeholders	1	
10. Make job offer and negotiate agreement	1–4	

ensure that their perspective of their performance is in line with the organization's. Unfortunately, a common situation in healthcare organizations is little or no feedback, followed by a discharge notice.

Noted coach and advisor to multimillion-dollar professional basketball players Phil Jackson provides this insight: "Provide positive and negative feedback on a regular basis for results" (Jackson and Delehanty 2002). The effective supervisor must provide feedback to even the best and brightest employees. In fact, top organizations tend to provide a culture that optimizes already-strong talent and gets rid of individuals who are not able to keep up. "Employers don't have time to waste with unproductive employees, or even people who have to be coddled, coaxed, and disproportionately supported to get their jobs done," says Roger E. Herman (Herman and Gioia 2000).

Effective management of employees is the employer's most important task. A *Harvard Business Review* article (Jackman and Strober 2003) provides a summary:

- Accountability is difficult; eliminating a nonperforming employee is comparatively easy.
- Provide regular and timely feedback to achieve results.
- Do not choose popularity over accountability.

Real accountability is difficult, as Carson Dye, senior vice president at Witt/Kieffer, recalls during an exchange of correspondence with the author.

> I was hired by the hospital board to recruit a new CEO. The board had recently fired the CEO due to poor performance and incompetence. In reviewing past annual evaluations, the dismissed CEO had glowing reports of exceptional leadership and performance. Then, on the day of his discharge he was found to be incompetent. The chairman replied that it was difficult for the board to provide honest feedback to the CEO throughout his tenure.

No feedback at all may be easier for the supervisor in the short term; however, this approach diminishes performance and eliminates the entire notion of an effective team.

A troubled organization has several challenges in developing a collaborative team. Atchison and Bujak (2001) provide the following insight:

> Individuals go through a predictable progression in working with an organization. First, an egocentric position, do I have a job—am I going to get fired? Only when that issue is worked out can the employee progress to a rolecentric situation, what is my job—where is my desk? If the person has a good grasp on her role then a missioncentric situation develops, what can I do to help—let's do good for the organization?

If an organization is undergoing substantial downsizing, it must be careful not to fall into the trap of having employees stuck in a largely egocentric position. Effective communication can limit these issues during a turnaround; however, it takes considerable effort to maintain employees at the missioncentric level of participation.

Thus, the employee must understand his or her job and expected objectives. Before the employee is hired, top organizations develop a position specification to detail the position, requirements, and expectations at specific time intervals. An ambiguous understanding of expectations cannot achieve optimal results for the organization. Thus, the supervisor must ensure that the employee clearly understands expectations before the first day and then provide effective and timely feedback during the entire employment relationship. Accountability will not happen without effort; it requires the tenacity and focus of real leadership.

Measure Just Enough to Confirm Improvement or Stagnation

Effective leadership and strategic planning both require measurement to better understand the organization and target markets. The challenge for effective executive teams is just how detailed and precise the information has to be before a decision is made to move forward. Information paralysis is a common problem in healthcare organizations. Despite the promise of data from powerful computers, the effective leader must act on trends rather than wait for statistical significance. It may take years to achieve statistical significance for critical management decisions. An executive who waits for perfect information may damage the organization's competitive position.

One must know what to measure. While the powerful data systems in most hospitals can churn out reams of data, only a few pieces of information are useful to implementing improvement. Michael Lewis (2003), in his book *Moneyball*, presents the story of how the Oakland A's created championship baseball seasons despite having one of the lowest-salaried teams in the major leagues. The manager of the team found that the traditional measures of batting average and home runs were not necessarily the most important measures correlated to winning baseball games; he understood that on-base percentage was far more important than these other measures. From this new way of thinking, the A's were able to recruit less-expensive players who could consistently get on base, which helped win games. Healthcare leaders can learn from this baseball story by looking at their data in a different way. By identifying the right measures to achieve the organizational vision, executives can better lead the organization to success.

While risk does exist in making decisions without full information, top leaders make decisions with the information available combined with their instincts. Sutcliffe and Weber (2003) suggest that "the returns on accurate knowledge are initially positive, taper off, and then turn negative. . . . The way executives interpret their business environment is more important for performance than how accurately they know their environment." The concept of leading with "good-enough information" is a challenge for executives and does go against several research principles; however, just as a physician sees the patient and makes a reasonably accurate, but not precise, judgment on the patient's condition and offers treatment, the executive must make decisions in a timely way given the information available at the time, without procrastination.

The executive must consider the effect of decisions from all perspectives. A decision to improve financial performance may have a downstream effect on clinical quality or patient satisfaction. Similarly, a program to improve patient satisfaction may have a negative effect on the bottom line. The effective executive must quickly understand the implications of these decisions and act accordingly (see Figure 15.1). Waiting for statistically significant information is not operationally feasible in the highly competitive healthcare environment. As executives ponder options and conduct further studies to make the best decision, the competitor may have already acted and eliminated the window of opportunity.

Expect and Encourage Productive Conflict

Change is difficult. If a meeting related to any change of a system goes easily, without any conflict, the participants have not presented their real opinions. If these conflicts do not get discussed, forward movement may never occur. Introducing a quality initiative attempts to create positive change; however, change will never occur without at least some challenge.

Productive staff meetings should be passionate, with critical discussions. Pleasant meetings—or even worse, boring ones—are indications that a proper level of overt and constructive ideological conflict is not taking place (Lencioni 1998). Team complaints about meetings taking up time needed for "real work" are a sign that those meetings are not as productive as they should be. Executives and change initiators need time and the forum to openly discuss issues that may facilitate change. If the forum does not at least discuss the inherent conflicts with the suggested change, nothing will improve. That is, harmony will not allow real improvement.

While many reports have been made public about medication errors, patient safety problems, and obvious surgical errors, many physicians and staff do not see any problem with the status quo. The common response is that the problems occur in someone else's clinic or operating room. The reality is that problems are pervasive throughout the healthcare system. Physicians are much less likely than the public to believe that quality of care is a problem and less likely to believe that a national agency is needed to address the problems of medical errors (Brennan and Berwick 1996). For improvement to occur, these physicians must be confronted with data and discussion (Bradley et al. 2003).

Consumers of healthcare services know that healthcare has problems beginning at the phone call to get an appointment. A patient calling his or her primary care office often waits several minutes to talk with the scheduler and is then asked the same questions as at the last visit. Healthcare has countless examples of huge errors, yet many healthcare workers cannot see the forest for the trees (see Figure 15.2).

Studies have shown the chasm between managers' perceptions and the objective reality of their businesses. Senior managers commonly surround themselves with yea-sayers who filter warnings from middle management. Similarly, Mezias (2003) found an astonishingly high prevalence of large errors in perception of their businesses among executives. One-third of specialists in fields other than quality and one-quarter of quality

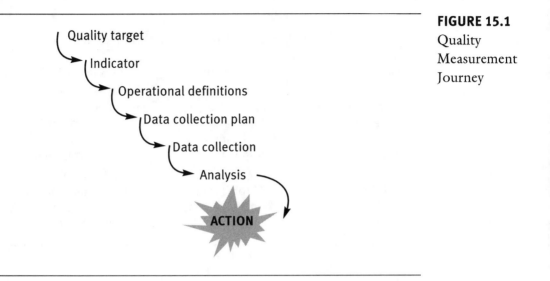

FIGURE 15.1
Quality
Measurement
Journey

specialists were off by at least 50 percent when tested on the meaning of basic outcome metrics (Mezias and Starbuck 2002). These errors in perception are a challenge for physicians. Physicians tend to focus on the specific task at hand, without an appreciation for the bigger system. Physicians have succeeded throughout medical school and postgraduate training largely because of their individual work ethic and find teamwork and the larger system of care to be a foreign concept. The change in perception from the individual physician's contribution to care and the larger system must be highlighted for physicians and other staff to facilitate quality improvement and change (Bujak 2003).

While difficult, organizations must create a climate and culture where the truth is heard and understood. Leaders must learn to lead with questions, not answers. The powerful must engage in dialog and debate, not coercion. Subordinates may find it difficult to engage in open dialog, thereby derailing the improvement process. Perlow and Williams (2003) highlight these change challenges by suggesting a blameless culture where staff can evaluate errors (conduct autopsies) without blame. They suggest the creation of red-flag mechanisms that turn information into information that cannot be ignored. Thus, successful change agents create a climate where the truth is really heard and cannot be ignored (Bottles 2003). Executives must encourage employees to present their uncomfortable perspectives. The understanding of these alternative views is critical to improve quality in the healthcare organization.

FIGURE 15.2
Comparison
to Other
Industries

Putting Performance in Perspective

Industry Excellence	Healthcare	Track Record
Federal Express	Medical records	1/M vs. 5%–10%
Banking transactions	Hospital billing	1/10M vs. 2%
Airline landing/takeoff	Medication administration	1/M vs. 7%–10%
Lands End	Appointment scheduling	Knows size, color vs. no recognition
Home Depot	Chronic care management	$3 purchase and advice vs. $500 visit and little advice

Engage Physicians and Other Key Clinical Staff

Executives must include key clinical leaders and staff in any change process. While executives can prod and support change, the real drivers of clinical change must be physicians, nurses, and other staff. Executives may attempt to inspire a shared vision through effective communication and finding common ground; however, key clinical leaders must lead improvement initiatives in patient care areas.

Example

For example, the associate director of University Hospital in Ann Arbor, Michigan, developed a business plan and proposal for a center of excellence in women's health. She was passionate about the project but did not find a clinical leader to provide support. She opted to place the proposal in a drawer and await stronger support from clinical leadership. Fortunately, a new chairman of obstetrics and gynecology was soon recruited and had the same motivation for the center of excellence program. Within weeks, the center of excellence was successfully implemented with strong support from clinical leaders and other providers. The chairman was able to diffuse support for the program throughout the organization, starting with a few key individuals and eventually spreading the enthusiasm to other physicians and nurses. Through the associate director's patience and timing, the program's implementation was successful.

The theory of tipping-point leadership hinges on the insight that in any organization, once the beliefs and energies of a critical mass of people are engaged, conversion to a new idea will spread like an epidemic, bringing fundamental change quickly (Kim and Mauborgne 2003). The theory of tipping-point leadership categorizes the members of any organization into the following rough groupings:

- Innovators (2.5 percent)
- Early adopters (13.5 percent)
- Early majority (34.0 percent)
- Late majority (34.0 percent)
- Laggards (15.0 percent)

This predictable process must be considered in implementing change. It took the right team of innovators to make the center of excellence work at University Hospital. All the hard work by the associate director would not have resulted in the project's fruition without proper support. That is, the chairman provided the clinical leadership required to convert other key clinical chairs, which led to the support of the division directors, which led to the support of the faculty and nursing staff, and then implementation was possible. Successful program development can be enhanced by a *rapid-results initiative*, which uses teams to achieve a miniature version of the overall goal. Team members draw on the work of all the parallel teams to have a successful program implementation (Matta and Ashkenas 2003).

Obstacles

Physicians will support change but are often skeptical at first. Change will only occur when the inadequacy of the current behavior or process is understood. Physicians often have divergent views based on past personal experience. A physician who has participated in a similar, but failed, program will be reluctant to spend time or lend support and may see the initiative as a waste of time. Physicians often have financial conflicts of interest in working on these projects. These conflicts can be direct, as with an internist who is paid for every day the patient is admitted while the hospital is paid on a diagnosis-related group fixed payment basis. The hospital that attempts to limit length of stay may present a direct conflict with the physician. It is important for the executive to understand that the private practice physician is an independent businessperson and does not see the hospital as anything but a place to admit patients. Hospital committee work and time spent on improvement initiatives take away from time the physician can see patients and earn money for the private practice. Providing medical services with a revenue stream is how the private practice physician survives. Thus, the hospital administrator must understand these direct and indirect conflicts when targeting physicians' participation in improvement and change programs.

Implementation Considerations

Nevertheless, physicians can and will change given the right situation. Emphasize personal communication with physicians. Personal meetings with credible messengers have the best chance to build rapport and credibility with these key individuals. Committee discussions can be effective; however, the key leaders need to be enthusiastic supporters of the change before the meeting begins. The process of effective change implementation can be very time consuming. It may appear to be more time efficient to present new initiatives to a group; however, unless key people have seen and support the information before the group meeting, the initiative is unlikely to move forward. Similarly, letters, phone calls, newsletters, bulletin board messages, and e-mail tend to be ineffective in moving projects forward. As an information source for the general medical staff, these impersonal methods of communication can be beneficial; however, the real work must be done through a series of one-on-one and small-group discussions to get the initiative moving.

Effective leaders must eliminate the "we versus them" mentality and work toward effective partnerships. Medical staff is infrequently homogenous and cannot generally be represented by one common voice. This is particularly important when working with medical staff leaders. It is not uncommon for elected leaders to assume that the physicians agree with both platform and direction. In reality, support must be tested through direct and open discussions with individuals on the medical staff. While the chief of staff may have clout, other practicing physicians do not necessarily recognize this individual as their representative.

Effective communication depends on a clear understanding of terminology and language. Healthcare has become increasingly specialized, which can impair effective communication. Physicians use a clinical and patient-specific lexicon, whereas administrators speak the language of teams, systems, and populations (Ransom, Tropman, and Pinsky 2001). Frequently, words used by an administrator may not convey the intended message to the physician. For example, an experiment was conducted with the leadership team of a large health system including more than 40 hospitals nationwide. The leadership team consisted of all site CEOs and chief medical officers. The team was asked to individually write ten words that describe or support the term *quality healthcare*. Fewer than 25 percent of the group had three or more of the same terms describing healthcare quality. In fact, only 60 percent of the group had just one of the same terms describing healthcare quality. While everyone in the room was an expert in leading their hospitals, the group had completely inconsistent definitions of healthcare quality. This simple experiment shows the difficulty with effective communication of even basic concepts to healthcare workers.

Effective communication is critical in gaining support for new initiatives. Specifically, developing a compelling reason for clinicians to support a program is essential. For example, an obstetrical clinical pathway was developed and implemented by a multidisciplinary team for a hospital system delivering more than 12,000 babies annually. The clinical pathway received much support from management, and most providers expressed agreement; however, as with most clinical pathway programs, the implementation was not widespread despite verbal support from clinicians. Simultaneously, a study demonstrated that care for 11.7 percent of all obstetrical patients and 43.2 percent of filed malpractice claims did not follow the clinical pathway (Mello 2001; Ransom et al. 2003). Only after collection of these data that demonstrated clinical pathway use with a reduction in medicolegal claims did the physicians support the pathway effort. While not said, the physicians originally saw the clinical pathway effort as a way for the hospital to save money. Only after the physicians saw a significant benefit to their practices was the pathway operationally supported. Thus, leading an improvement initiative is optimized when clinicians can be shown that the change will improve their situation (Elsbach 2003).

It is imperative to engage clinical staff on quality initiatives. While it may seem more efficient to garner support after the program is nearly complete and ready to implement, this approach often results in unforeseen delays. Physicians will support programs that have had their real commitment and involvement, and they should be involved in the initiative from the beginning for meaningful change. Another advantage of early involvement is effective communication. The physician will be a better translator to other providers if the initiative is presented in clinically oriented language. A program that is ready to implement, with an executive hoping to get last-minute support from a token physician, is often met with opposition. The astute physician will frequently understand the operational issues that will hinder implementation of the program and thereby address or even avert them. That is, until the individual physician can understand how his or her practice style or behavior affects the whole, change is often difficult. Following are some of the possibilities of modifying physician behavior (see Chapters 3 and 8) (Ransom and Pinsky 1999):

- Physician profiling
- Practice guidelines
- Disease management programs
- Academic detailing
- Alerts and reminders
- Standard order sets
- Compensation programs

- Effective credentialing
- Clinical leadership commitment

Implementing quality as a core organizational strategy requires substantial leadership from the top. While very few healthcare organizations have made the commitment to focus on quality as the core objective, more and more hospitals are individually pursuing this course. IHI has facilitated a group of highly committed hospitals interested in achieving top quality through its IMPACT group. Similarly, the Solucient top 100 hospital list has presented an opportunity to recognize organizations that have achieved the highest levels for measurable quality. Lastly, many hospitals are going through the long and arduous process to be considered for the Malcolm Baldrige National Quality Award.[6] While few will receive the award, the process and additional focus on quality will improve performance in these inspired organizations.

Case Study: Entering the Digital Era

Within the last 15 years, a sustained commitment has existed within the healthcare industry to adopt technologies that enable the electronic medical record to become a reality. The obvious first steps were within the business office functions. The admission/discharge/transfer (ADT) function has matured, and the demographic, identifier, and billing data are routinely handled electronically. In fact, payment mechanisms now emulate the best-of-breed environment in which claims processing and payment are fully automated. In conjunction, the ancillary environment of laboratory, pharmacy, radiology, and pathology has also evolved through niche best-of-breed vendors maturing into robust systems that have seen at least three product cycles. These form the foundation of the legacy systems present in healthcare today. This fact brings formidable challenges to interface issues, especially when one realizes that most of these systems are highly configured to the adopting institution's needs.

Within the clinical environment, defined by imaging, waveform, and actual patient care units, the picture changes significantly. The paper-based, nonlongitudinal record, coupled with a prevalent "art of medicine approach," is not sufficient to enhance the quality of care. Immediate clinical access to standard protocols has been shown to reduce the variation in patient care.

The decision to go digital is still a challenging one given the state of the legacy systems in place and the experience with them. An air of skepticism is often prevalent in the senior executive suite. While there is vigorous debate that going digital is largely an unfunded mandate, the perception of the consumer and pressure from quality organizations such as the Leapfrog Group have made the conversion to a digital environment a top priority. National databases show that clinical applications such as computerized physician order entry (CPOE), the clinical data repository, pharmacy integration, and electronic medical records are high on hospital budget request lists. The following case describes the evaluation and implementation process for a large academic tertiary care children's hospital that had a mix of paper and electronic systems.

Diary of an Academic Medical Center

The Children's Hospital of Wisconsin is located in Milwaukee, where a fair degree of managed care penetration has occurred over the last decade. The hospital is affiliated with a medical school, with faculty physicians on staff in addition to private medical staff. The legacy system includes a hospital information system with an ADT module, outpatient scheduling, complete billing and collection system, charge system, and demographics module. In addition to various administrative systems, a host of applications manage individual department functions such as the laboratory, radiology, pharmacy, dietary, facilities, and environmental services.

The main documentation system for medical records is a combination of electronic and paper, whereas radiology is primarily film. Dictation is available in specific departments such as radiology, ICU, emergency, and operating room. Monitors are capable of sending telemetry data to central stations inside the hospital. Electrocardiograms are currently paper based. Clinicians can view summary discharge data; laboratory, pathology, and radiology reports; as well as medication administration summaries on workstations and remotely through a secure virtual private network.

A CPOE system was implemented approximately three years ago; it has resulted in more than 98 percent of inpatient orders being entered electronically by physicians. The exceptions are the outpatient clinics and emergency department, where unit secretaries are responsible for entering the orders. To complete the picture, there are various decision support applications supporting quality improvement, utilization management, risk management, a trauma registry, and finance.

Exploring the human factor against this backdrop, a few facts are relevant. The medical staff is an open staff, with a large number of private physicians admitting to the hospital. Apart from the approximately 250 faculty physicians, at various times during any month about 100 residents and fellows, 60 to 80 medical students, and an equal number of allied health students are rotating through the various services. Approximately 100 private physicians account for a large percentage of the overall admissions.

Implementation of New Technology

This hospital has benefited from the presence of a mature information technology department. Regardless, the experience implementing a CPOE system highlights that physician resistance can be considerable if there is no perceived value to the practitioner. Cultural factors were actually more significant than technology issues in the acceptance of the new system. With the implementation of bar coding and other safety-related technologies such as medication cabinets and a unit dose pharmacy robot, as well as an ever-increasing array of services and high-technology devices, the volume of data needed for patient care was obviously overwhelming the remaining paper and film media.

The evaluation process to decide on a total digital environment was a long and challenging one. Over a period of two years, the present legacy system infrastructure was thoroughly analyzed. It became obvious from this exercise that the issue of data standards for coding items, such as problems, was critical because information was generated and passed between various vendor products. Even with the HL-7 standard, enough ambiguity existed that additional standards or highly customized interfaces were needed to achieve this goal. An enterprisewide data repository that could be accessed by the various clinical applications was also clearly needed. A filmless digital radiology and cardiology system would also be needed to complete the medical record.

When the issue of monitoring data was reviewed, an even more interesting fact emerged. Waveform data are transmitted in primarily proprietary formats, so integrating monitors and information systems is difficult if this fact is not considered beforehand. The case worsens when other devices such as intravenous pumps, anesthesia machines, and ventilators are examined.

The major consideration was user needs and requirements. Nurses comprise the majority of clinicians in hospitals. Documentation, results review, and communication essentially define their requirements of the system. One of the more demanding sets of tasks for the nurse clinician is capturing data from devices and documenting it in flowsheets that are part of the medical record. Enabling automatic capture of this data stream would have positive consequences for workflow. In addition, it would enable real-time review by physicians, thus reducing communication requirements between clinicians.

Physicians had the additional issues of order entry and note completion. Given the extreme variations in comfort level with a digital environment, it was necessary to select systems that would be acceptable to the least-savvy group. Sign-on and system navigation ("clickology") were identified as major issues relating to acceptance for busy practitioners, who saw the initiative as an increased time commitment without a demonstrable value.

In addition, there was an unrelenting demand for clinical content and decision support as subjective measures of quality and safety. With the addition of a patient safety officer at this institution, new safety issues related to alerts as well as timeliness of information were raised.

Also emerging as part of this evaluation was an interesting phenomenon, the "feature and functionality" perception. Various groups of specialty physicians expected features and functions in the system's components based on their perceptions of what and how a digital system should perform. On closer examination, this was based on a mix of what they had seen in various products as well as individual perceptions of what computers were supposed to do. This was a valuable lesson learned, in that expectations needed to be firmly managed to achieve success.

Evaluation Phase

Evaluation began with an assessment of commercial systems in existence and their classification. Three major groups could be identified:

1. Best-of-breed applications that offered superior features and functionality in a specific care area but required significant interfaces to other parts of the enterprise as well as the data repository.
2. Enterprisewide information systems that had clinical, financial, support, and resource management systems. These required a significant investment in the basic architecture as well as reinvestment in the legacy infrastructure.
3. Enterprisewide clinical information systems that offered features and functionality across care areas and the capability to store data in a single repository as well as the capability to interface with existing support and legacy systems.

Each group offered varying degrees of capability in terms of integration with medical devices. In addition, when the experience of installation, maintenance, and upgrades was examined, significant differences existed among the groups. One would logically assume that more interfaces and customization would require more resources from the health system information technology department as well as more extensive support from the vendor. The best-of-breed group was eliminated first because of the sheer number of interfaces, patient safety issues with inconsistent alerts and coding standards between systems, and long-term maintenance challenges. The other two groups were much harder to differentiate. This work required another look at the vision. If one were to characterize it as enabling the hospital to provide the best care possible using the most recent information generated from any source, with maximum decision support from the system, what would be the determining factor in the direction? The answer lay in the needs of the user. The system that enabled an integrated, clinically relevant record to be used by physicians and nurses in an efficient manner would provide the best solution. Issues such as single sign-on; graphical user interface; and availability of information in a wired, wireless, and remote fashion were also critical factors for the eventual direction.

Based on the analysis described above, it was decided that the present legacy medical equipment and information systems were most compatible with an enterprise clinical information system. Accordingly, a system was selected that offered a clinical data repository, ambulatory medical record, care area models for documentation and flowsheet capture, enterprisewide portal, and digital systems for cardiology and radiology, including a filmless capability. A digital electrocardiograph repository was also purchased. A successor-integrated order entry module was also included. The vendor commitment to enhance the features and functionality of the various modules was also essential in satisfying the clinicians' requirements.

The final decision was the order of implementation. Modules that presented immediate benefit to clinicians by providing new functionality were implemented first, working toward progressively more complex applications and replacement of current applications. The first applications listed for installation were the emergency department digital tracker and documentation modules, a portal to accommodate remote access and single sign-on, and modules supporting cardiology. This was, by experience, the path of least resistance from a cultural and learning point of view. It also took into account the most pressing clinician needs from a workflow perspective. The recognition of which specialty physicians required the most convincing also played a role in the order of installation.

In summary, the conversion, although long in the making, is just beginning. A tremendous amount of perspective has been gained in the process of planning a digital conversion to a mixed legacy infrastructure. The future holds great promise for safe, effective, and high-quality care, and a lot of hard work remains.

Study Questions

1. Did the executive team of the Children's Hospital of Wisconsin develop a clear vision for implementing the more comprehensive clinical information system?
2. What should the executive team consider in developing an effective implementation team to achieve its vision?

3. What type of metrics may provide value in ensuring that the vision was achieved and implementation was successful?
4. How can the clinical information systems implementation team engage physicians and other key clinical staff in the implementation?

Notes

1. See IOM's web site at www.iom.edu.
2. See the group's web site at www.leapfroggroup.org.
3. See IHI's web site at www.ihi.org.
4. See NQF's web site at www.qualityforum.org.
5. For more information, see www.solucient.com.
6. See www.quality.nist.gov.

REFERENCES

Atchison, T. A., and J. S. Bujak. 2001. *Leading Transformational Change: The Physician-Executive Partnership.* Chicago: Health Administration Press.

Bottles, K. 2003. "Wandering in the Desert: Lessons from a Life in Health Care." *Physician Executive* 29 (3): 14–17.

Bradley, E. H., E. S. Holmboe, J. A. Mattera, S. A. Roumanis, M. J. Radford, and H. M. Krumholz. 2003. "The Roles of Senior Management in Quality Improvement Efforts: What Are the Key Components?" *Journal of Healthcare Management* 48 (1): 15–29.

Brennan, T. A., and D. M. Berwick. 1996. *New Rules: Regulations, Markets, and the Quality of American Health Care.* San Francisco: Jossey-Bass Publishers.

Bujak, J. S. 2003. "Service and Collaboration: Keys to Physician Control." *Physician Executive* 28 (3): 22–25.

Collins, J. 2001. *Good to Great: Why Some Companies Make the Leap . . . and Others Don't.* New York: Harper Collins.

Collins, J., and J. Porras. 1997. *Built to Last: Successful Habits of Visionary Companies.* New York: Harper Collins.

Dye, C. F. 2002. *Winning the Talent War: Ensuring Effective Leadership in Healthcare.* Chicago: Health Administration Press.

Elsbach, K. D. 2003. "How to Pitch a Brilliant Idea." *Harvard Business Review* 81 (9): 117–23.

Herman, R. E., and J. L. Gioia. 2000. *How to Become an Employer of Choice.* Greensboro, NC: Oakhill Press.

Jackman, J. M., and M. H. Strober. 2003. "Fear of Feedback." *Harvard Business Review* 81 (4): 101–108.

Jackson, P., and H. Delehanty. 2002. *Sacred Hoops*. New York: Hyperion.

Kim, W. C., and R. Mauborgne. 2003. "Tipping Point Leadership." *Harvard Business Review* 81 (4): 60–69.

Langley, G. J., K. M. Nolan, T. W. Nolan, C. L. Norman, and L. P. Provost. 1996. *The Improvement Guide: A Practical Approach to Enhancing Organizational Performance*. San Francisco: Jossey-Bass Publishers.

Lencioni, P. 1998. *The Five Temptations of a CEO*. San Francisco: Jossey-Bass Publishers.

Lewis, M. 2003. *Moneyball*. New York: W.W. Norton.

Matta, N. F., and R. N. Ashkenas. 2003. "Why Good Projects Fail Anyway." *Harvard Business Review* 81 (9): 109–16.

Mello, M. 2001. "Of Swords and Shields: The Role of Clinical Practice Guidelines in Medical Malpractice Litigation." *University of Pennsylvania Law Review* 149: 645–710.

Mezias, J. 2003. "What Do Managers Know, Anyway?" *Harvard Business Review* 81 (3): 101–104.

Mezias, J. M., and W. H. Starbuck. 2002. "Opening Pandora's Box: Studying the Accuracy of Managers' Perceptions." *Journal of Organizational Behavior* 17: 99–117.

Michaels, E., H. Handfield-Jones, and B. Axelrod. 2001. *The War for Talent*. Boston: Harvard Business School Press.

National Committee for Quality Assurance. 2003. *The State of Health Care Quality: 2003. Quality Compass*. Washington, DC: NCQA.

Perlow, L., and S. Williams. 2003. "Is Silence Killing Your Company?" *Harvard Business Review* 81 (5): 52–58.

Ransom, S. B., M. P. Dombrowski, D. Studdert, M. Mello, and T. A. Brennan. 2003. "Reduced Medico-Legal Risk by Compliance with Obstetrical Clinical Pathways: A Case-Control Study." *Obstetrics and Gynecology* 101 (4): 751–55.

Ransom, S. B., S. G. McNeeley, G. Doot, and D. B. Cotton. 1996. "The Effect of Capitated and Fee-for-Service Remuneration on Physician Decision Making in Gynecology." *Obstetrics and Gynecology* 87 (5): 707–10.

Ransom, S. B., and W. W. Pinsky. 1999. *Clinical Resource and Quality Management*. Tampa, FL: American College of Physician Executives Press.

Ransom, S. B., J. Tropman, and W. W. Pinsky. 2001. *Enhancing Physician Performance*. Tampa, FL: American College of Physician Executives Press.

Slater, R. 1999. *Jack Welch and the GE Way*. New York: McGraw-Hill.

Sutcliffe, K. M., and K. Weber. 2003. "The High Cost of Accurate Knowledge." *Harvard Business Review* 81 (5): 74–82.

Thompson, C. B., and J. W. Ware. 2003. *The Leadership Genius of George W. Bush*. New York: John Wiley & Sons.

IMPLEMENTING HEALTHCARE QUALITY IMPROVEMENT: CHANGING CLINICIAN BEHAVIOR

Valerie Weber and John Bulger

This chapter guides the healthcare leader, armed with a well-designed quality improvement initiative, toward success in implementation and diffusion of the initiative. The literature of change management as it pertains to healthcare is summarized. A framework for leadership of change initiatives within healthcare organizations is presented. This framework is then applied in a practical sense to guide the learner through key steps toward successful implementation of these initiatives. Case studies of three quality improvement initiatives and lessons learned are described.

Understanding Change Management in Healthcare

Preceding chapters have exposed readers to the important elements of healthcare quality and many of the latest strategies to bridge the "chasm of quality" in healthcare. Yet, without a solid knowledge of change management, healthcare leaders will not be able to improve the quality of healthcare in their organizations at the rate needed to bring about substantial improvement. Skills in change implementation are a necessary ingredient in the toolkits of current and future healthcare leaders. Understanding how physicians behave with respect to initiatives such as clinical pathways and the adoption of best practices is necessary to implement strategies that will actually be effective and to avoid repeated cycles of new initiative failure. In the field of healthcare quality, it is often not the strength of the initiatives, but rather the lack of leadership for change management and lack of focus on implementation that have led to much slower progress than should have been the case.

In examining healthcare in the context of other industries, it is ironic that healthcare systems do not pay more attention to change management. Healthcare has undergone a more dramatic technological explosion in the past few decades than perhaps any other industry; yet our healthcare organizations have not reacted with the same speed and agility to improve quality processes and decrease error as other industries such as airlines or manufacturing. While Motorola, Allied Signal, and other manufacturers have made great strides in Six Sigma quality programs, many in healthcare are still using the same care models and approaching patient care using the same outmoded paradigms despite the inefficient and error-prone nature of these systems. The ability to embrace change will be the distinguishing feature of the successful healthcare organization—and the successful healthcare leader—in the twenty-first century.

No matter how well a system or solution is conceived, designed, and executed, if people do not like it, it will fail. Conversely, no matter how poorly a system or solution is conceived, designed, and executed, if people want it to work, it will succeed (Shays 2003). The goal of the change leader is to do both things well: create well-designed solutions that will gain wide acceptance.

Diffusion of Innovations and Other Change Theories

How do some new ideas in healthcare, such as a new drug or treatment, gain broad acceptance, while other changes with equally strong—or even stronger—evidence bases never catch on? An often-cited example in healthcare is the use of laparoscopic surgery. Within a few years of its invention, it became widely used and is now considered the standard of care for most routine surgery. However, simpler innovations, such as the use of beta-blockers and aspirin after myocardial infarction, for which strong evidence has been available for years, are still not widely used.

The science of *diffusion of innovations* focuses on the study of how quickly change spreads and can help to explain these differences. These theories center on three basic themes: the perception of the innovation; characteristics of the people who choose to adopt or not adopt an innovation; and context, that is, how the change is communicated and led (Berwick 2003).

How an innovation is perceived is an important predictor of the rate of spread of the variation. Why do certain innovations spread more quickly than others? The characteristics that determine an innovation's rate of adoption are relative advantage, compatibility, complexity, trialability, and observability.

- *Relative advantage* is the degree to which the innovation is seen as better than that which it replaces. The greater the perceived relative advantage of an innovation, the more rapid its rate of adoption will be. Most of the time in medicine, this results from a risk-benefit calculation made by the individual physician. For example, most physicians will make the decision to try a new medication by weighing its efficacy against the need for monitoring, potential side-effects, and cost. A physician will prescribe a new medication if it is cheaper, easier for the patient to take (e.g., once a day as opposed to multiple doses), or safer or requires less monitoring.

- *Compatibility* is the degree to which the innovation is perceived as being consistent with the values, past experiences, and needs of potential adopters. It is less risky to trial a new drug that is similar to one a physician has tried with success in the past. An example is the plethora of "me-too" medications on the market today. These drugs are easy to introduce successfully into the market because of the compatibility factor.
- *Complexity* is the perception of the ease of application of the innovation. The simpler the change, the more likely it is to take root. Again using a medication example, a physician is unlikely to try a new drug if a letter needs to be written to a health maintenance organization (HMO) for approval because the drug is not on that HMO's formulary. This would make trying the new drug too complex and make it unlikely that it would be used.
- *Trialability* implies that the innovation can be used on a trial basis before the decision to adopt is made and enhances the perception that trying the innovation is low risk. If the medication is immediately available in a trial form in the office (pharmaceutical sampling), this will increase its likelihood of use by the physician.
- *Observability* is the ease with which a potential adopter can view others trying the change first. Pharmaceutical companies, in marketing new drugs to physicians and patients, use the observability and trialability concepts extensively. The use of in-office pharmaceutical samples decreases complexity, increases trialability and observability, and allows for compatibility once the physician gains success with the new drug.

Social science helps us to understand how individual characteristics of the members of a social group can in part explain the spread of a potential innovation. Everett Rogers's (1995) theory of diffusion of innovations explains that any innovation within a social group is adopted over time by a process he terms *natural diffusion*. These processes were first described in a group of Iowa farmers adopting a new form of hybrid seed corn. Over time, it has been recognized that this theory can be widely applied to any institution, societal fad, or organization, including healthcare. The change process is generally initiated by just a few adopters, whom Rogers terms *innovators*, who are excited by change and cope well with uncertainty. They often perform a gate-keeping role for new ideas into a system. Although this role is important, innovators are regarded by much of the group as somewhat radical and do not help the majority of the group to enact an innovation, but rather are the first to introduce it.

The next, and most important, group of individuals to adopt an innovation is the *early adopters*. This group includes the opinion leaders. These individuals are those to whom others look for guidance about the innovation. They often are the informal leaders and are key to decreasing uncertainty about the innovation by networking with their peers.

Innovations generally begin to take off when members of the *early majority*, hearing from satisfied adopters of the new idea, begin to create a critical mass for change. The *late majority* will eventually follow the lead of others after increasing pressure from their peers. The *laggards*, the last group of individuals in a system to adopt, remain suspicious of change agents and innovations. They tend to be socially isolated and are resistant to change efforts. These groups tend to be represented in a social group over a normal distribution (see Figure 16.1).

The rate of diffusion of innovations has much to do with organizational context, that is, those characteristics of an organization's culture that tend to support (or discourage) innovation and spread. The clear setting of goals, strong administrative support, support from physicians and nurses, and the use of high-quality feedback data are important factors leading to success (Bradley et al. 2001).

In his book *The Tipping Point*, Malcolm Gladwell (2000) makes several observations regarding change that can provide useful tools to guide those leading within organizations. Some ideas, behaviors, or products start epidemics, whereas others do not. The *tipping point* is that moment of critical mass, a threshold or boiling point for change with three identified agents, including the law of the few, the stickiness factor, and the power of context.

The *law of the few* describes three important types of persons critical to spreading epidemics—connectors, mavens, and salesmen. *Connectors* are important for both the numbers and kinds of people they know. They have an ability to maintain this high connectedness by spanning many different worlds. The connectors use the power of weak ties (i.e., word of mouth) to spread ideas with which they become enamored. Other key individuals, termed *mavens*, have a talent for accumulating and passing on knowledge. *Salesmen* help to create epidemics through their power to persuade others. Acting in concert, these individuals can rapidly spread an innovation. The implication is that the identification of these individuals in an organization enables them to be enlisted as champions of the change process.

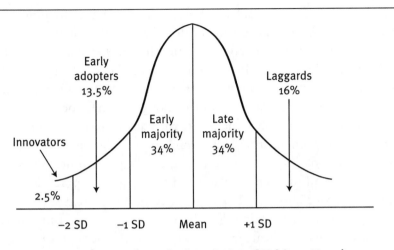

FIGURE 16.1
Rogers's
Adopter
Categories
Based on
Degree of
Innovativeness

Time to Adoption (Standard Deviations [SD] from Mean)

Source: Rogers (2003). Reprinted with the permission of The Free Press, a Division of Simon & Schuster Adult Publishing Group, from DIFFUSIONS OF INNOVATIONS, 5th Edition by Everett M. Rogers. Copyright © 1995, 2003 by Everett M. Rogers. Copyright © 1962, 1971, 1983 by The Free Press. All rights reserved.

The *stickiness factor* relates to the innovation or characteristics of the message itself that determine the rapidity with which an innovation or change "tips"(Gladwell 2000). Anything a change agent can do to enhance the "stickiness" of the message will increase the rate at which the change will tip. The power of context again addresses the framework for delivery of the message. Gladwell discusses what he calls the broken-window theory: "If a window is broken and left unrepaired, people walking by will conclude that no one cares . . . soon more windows will be broken and the sense of anarchy will spread from the building to the street on which it faces." This implies that quality initiatives will be more effectively received in a background of quality that pervades a healthcare organization. Literature regarding organizational culture and change discusses such issues in detail; such a discussion is beyond the scope of this chapter.

Physician-Specific Research

Understanding why and how physicians change is key to a mastery of how to implement changes in healthcare quality. A behavioral study targeted at general practitioners in London showed that rarely did a single trigger for behavior change exist, but rather an accumulation of evidence that change was possible, desirable, and worthwhile. These cues came from educational interactions in some cases, but more importantly from contact with professional colleagues, particularly those who were especially influential or respected (Armstrong, Reyburn, and Jones 1996). When enough of these cues accumulated, the behavior would change *(accumulation model)*. Furthermore, there seemed to be a limited number of changes that could be made over a fixed period, with three to four changes over a six-month period being the norm. At other times, though, changes occurred abruptly in the face of an immediate challenge; the authors term this the *challenge model* of change. One particularly strong source of influence was the practitioner's personal experience of a drug or illness. Another was a clinical disaster, or a bad outcome that tended to change the practitioner's prescribing behavior abruptly. The experience of one patient with a particularly serious or life-threatening side-effect could cause long-lasting avoidance of the use of that medication and was one of the strongest effects seen.

The *continuity model* of change describes how sometimes practitioners change readily based on a level of preparedness for a particular change (e.g., the provider was waiting for a more acceptable treatment because of the difficulty of use of the currently available treatment or the cost of the current therapy). The strongest reinforcer to continue the change is the feedback of patients. A patient's positive report reinforces the behavior change; conversely, a negative result such as a major side-effect is often enough to stop the experiment. In the initial stages of the change, a high risk of reverting to the original prescribing patterns exists. Ironically, though, many clinicians espouse evidence-based medicine, which emphasizes the importance of proving effectiveness in large numbers of patients; in this study, most physicians seemed to base changes in prescribing on the results of a few initial experiments with a small number of patients (Armstrong, Reyburn, and Jones 1996). Most changes appeared to require a period of preparation through a process of educational cues and contact with opinion leaders. Educational efforts were necessary, but by no means sufficient, to produce the needed change.

Physicians often fail to comply with best practices. One study analyzed self-reports by physicians explaining why in particular instances, after chart review, best practices in diabetics such as screening for microalbuminuria, hyperlipidemia, and retinopathy were not followed. Reasons found were less-than-optimal oversight (it slipped through the cracks), systems issues, and patient nonadherence, but in a surprising number of cases, physicians made a conscious decision not to comply with the recommendation (Mottur-Pilson, Snow, and Bartlett 2001). Individual physicians have often balked at the idea of practice guidelines as inherently "cookbook medicine." Many physicians view themselves in the craftsperson or artist mode and consider individual variation as acceptable or even desirable. As a group, physicians have seen their practices increasingly scrutinized by the government, third-party payers, and consumers. When viewing the quality improvement movement from this direction, the lack of championing by the medical profession, although improved in recent years, has clearly slowed the pace of change.

Leading Change

Change within organizations cannot occur in the absence of skilled leadership. Leadership can be defined in many ways and has been described as "a set of processes that creates organizations . . . or adapts them to significantly changing circumstances. Leadership defines what the future should look like, aligns people with that vision, and inspires them to make it happen, despite the obstacles" (Kotter 1996). Many feel that leadership is entirely about creating change. While managers create order and predictability, leaders establish direction and motivate and inspire people. While both management and leadership are necessary, change depends on skilled leadership.

Reinertsen (1998) describes leaders as "initiators," who "define reality, often with data . . . they develop and test changes, persuade others, are not daunted by the loud, negative voices, and are not afraid to think and work outside their immediate areas of responsibility." Similarly, John Kotter (1996) has proposed a road map to create change that includes establishment of a sense of urgency, creation of a guiding coalition, creation of a vision, effective communication of the vision, and creation of short-term wins to show success can be achieved (see Figure 16.2).

Leaders of change find it necessary to remove structural barriers to ensure that the needed changes are possible. For example, if resources of time are an issue, it may be necessary to dedicate a percentage of time to key employees to direct quality initiatives or to restructure reward and incentive systems to promote quality improvement. Increasingly, physicians are taking on leadership roles; these roles are important in serving as boundary spanners to champion quality initiatives in healthcare (Zuckerman et al. 1998). Developing this leadership within healthcare organizations is key to maximize cooperative leadership between physicians and administration.

Reducing Variation: The Example of Clinical Practice Guidelines

It has been increasingly recognized that large variations in the standards of care exist for many healthcare conditions. The literature (Jencks, Huff, and Cuerdon 2003) has demonstrated that extremes of variation in the amount of expenditures on care in Medicare populations have not resulted in better quality, increased access to services, improved satisfaction, or better health outcomes in these populations. Underuse, overuse, and misuse

FIGURE 16.2

Kotter's
Stages of
Creating
Major Change

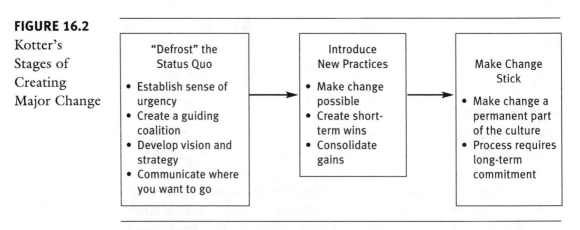

"Defrost" the Status Quo	Introduce New Practices	Make Change Stick
• Establish sense of urgency • Create a guiding coalition • Develop vision and strategy • Communicate where you want to go	• Make change possible • Create short-term wins • Consolidate gains	• Make change a permanent part of the culture • Process requires long-term commitment

Source: Weber and Joshi (2000). © Joint Commission Resources: *Joint Commission Journal on Quality Improvement.* Oakbrook Terrace, IL: Joint Commission on Accreditation of Healthcare Organizations, 2000, Figure 1. Reprinted with permission.

all clearly abound in U.S. medicine (Chassin 1998). Again, industry has been the leader in the concept of achieving quality by reducing variation.

From this concept, the clinical practice guideline movement was born in the last decades of the twentieth century. Since the 1980s, the knowledge base required to practice high-quality medicine has increased dramatically. Each month, thousands of articles in the medical literature could potentially result in changes in practice. It is estimated that within five to ten years of the completion of training, more than 50 percent of the knowledge learned by physicians has become obsolete. The clinical practice guideline movement arose as a means of helping to translate the medical literature into concise statements meant to change practice. By 1995, more than 60 organizations in at least ten countries were producing clinical practice guidelines (Rogers 1995). Although this movement continues, observations show that its basic mission has largely been unsuccessful. Clinical guidelines are gathering dust on every clinician's bookshelf because of a lack of attention to implementation.

During the development of most guidelines, data are synthesized from the literature by the sponsoring body, often a national specialty organization; experts review the quality of the evidence; then the information is collated as guidelines. Often, these guidelines are published or disseminated to providers. Although these guidelines are widely available, most practitioners are not using them in everyday practice. The gap between the knowledge and practice is complex, and a growing literature regarding this issue exists.

First, some qualities of the guidelines themselves may influence their adoption by clinicians. In the implementation of disease management strategies, clinicians insist that they (1) be simple, (2) be practical, and (3) not increase their workload or their staff's. The less complicated the guideline, the more compatible the recommendation with existing beliefs or values; the greater the ease of use of the guideline, the more likely it is to be adopted. Other variables, such as the characteristics of the healthcare professional (age and country of training in particular), characteristics of the practice setting, and use of incentives and imposed regulations, can also influence their adoption. A review by Cabana et al. (1999) discussed other barriers to guideline implementation, including physician knowledge (e.g., lack of awareness, lack of familiarity), attitudes (e.g., lack of agreement, lack of self-efficacy, lack of outcome expectancy, inertia of previous practice), or behavior (e.g., external barriers) (see Figure 16.3).

The literature has continued to examine why physicians do not adhere to clinical practice guidelines. One report studied the use of a pneumonia practice guideline in an emergency department. The authors report influence of a variety of patient factors, including age greater than 65, comorbidities, and social factors; and physician factors, most notably, the more experience treating pneumonia reported by the physician, the less likely the physician was to adhere to the guideline (Halm et al. 2000).

Active Implementation Strategies

Greco and Eisenberg (1993) note that at times changes in medical practice are rapid and dramatic, as with the replacement of many open surgical procedures with laparoscopic procedures in the span of just a few years, and at times slow to proceed, as with the use of beta-blockers for patients after myocardial infarction. The traditional, time-honored approach of continuing medical education (CME) is the most often used method to attempt to improve the dissemination of new medical knowledge, yet this approach has consistently been shown to have little effect in the absence of enabling or practice-reinforcing strategies (Davis 1998). In particular, most studies that used only printed materials failed to demonstrate changes in performance or health outcomes, a finding that has also been associated with the distribution of guidelines (Oxman et al. 1995). Similarly, conferences, particularly those during which no explicit effort was made to facilitate practice change, failed to demonstrate change in performance or health outcomes. More interactive workshops have demonstrated some positive, but overall mixed, results. One publication demonstrated that the exposure of Canadian family practice physicians to a 90-minute workshop on the ordering of preventive tests did not increase the ordering of items recommended for inclusion but did decrease unnecessary test ordering (Beaulieu et al. 2002).

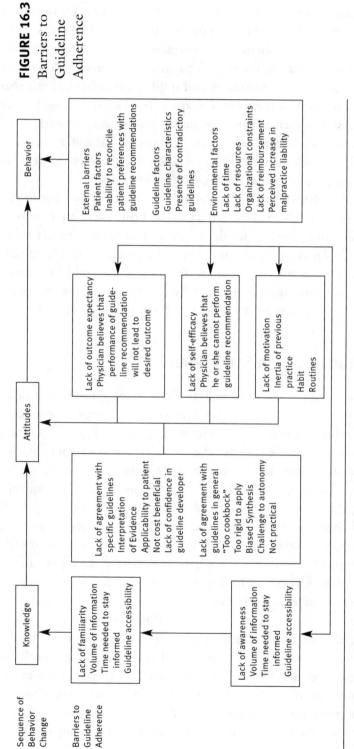

FIGURE 16.3
Barriers to
Guideline
Adherence

Other, more active strategies of diffusing medical knowledge have shown more promise. The use of opinion leaders, locally influential physicians whose opinions hold sway with their peers, has been shown to be effective in improving outcomes (Davis 1998). Other studies have shown that the recruitment of these leaders to disseminate information via local implementation of clinical practice guidelines can effectively change prescribing patterns and health outcomes (Davis 1998).

A strategy termed *academic detailing*, which involves outreach visits to a practice site by opinion leaders, has been found to be effective in accelerating the dissemination of best practices. This strategy was modeled on the methods of pharmaceutical sales representatives. A trained physician or pharmacist would deliver one-on-one education or feedback sessions. Evidence from controlled trials shows that academic detailing alters prescribing, affects blood pressure blood product transfusion practices, and improves hypertension control (Goldberg et al. 1998). These studies suggest that, although the content of the guidelines is indeed important, the presentation of the guidelines (i.e., in a weak fashion—mass mailings, didactic, CME—or by methods that are of proven benefit—academic detailing, the use of opinion leaders) is critical to their success.

The use of reminders involves any intervention (manual or computerized) that prompts the healthcare provider to perform a clinical action. Examples include concurrent or intervisit reminders to professionals regarding desired actions or enhanced laboratory reports or administrative systems that can prompt a desired action (e.g., follow-up appointment reminders). These methods are moderately effective in some settings (Oxman et al. 1995).

The use of audit and feedback systems is an additional strategy that has been examined. Such systems generally involve providing clinicians with information comparing their practices and outcomes with those of other physicians in their group or an external benchmark. Such methods have demonstrated decreased laboratory ordering (Ramoska 1998), increased compliance with preventive care or cancer-screening guidelines (Mandelblatt and Kanetsky 1995), and more appropriate drug-prescribing behavior (Schectman et al. 1995).

Administrative interventions that implement rules or barriers to test ordering have also been shown to be effective in various settings. For example, evidence shows these interventions to decrease the utilization of certain laboratory studies by simple modifications of the laboratory ordering form or changes in funding policy (Van Walraven, Goel, and Chan 1998).

The use of continuous quality improvement teams has also been described. Practice sites are trained in quality improvement techniques including the Plan-Do-Study-Act methodology. Although healthcare has shown a great deal of enthusiasm for the adoption of Six Sigma methodology, exported from successful initiatives for quality improvement in industry, the use of such strategies in healthcare to improve outcomes has a limited track record. One report using local team-based quality improvement practices found variable success in improving guideline conformity but increased effectiveness when used in conjunction with other techniques such as academic detailing (Goldberg et al. 1998).

The use of multifaceted interventions, including combinations of audit and feedback, reminders, academic detailing, and opinion leaders, has demonstrated changes in professional performance and, less consistently, changes in health outcomes. A systematic review of interventions intended to change clinician behavior found that 62 percent of interventions aimed at one behavioral factor were successful in changing behavior, whereas 86 percent of interventions targeted at two or more behavioral factors reported success (Solomon et al. 1998). Healthcare leaders must combine strategies to produce effects that are cumulative and significant (see Figure 16.4).

Decision Support

The use of reminder systems has long been suggested as a method of increasing guideline adherence by clinicians. Many early studies used manual chart review strategies with reminders to physicians during the actual visit. Such strategies included chart stickers or tags, medical record checklists, flowsheets, and nurse-initiated reminders. Patient-directed reminders have also been tried and include letters, telephone calls, and questionnaires. Proven efficacy exists for many of these interventions (McPhee et al. 1991). Limitations of these efforts center on the labor-intensive nature of these processes and their unsustainability over time.

The promise of information technology and electronic medical records to streamline this process is immense. Beginning in the early 1990s, reports of computerized reminder systems began to appear in the literature. Early trials showed significant differences in performance of cancer prevention activities (McPhee et al. 1991) and surveillance activities (McDonald, Wilson, and McCabe 1980). More recent trials have demonstrated that computerized reminders can increase the performance of preventive care activities in hospitalized patients (Dexter et al. 2001) as well as improve adherence to guidelines for the prophylaxis of deep venous thrombosis (Durieux et al. 2000).

There is a burgeoning literature regarding the use of electronic medical records to influence physician behavior through the implementation of more advanced decision support systems. Thus far, computerized test ordering systems with embedded clinical practice guidelines have demon-

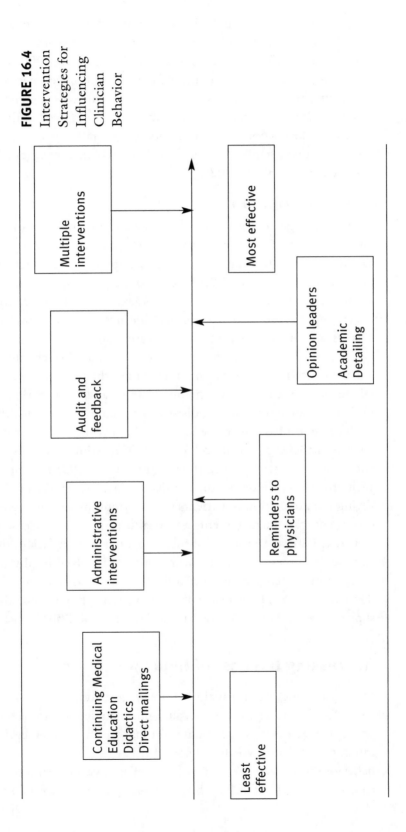

FIGURE 16.4 Intervention Strategies for Influencing Clinician Behavior

strated the ability to reduce laboratory test ordering by primary care physicians (Van Wijk et al. 2001) and increase the use of aspirin in patients with
coronary artery disease in the outpatient setting (Walker 2003). Preliminary
work in this area shows that alerts for aspects of preventive medicine vary
in effectiveness depending on where in the course of the encounter such
prompts appear. For example, if the physician is reminded during the wrong
portion of the encounter, the prompts are generally ignored. Alerts are also
more effective when supported by other enabling strategies such as audit
and feedback (Walker 2003).

Disease Management

Disease management has been one answer to the question of how to drive
physicians to conform to best practices. Disease management can be defined
as any program devoted to the care of populations characterized by the
presence of a chronic disease. Most of these programs have been designed
by third parties such as managed care organizations to reduce costs through
decreasing variation. Improving health outcomes while lowering use and
costs is the underlying strategy of disease management.

Many believe that the most effective method of changing physician
behavior is to make "doing the right thing" the path of least resistance by
taking the guideline out of the physician's hands and sharing the responsibility of managing chronic diseases with an expanded healthcare team.
Such programs have proven effective in improving outcomes and reducing
costs of diabetes care (Sidorov et al. 2002), asthma (Bolton et al. 1991),
and congestive heart failure (CHF) (Rich et al. 1995). Characteristics of
such programs include population disease management, a method of identifying the population of patients with a symptom management plan, education and case management, and health promotion/disease prevention
activities. Barriers to the use of such programs include lack of financial and
staffing resources as well as cultural barriers involved in physicians evolving to a more team-based method of disease management. As with any
implementation, adequate attention to physician buy-in and administrative
support and involvement are crucial (Waters et al. 2001).

Addressing the Cost of Implementation

Many guidelines do not include information about how implementation
will affect health resources. Because most guidelines do not address this
issue, one barrier to implementation may be the misperception that the
value gained is not worth the cost. Efforts to change physicians' clinical
behavior should be in accord with administrative and reimbursement policies. For example, if an organization asks physicians to spend more time

identifying and treating depression and at the same time pressures them to see more patients, depression care is unlikely to improve. If the structure of the healthcare system, in particular its reimbursement structure, runs counter to medical guidelines, even the best guidelines will not likely be implemented successfully (Brook 1995).

It is necessary to distinguish between *treatment cost effectiveness*, that is, the incremental costs and benefits of a treatment, and *policy cost effectiveness*, the cost when taking into account treatment cost effectiveness and the cost and magnitude of the implementation method needed to enact the change. Having to invest resources to change physician behavior imposes an additional cost on treatment cost effectiveness. Policy cost effectiveness will only remain attractive when effective but inexpensive implementation methods exist, or if large health gains per patient exist for a high-prevalence disease. For example, the use of angiotension converting enzyme (ACE) inhibitors for heart failure is considered cost effective at $2,602 per life year gained. Estimates of successful implementation based on academic detailing programs used in England by the National Health Service, which had a significant effect at a small cost per patient ($446 per life year gained) would allow the intervention to retain its cost effectiveness. However, the cost of academic outreach to promote a reduction in newer classes of anti-depressants in favor of less-expensive tricyclic antidepressants is not cost saving, as the cost per patient for outreach exceeds the cost saving from behavioral change. Thus, the cost and efficacy of the implementation method must be added to the cost effectiveness of the treatment to make a policy decision based on cost effectiveness (Mason et al. 2001) (see Figure 16.5).

Furthermore, whether quality improvement initiatives make financial sense for an organization is a complex problem. A healthcare organization operating under capitated payment structures is likely to benefit from any strategy that reduces utilization or hospital admissions. A health system that is largely reimbursed under fee-for-service plans or relies on diagnosis-related group payments from Medicare would lose money from any program that reduced hospital admissions. Successful chronic care programs have been discontinued because financial incentives did not exist to support the expense of such programs (Rich et al. 1995). In the ambulatory setting, the tables are reversed. Incurring utilization of ambulatory resources for largely unreimbursed chronic disease management results in decreased revenue per visit in a capitated managed care setting. Thus, to create a favorable business case for quality improvement initiatives, the savings or increased revenues from improved care must accrue to the organization paying for the improvements. External incentives are likely to play an increasingly dominant role in moving quality improvement and clinical guideline use, along with chronic disease models, forward.

FIGURE 16.5
Evaluating
Cost
Effectiveness

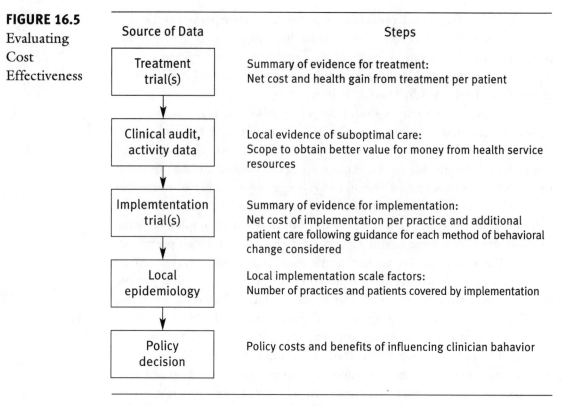

Source of Data	Steps
Treatment trial(s)	Summary of evidence for treatment: Net cost and health gain from treatment per patient
Clinical audit, activity data	Local evidence of suboptimal care: Scope to obtain better value for money from health service resources
Implemtentation trial(s)	Summary of evidence for implementation: Net cost of implementation per practice and additional patient care following guidance for each method of behavioral change considered
Local epidemiology	Local implementation scale factors: Number of practices and patients covered by implementation
Policy decision	Policy costs and benefits of influencing clinician bahavior

Source: Mason et al. (2001). Reprinted with permission of the American Medical Association. *Journal of the American Medical Association* 286 (23): 2988–92, figure. Copyright © 2001, American Medical Association. All rights reserved.

Keys to Successful Implementation and Lessons Learned

From the above discussion, readers should have gained knowledge of specific tools to improve dissemination of healthcare quality initiatives. This section summarizes key steps to the successful implementation of such initiatives.

1. *Focus on high-impact interventions.* What disease processes are most prevalent in your population? For most adult populations, diabetes, hypertension, and CHF will be the big three. What is your goal? If your goal is to reduce hospitalizations in patients with CHF, this will be attainable in the short term, whereas if your goal is to reduce the number of amputations in diabetics, expect a longer period for attainment.

2. *How are you performing now?* To know what to focus on, you need to know your current performance relative to benchmarks. Initially, it

will be easiest to correct those things that are furthest from benchmarks, often termed the "low-hanging fruit." Keep in mind the Pareto principle, or 80/20 rule, recognizing that the greatest amount of effort will be expended trying to accomplish that final 20 percent.

3. *For every hour spent discussing the content of the initiative, spend four hours planning its implementation.* Your practice guideline will do no good in your organization unless it is used. Emphasizing the structural or developmental phase without adequate attention to implementation is a sure recipe for failure. Use proven implementation methods, not merely passive education and dissemination, and use multiple interventions simultaneously.

4. *Who needs to change?* Analyze which individuals in the organization must respond to the proposed change and what barriers exist. Invest in the innovators and early adopters. Know who your opinion leaders are, and enlist them as your champions. Spend little time with the laggards, recognizing that in an era of constrained resources, change leaders must direct efforts at those who are on board or coming aboard.

5. *Do a cost-benefit analysis.* The costs of implementation, taking into account the implementation method, must be weighed against both the costs of inaction and the gains of a successful result. Too often, leaders fail to factor in the cost of a change early enough into the process. As a result, a great deal of work is done in an area that in the long run will not be sustainable. As described previously, the party who is expending the resources must generally be the same party reaping the financial benefits of the change.

6. *Enlist multidisciplinary teams.* Teams should consist of those who actually do the work, not the formal leadership. For example, an office redesign project should include representation from the front desk personnel, secretaries, nursing staff, and operational leadership, not just physicians.

7. *Think big, but start small.* The old saw "Rome wasn't built in a day" applies here. Projects that are too ambitious may cause an early failure—you need to achieve an early short-term gain to keep the bosses on board and silence the nay-sayers. Is your real goal to convert your practice from a traditional scheduling scheme to an open-access scheduling system? Start with a small project—either piloting this with one physician or working on a smaller, related project—before redesigning the entire system.

8. *Construct a timeline and publicize it.* Teams may sometimes spin their wheels and grind on forever without accomplishing anything. Once your goal has been determined, a timeline or road map should be constructed and publicized. This will give the team accountability

to keep moving along in the process. This is not to say that things cannot be changed midstream—flexibility is important—but procrastination cannot be an excuse.

9. *Change must be well communicated.* Many an initiative has failed because the change was poorly communicated. Make use of multiple and informal forums, everything from meetings to e-mail to water-cooler conversations. Make sure your vision can be clearly articulated in 30 to 60 seconds—if the new way is transparent, seems simple, and makes sense, it will be easier to spread its adoption.

10. *Leaders should back up their talk with actions.* Leaders not only should *not* be exempt from following the new path but they must also be perfect role models of the new process. Do you want to implement open access in your practice? Do it yourself first. Have you reconstructed a new patient-identification process to reduce the chance of wrong-site surgery? Do it yourself, 100 percent of the time.

11. *Is your change working? Celebrate its success.* Hold systemwide meetings (such as a quality grand round) highlighting how your new medication error reduction system is reducing errors. Making sure everyone in your organization is aware of the successes makes change less threatening the next time around. Moreover, publishing and speaking outside your organization about your successes can lead to the spread of successful techniques outside your organization. In exchange, you may learn of successful approaches from others to apply in your organization.

12. *Create a culture of continual change within your organization.* Successful organizations and industries understand that their survival is dependent on a continual reinvention of themselves—continuous quality improvement. Many who have been along on the bumpy ride will be asking "Are we almost there yet?" The answer is a resounding "No." Like viewing an object on the distant horizon, our organizations should always be striving for a state of perfection, to which we may get close but likely can never reach. Figure 16.6 summarizes common pitfalls encountered in the change process.

Case Studies

Case 1: A Good Strategy at the Wrong Time

A large East Coast healthcare organization rooted in an academic medical center was located in a highly competitive market. A rising number of managed care organizations in the marketplace were approaching the organization to negotiate full-risk contracts. An early experiment showed this to be very costly to the organization.

FIGURE 16.6
Common
Implementation
Pitfalls

- Lack of attention to implementation
  - ○ Overemphasis on guideline development
  - ○ No knowledge of effective implementation strategies

- Involvement of the wrong people
  - ○ Lack of recognition of informal leadership
  - ○ Failure to enlist opinion leaders

- Failure to commit adequate resources to implementation process
  - ○ Lack of commitment of time and staffing
  - ○ Lack of visible leadership support

- Inadequate communication
  - ○ Message too complex
  - ○ Lack of establishing a sense of urgency

- Implementation too costly/failure to assess cost effectiveness
  - ○ Program too expensive or incentives misaligned

- Competing crises or uncontrollable factors in the external environment

To prepare for what was felt to be the coming wave of risk contracting, the CEO and chief quality officer embarked on a major endeavor to make quality the driving force of the organization. The belief was that a strategy of providing the best care with assistance from disease management programs throughout the organization's practice network would allow the organization to engage in full-risk capitation, earn the organization a competitive advantage of offering the best quality, and thus help the organization negotiate favorable contracts in the healthcare marketplace.

The program addressed high-volume chronic conditions for which there were known gaps from best practice, such as CHF, diabetes, and asthma. Clinical champions—well-known physicians respected by their peers—led teams in designing outpatient clinical guidelines according to evidence-based best practices. A multipronged effort included educational strategies, academic detailing to individual physician practices, clinical decision support with prompts and reminder systems, and office-based coordinators to disseminate the guidelines.

At its peak, the department contained three medical directors, employed 70 persons, and enrolled more than 14,000 patients in 28 programs. It was successful in demonstrating improved outcomes in asthma care, including reduced hospitalizations and emergency room visits, as well as improved compliance to best practices in CHF and asthma care. The program was successful because of its intense focus on implementation.

Particularly effective was the focus on the use of opinion leaders and clinical champions as well as the use of multiple interventions to increase physician enrollment and buy-in. In addition, the system's leadership communicated a strong mandate for quality improvement and disease management, and strong physician leadership for the programs existed. Initial programs in high-impact areas were able to demonstrate short-term wins.

However, the organization began suffering financial losses, and the entire program was abruptly dismantled during a round of consultant-driven expense reduction. The expected rush to full-risk capitation never occurred, and the organization's emphasis on quality did not seem to garner it a special place in the crowded marketplace. In reality, the party incurring the cost was not the party obtaining the financial benefit. Who benefited financially from the program? The insurers and managed care organizations. Who paid the expense? The health system. Thus, the cost of the program was not sustainable over time.

Case 2: A Novel Approach

An integrated healthcare delivery system implemented a disease management effort that emphasized both short- and long-term goals. The system included two acute care hospitals, a large academic physician group practice, and an HMO. The leadership of the disease management effort established goals to drive the process; they included improving the quality of patient care (appealing to the providers in the group practice), decreasing the variation in care (appealing to health system leadership, who realized that decreased variation means increased cost efficiency), and decreasing long- and short-term utilization by health plan members (appealing to the HMO by decreasing medical loss ratios). These goals led to a viable financial model, with each stakeholder gaining ownership in the success of the endeavor.

Physicians actively engaged in the group practice led the disease management program, although it was centered in the HMO. These leaders were respected clinicians and continued to practice at the grass-roots level, helping to sell the program to peers and creating instant credibility for the program.

The model began with the diseased population and sought to find strategies to affect this group. The populations chosen were high-prevalence, high-impact areas including tobacco cessation, asthma, diabetes, CHF, hypertension, and osteoporosis. Each disease was rolled out individually in a stepwise manner. This mix of diseases offered both short-term (decreased hospitalizations for asthma and CHF) and long-term (decreased lung disease from smoking and decreased complications from diabetes) gains. The implementation team included physicians, case management nurses, information systems, triage systems, physician office staff (e.g., nurses, medical records personnel, scheduling coordinators), and patients themselves.

Specific strategies included the following:

- Place health plan–employed care coordination nurses in local physician offices to coordinate care and assist the primary care physician and his or her staff;
- Establish evidence-based guidelines by employing nationally recognized seed guidelines and engaging opinion leaders from the academic group practice to review and disseminate the data;
- Enroll all members of a population in the program and allow them to opt out if they choose;
- Risk stratify patients and target the highest-risk members of the population first, thereby achieving early successes;
- Use regional case managers to help oversee management of difficult or high-acuity cases;
- Employ electronic just-in-time decision support to allow providers a greater opportunity to follow guidelines (providers were given up-front input on the content, and each new intervention was pilot tested on a small group);
- Promote member self-management, allowing the patient, the true consumer of the service, to become a stakeholder;
- Provide frequent member and provider education in multiple media and forums, including regional group sessions, face-to-face contact, and print and electronic active and passive communication; and
- Maintain an active data acquisition and processing department to measure progress, fine tine procedures, and enable celebration of successes.

The health plan had approximately 250,000 members in more than 1,200 primary care providers' offices. These physicians included both those employed by the health system and those contracted by the health plan. The disease management program employed more than 70 full-time equivalent staff, with more than two-thirds in direct patient care at the point of service. The health plan received "excellent" accreditation status from the National Committee for Quality Assurance (NCQA), and NCQA and the American Diabetes Association recognized the disease management program for excellence and innovation. Realization of tangible benefits included increased quality of care, decreased variation in practice, decreased cost to the system, and decreased utilization for the health plan.

Why did this disease management system succeed? First, a stepwise approach ("think big, but start small") was used, with pilot projects prior to large-scale rollouts. Attainable goals were set using high-impact diseases, outcomes were measured, and successes were celebrated. Second, all constituencies were stakeholders in the change process. A global, multifaceted approach to implementation was enlisted, involving as many different resources and tools as possible. Thought leaders from each affected area were enlisted. Innovative approaches were used to implement, maintain, publicize, and remediate processes. Most important, the downstream cost savings produced by the program were accrued by the same system as the costs of the programs, which allows for sustainability over the long term.

Case 3: System Implementation of Clinical Office Redesign

One mid-Atlantic region integrated health system, heeding complaints from referring physicians and patients regarding access issues, joined a collaborative initiated by the Institute for Healthcare Improvement called the Idealized Design of Clinical Office Practices. This initiative centered on multiple facets of office practice, including access (the ability to get into the system), interaction (the experience of the patient in the system), reliability (practicing state-of-the-art medicine), and vitality (financial sustainability). This healthcare system chose to focus its early efforts on redefining access as a means of gaining market share, increasing patient satisfaction, and enhancing clinical and financial performance. The system began with implementation in two practice sites, with rapid-spread methods for implementing successful processes across multiple sites. Lessons learned from these early sites were then used to spread the process to the entire system and medical center specialties.

The deployment model included a team of dedicated, trained staff to support the rollout. These staff were trained in change management and quality improvement and taught local leadership how to lead the practice through these changes. Local teams took ownership of the process and tailored it to fit their needs. The support team worked with sites for eight to ten weeks to assist with team formation, facilitate team leadership, introduce data collection tools, and encourage change. There was periodic follow-up support and review. Positive early prototype results built interest throughout the rest of the system practices. Rolling, scheduled spread then occurred across community practice sites, followed by sites at the medical center. Sites were able to markedly improve access, demonstrate improved patient satisfaction, and increase market share.

Key components of success included the following:

* Visible support from leadership for the process;
* Demonstrating short-term wins with early results from the prototype sites;

- Using multidisciplinary, local teams;
- Providing structural support for the teams;
- Actively communicating the process through multiple forums;
- Developing a structured timeline for the rollout;
- Leaving accountability at the local leadership level; and
- Celebrating successes both locally and nationally.

The success of this initiative has been a model for other quality improvement initiatives within the organization.

Conclusion

In this chapter, practical methods of leading healthcare organizations through change have been reviewed. The need for leaders in healthcare to master skills that will lead to effective quality improvement is critical at a time when American healthcare is in substantial need for such improvement in care delivery. Future research in the use of informatics, pay for performance, and other strategies is needed to expand our knowledge and discover additional strategies that can induce change in the healthcare system.

Study Questions

1. You are the chair of the hospital performance improvement committee at Community Hospital. You learn that only 40 percent of acute myocardial infarction admissions appropriately receive beta-blockers, and 50 percent receive aspirin. Outline the steps you would take to improve this situation to at least 90 percent compliance.
2. You are in charge of pharmaceutical utilization for a large HMO. Outline steps necessary to decrease pharmacy utilization by 20 percent over the next three years while maintaining high-quality care.
3. You are hired to lead a large, missioncentric department within a multispecialty group practice. This department is historically conservative, with a stable staff that are perceived to be "set in their ways." Discuss methods that will help you implement change during your tenure.

REFERENCES

Armstrong, D., H. Reyburn, and R. Jones. 1996. "A Study of General Practitioners' Reasons for Changing Their Prescribing Behaviour." *British Medical Journal* 312: 949–52.

Beaulieu, M. D., M. Rivard, E. Hudon, C. Beaudoin, D. Saucier, and M. Remondin. 2002. "Comparative Trial of a Short Workshop Designed to Enhance Appropriate Use of Screening Tests by Family Physicians." *Canadian Medical Association Journal* 167 (11): 1241–46.

Berwick, D. M. 2003. "Disseminating Innovations in Health Care." *Journal of the American Medical Association* 289: 1969–75.

Bolton, M. B., B. C. Tilley, J. Kuder, T. Reeves, and L. R. Schultz. 1991. "The Cost and Effectiveness of an Education Program for Adults Who Have Asthma." *Journal of General Internal Medicine* 6: 401–407.

Bradley, E. H., E. S. Holmboe, J. A. Mattera, S. A. Roumanis, M. J. Radford, and H. M. Krumholz. 2001. "A Quality Study of Increasing Beta-Blocker Use After Myocardial Infarction: Why Do Some Hospitals Succeed?" *Journal of the American Medical Association* 285 (20): 2604–11.

Brook, R. H. 1995. "Implementing Medical Guidelines." *Lancet* 346 (8968): 132.

Cabana, M. D., C. S. Rand, N. R. Powe, A. W. Wu, M. H. Wilson, P. A. Abboud, and H. R. Rubin. 1999. "Why Don't Physicians Follow Clinical Practice Guidelines? A Framework for Improvement." *Journal of the American Medical Association* 282 (15): 1458–65.

Chassin, M. R. 1998. "Is Health Care Ready for Six Sigma Quality?" *Milbank Quarterly* 76: 565–91.

Davis, D. 1998. "Does CME Work? An Analysis of the Effect of Educational Activities on Physician Performance or Health Care Outcomes." *Journal of Psychiatry in Medicine* 28 (1): 21–39.

Dexter, P. R., S. Perkins, J. M. Overhage, K. Maharry, R. B. Kohler, and C. J. McDonald. 2001. "A Computerized Reminder System to Increase the Use of Preventive Care for Hospitalized Patients." *New England Journal of Medicine* 345 (13): 965–70.

Durieux, P., R. Nizard, N. Ravaud, and E. Lepage. 2000. "A Clinical Decision Support System for Prevention of Venous Thromboembolism: Effect on Physician Behavior." *Journal of the American Medical Association* 283 (21): 2816–21.

Gladwell, M. 2000. *The Tipping Point: How Little Things Make a Big Difference.* New York: Little, Brown.

Goldberg, H. I., E. H. Wagner, S. D. Fihn, D. P. Martin, C. R. Horowitz, D. B. Christensen, A. D. Cheadle, P. Diehr, and G. Simon. 1998. "A Randomized Controlled Trial of CQI Teams and Academic Detailing: Can They Alter Compliance with Guidelines?" *Joint Commission Journal of Quality Improvement* 24 (3): 130–42.

Greco, P., and J. Eisenberg. 1993. "Changing Physician Practices." *New England Journal of Medicine* 329: 1271–73.

Halm, E. A., S. J. Atlas, L. H. Borowsky, T. I. Benzer, J. P. Metlay, Y. C. Change, and D. E. Singer. 2000. "Understanding Physician Adherence with a Pneumonia Practice Guideline: Effects of Patient, System and Physician Factors." *Archives of Internal Medicine* 160: 98–104.

Jencks, S. F., E. D. Huff, and T. Cuerdon. 2003. "Change in the Quality of Care Delivered to Medicare Beneficiaries, 1998–1999 to 2000–2001." *Journal of the American Medical Association* 289 (3): 305–12.

Kotter, J. P. 1996. *Leading Change.* Boston: Harvard Business School Press.

Mandelblatt, J., and P. A. Kanetsky. 1995. "Effectiveness of Interventions to Enhance Physician Screening for Breast Cancer." *Journal of Family Practice* 40: 162–67.

Mason, J. M., N. Freemantle, I. Nazareth, M. Eccles, A. Haines, and M. Drummond. 2001. "When Is It Cost-Effective to Change the Behavior of Health Professionals?" *Journal of the American Medical Association* 286 (23): 2988–92.

McDonald, C. J., G. A. Wilson, and G. P. McCabe. 1980. "Physician Response to Computer Reminders." *Journal of the American Medical Association* 244 (14): 1579–81.

McPhee, S. J., J. A. Bird, D. Fordham, J. E. Rodnick, and E. H. Osborn. 1991. "Promoting Cancer Prevention Activities by Primary Care Physicians: Results of a Randomized, Controlled Trial." *Journal of the American Medical Association* 266: 538–44.

Mottur-Pilson, C., V. Snow, and K. Bartlett. 2001. "Physician Explanations for Failing to Comply with 'Best Practices.'" *Effective Clinical Practice* 4: 207–13.

Oxman, A. D., M. A. Thomson, D. A. Davis, and R. B. Haynes. 1995. "No Magic Bullets: A Systematic Review of 102 Trials of Interventions to Improve Professional Practice." *Canadian Medical Association Journal* 153 (10): 1423–27.

Ramoska, E. A. 1998. "Information Sharing Can Reduce Laboratory Use by Emergency Physicians." *American Journal of Emergency Medicine* 16: 34–36.

Reinertsen, J. L. 1998. "Physicians as Leaders in the Improvement of Health Care Systems." *Annals of Internal Medicine* 128: 833–38.

Rich, M. W., V. Beckham, C. Wittenberg, C. L. Leven, K. E. Freedland, and R. M. Carney. 1995. "A Multidisciplinary Intervention to Prevent Readmission of Elderly Patients with Congestive Heart Failure." *New England Journal of Medicine* 333: 1190–95.

Rogers, E. M. 1995. "Lessons for Guidelines from the Diffusion of Innovations." *Joint Commission Journal of Quality Improvement* 21: 324–28.

Schectman, J. M., N. K. Kanwal, W. S. Schroth, and E. G. Elinsky. 1995. "The Effect of an Education and Feedback Intervention on Group-Model and Network-Model Health Maintenance Organization Physician Prescribing Behavior." *Medical Care* 33 (2): 139–44.

Shays, M. 2003. "Helping Clients to Control Their Future." *Consulting to Management* 14 (2): 1.

Sidorov, J., R. Shull, J. Tomcavage, S. Girolami, N. Lawton, and R. Harris. 2002. "Does Disease Management Save Money and Improve Outcomes?

A Report of Simultaneous Short-Term Savings and Quality Improvement Associated with a Health Maintenance Organization–Sponsored Disease Management Program Among Patients Fulfilling Health Employer Data and Information Set Criteria." *Diabetes Care* 25 (4): 684–89.

Solomon, D. H., H. Hashimoto, L. Daltroy, and M. H. Liang. 1998. "Techniques to Improve Physicians' Use of Diagnostic Tests: A New Conceptual Framework." *Journal of the American Medical Association* 280 (23): 2020–27.

Van Walraven, C., V. Goel, and B. Chan. 1998. "Effect of Population-Based Interventions on Laboratory Utilization: A Time Series Analysis." *Journal of the American Medical Association* 280: 2028–33.

Van Wijk, M. A. M., J. van der Lei, M. Mosseveld, A. M. Bohnen, and J. H. van Bemmel. 2001. "Assessment of Decision Support for Blood Test Ordering in Primary Care: A Randomized Trial." *Annals of Internal Medicine* 134: 274–81.

Walker, J. 2003. Personal communication, May 13.

Waters, T. M., P. P. Budett, K. S. Reynolds, R. R. Gillies, H. S. Zuckerman, J. A. Alexander, L. R. Burns, and S. M. Shortell. 2001. "Factors Associated with Physician Involvement in Care Management." *Medical Care* 39 (7 Suppl.): 19–91.

Weber, V., and M. Joshi. 2000. "Effecting and Leading Change in Health Care Organizations." *Joint Commission Journal on Quality Improvement* 26 (7): 397.

Zuckerman, H. S., D. W. Hilberman, R. M. Andersen, L. R. Burns, J. A. Alexander, and P. Torrens. 1998. "Physicians and Organizations: Strange Bedfellows or a Marriage Made in Heaven?" *Frontiers of Health Services Management* 14 (3): 3–34.

ENVIRONMENT

MEDICAL MALPRACTICE AND MEDICOLEGAL IMPLICATIONS OF QUALITY

Troyen A. Brennan, Ann Louise Puopolo, John L. McCarthy,

Robert Hanscom, and Luke Sato

Medical malpractice is one of the oldest impulses for quality improvement in healthcare. However, it remains an area somewhat hidden from the view of practicing physicians, largely because tort claims create shame and are associated with great secrecy. Nevertheless, it is important to understand how tort law operates generally, and in healthcare in particular, if one is to understand the relationship of the law to quality improvement. Moreover, it is possible, given certain institutional arrangements between providers and insurers, to use information from tort claims to improve the quality of care, as the case studies in this chapter demonstrate.

Background and Terminology

Tort law is part of the common law. This means that the principles of tort law are enunciated in the precedent of various court decisions, rather than through legislative activity or regulatory oversight. In essence, tort law is judge-made law. Depending on the previous court decisions, the tort law of a particular state may be more favorable to those bringing claims (plaintiffs) or those against whom claims are lodged (defendants).

To successfully bring a tort claim, a plaintiff must demonstrate four critical points. First, the plaintiff must demonstrate that the defendant owed the plaintiff duty of care. This is not usually an issue in the area of tort law that deals with physicians, that is, medical malpractice law. Second, the plaintiff must show that he or she was injured by the defendant. Tort law is first and foremost a form of a method for compensation for injury. Third, the plaintiff must show that the injury was the result of the behavior of the defendant, not a natural occurrence or caused by another external agency. The latter is referred to as the *causation requirement*; the defendant must have caused the plaintiff's injury. Fourth, the defendant must have engaged in negligent activity below the standard expected of a reasonable person before a successful claim can be brought. In medical malpractice, the *negligence standard* is the standard expected of the reasonable medical practitioner, and it is set by testimony by physicians. This is known as the *rule of medical custom.*

The plaintiff has the burden of proof and initiates litigation by lodging a claim against the defendant. These claims are typically brought on behalf of the plaintiff by the plaintiff's lawyer. The plaintiff may simply request payment of money damages or may formally file a suit in court. In most circumstances, the litigation is mediated on behalf of the defendants by their insurance companies. The insurance company lawyers review the claim, make a determination as to whether all four elements were met, and engage in negotiation.

In the meantime, the plaintiff's attorney may be seeking more information about the case from the plaintiff. The plaintiff's attorney may request that interviews of individuals associated with the case be completed, so-called *depositions,* or the attorney may provide lists of questions that the defendant must answer, so-called *interrogatories.* Eventually, the case will be scheduled for trial in a civil court or will be settled by the insurance company attorneys and the plaintiff's attorney.

This operation performs several social functions. First, as noted above, the tort law is a mechanism for compensation of injuries. Other forms of compensation of injuries, primarily worker's compensation, do not involve fault-based systems. In worker's compensation, there is no need to prove negligence; an injury arising out of the workplace is sufficient cause for compensation. As a result, the administrative costs of worker's compensation are much lower than those associated with the litigation process under medical malpractice, for example. Because so many of the premium dollars paid to the insurer go toward administrative costs, that is, primarily defendants' and plaintiffs' attorneys, the tort system is thought to be an inefficient form of compensation.

The other major social function of tort law is deterrence. The theory of tort law is that the injurer who is successfully sued pays the economic penalty of the award to the injured individual. This payment will in the future create incentives for safety. The economic theory underlying tort law is that defendants will become more careful as they face an increasingly costly litigation signal. The more unsafe defendants will have higher litigation costs than safer defendants, and in competition between defendants, those who are safer will prosper comparatively. Thus, tort law creates incentives for safety.

Unfortunately, while the theory works well, there is little empirical evidence that a deterrent effect is associated with tort law (Mello and Brennan 2002). Few insurers, or their insureds, have made the vital connections among safety, malpractice litigation, and quality improvement. Most physicians deny any quality improving potential of malpractice or risk-management systems. Nevertheless, it is possible to see how, at least theoretically, tort law integrates nicely with quality improvement. Especially with regard to the domain of quality improvement known as enhancing safety, tort law could be an important influence, given that malpractice claims are likely the most carefully reviewed error episodes in healthcare.

Scope and Use of Medicolegal Implications of Quality in Healthcare

As noted above, chronic defendants usually have insurance policies and insurance mechanisms for dealing with the costs associated with accidents. This is particularly true in the healthcare industry. Both doctors and hospitals are all well represented by insurers. Indeed, malpractice liability insurance is ubiquitous in healthcare, with more than 99 percent of physicians, and virtually all hospitals, insured. These policies have long been in place and were nearly universal by the early 1970s.

Insurers should feature strong risk-management programs. It only makes sense, as a successful insurer, to work with clients on ways in which to reduce risk and improve defensibility, and hence reduce litigation. This is sensible for both the purchaser of the policy and the insurer, who is extremely interested in ensuring predictability and reasonable actuarial estimates of losses. Unfortunately, most malpractice insurers do little to address risk.

Nevertheless, it is reasonable to state that by 1975, the critical quality signals in healthcare came from medical malpractice and the Joint Commission on Accreditation of Healthcare Organizations (Brennan and Berwick 1996). By the late 1970s, almost all hospitals had risk-management offices that related closely to their insurers. These risk managers intervened whenever injuries were recognized as having been suffered by patients. They provided liaison with the insurers and worked to identify high-risk areas in hospitals. The more successful risk managers probably significantly decreased the risk of injury to patients by improving safety practices. In many hospitals, long before there was a quality assurance office there was a risk-management team.

It stands to reason theoretically that long-term risk-management processes, combined with a reasonably functioning tort system, would have led to much safer institutions. If hospitals and physicians were paying premiums based on the number of injuries they caused, they would have a strong financial signal, mediated by their insurers, to incorporate better safety measures into their practices. Moreover, they would be coached by seasoned risk managers, who would be privy to a large number of claims and be able to recognize patterns of injuries that could potentially be prevented.

This sunny prospect is, however, undermined by the true operation of medical malpractice law. Research since the mid-1980s has demonstrated that the tort system does not work in any way as theory would predict (Weiler et al. 1993).

This research contains several key elements. First, many more injuries occur in hospitals than lead to malpractice claims. The Harvard Medical Practice Study and the Utah Colorado Medical Practice Study, both completed because of interest in malpractice reform, demonstrated that between 3 percent and 4 percent of patients entering hospitals end up with some sort of iatrogenic injury, and approximately 1 percent of individuals entering hospitals have an iatrogenic injury because of negligence. These numbers, when extrapolated to national figures, gave rise to the Institute of Medicine's (IOM 1999) clarion call regarding the 44,000 to 98,000 deaths per year in U.S. hospitals.

The same research showed that while in New York, for example, as many as 27,000 negligent medical injuries occur, only 3,600 medical malpractice claims are brought (IOM 1999). This means a huge reservoir of potential claims are not reaching insurance companies or their risk managers. The relative lack of claims has to suboptimize the performance of the risk managers, as they do not even get to see a huge part of the iceberg.

But that is not the whole story. In New York in 1984, 3,600 malpractice claims were brought, but subsequent research suggested that only approximately 600 to 700 of these claims were brought in cases in which a negligent medical injury had occurred. The rest involved injuries that were not negligent or cases in which no injury at all could be identified in the particular episode of medical care that gave rise to the claim. A reasonable number of the latter category reflect instances in which the plaintiff's attorney brings the case but, in subsequent discovery, finds the case is not viable. This means that while many injuries do not lead to claims, many of the claims are brought in cases in which no negligent injury has occurred. As Paul Weiler has noted, this is akin to a traffic cop who is giving lots of tickets to people who are not speeding but letting lots of speeders go past (Weiler et al. 1993).

The results of such a system are relatively corrosive. Many physicians can justifiably claim that the suits brought against them are not reasonable, specifically that they do not involve negligent injury. As well, risk managers only get to see a small portion of the truly negligent injuries.

The system itself is thus discredited as a quality improving device, and most physicians, even some risk managers, do not see medical malpractice as having much to do with quality assurance. Thus, a great deal of resources are squandered.

At some U.S. insurance companies, however, experienced claims adjusters and risk experts have continued to push, believing that they can reduce the number of claims and injuries by setting up reasonable programs. They have been convinced that long-term safety can be accomplished, and that reasonable evidence exists in malpractice claims to help. Their efforts have been reinvigorated by the IOM report (1999), which has put safety on the policy map as an important issue. Indeed, many hospital risk-management offices have changed their names to *patient safety offices*, and some now work closely with insurers to mine the information they receive on medical injuries to develop safety-enhancing mechanisms.

The Risk Management Foundation (RMF) of the Harvard Medical Institutions can justifiably claim to be one of these more enlightened organizations. Indeed, RMF provided much of the initial funding and support for the original Harvard Medical Practice Study. RMF has also been a leader in developing—for physicians across the Harvard system—educational materials, risk management techniques, and safe practice models.

In certain cases, RMF has engaged in long-term projects aimed at improving the safety of care of patients in specific target areas. Motivated by its own malpractice claims data and developing hypotheses on where the most serious vulnerabilities to patient care lie, RMF has repeatedly brought together collaborating clinicians from the Harvard hospitals it serves to assist them in undertaking appropriate quality measure and improvement methods. Ironically, many of these institutions are otherwise competitive, and it is the unique ability of their self-insured captive—RMF, also known as CRICO—to convene them and trigger systemwide collaboration.

Since the mid-1990s, two such improvement efforts have borne significant fruit. Another did not prove to be as helpful. Each effort embodies important lessons discussed in this chapter.

Clinical and Operational Issues

RMF efforts have included, among others, three particular projects, giving rise to three different types of interventions. The first involved emergency department care. In the early 1990s, RMF noted that the number of claims arising in emergency departments, especially failure to diagnose, were increasing quickly. RMF requested leadership from the Harvard teaching hospitals and brought together the emergency department directors to understand and cope with these rising risks.

Similar motivations led to an effort to improve the safety of ambulatory care. Failure to diagnose cases had begun to lead to significant increase in risk, and therefore high premiums, for general medicine physicians. Again, RMF was interested in quality improvement mechanisms based on a Plan-Do-Check-Act (PDCA) methodology.

Finally, attention focused on diagnosis of breast care. Here, RMF wanted a specific approach, that is, an appropriate guideline for the care of breast problems. This issue was undertaken by the loss-prevention staff at RMF in association with researchers and quality improvement experts at the Harvard hospitals.

Project 1: Emergency Department

Perhaps the most comprehensive effort involved the emergency department directors. As noted above, RMF had recognized an increased number of emergency department claims. However, it was not clear how to prevent these claims other than by improving the quality of care generally in the emergency department. Therefore, RMF drew together the directors of each of the emergency departments as well as health services researchers from the Harvard hospitals to identify a series of quality measures. The plan was to engage in measurement, analyze the data, put improvement methods in place, and then remeasure. The Harvard Emergency Department Quality Study team members were explicitly following the advice of quality improvement experts in this regard (Berwick 1994).

The investigators chose to concentrate on quality in three areas. First, they designed process-of-care guidelines for six chief complaints including abdominal pain, shortness of breath, chest pain, hand laceration, head trauma, and vaginal bleeding. Methods were designed for reviewing medical records to understand compliance with these guidelines.

Second, the investigators focused on patient-reported problems, in particular patient satisfaction and patient health status reports. In this area, the focus was on questions similar to those used by the Picker Commonwealth Study of Patient Care, which were explicitly modified for use in emergency departments (Cleary et al. 1991).

Chart review and a survey of patients were done in the first five months of 1993. The emergency department leadership reviewed the outcomes of this study and put in place a host of interventions. At five hospitals, more than 30 different interventions were used. All were designed to improve patient reports of problems or compliance with clinical guidelines (Burstin et al. 1999). Again, the theme was to act, then check once again.

Subsequent follow-up of emergency department quality occurred in the first five months of 1997. It was heartening to find a statistically significant improvement in five of six overall patient problem areas. Moreover, both patient reports of problems and patient satisfaction improved significantly after the interventions were put into place. Thus, the focus on emergency department claims gave rise to a general improvement in quality of care at emergency department hospitals.

The other interesting thing, at least from the point of view of a large malpractice carrier, was the degree of collaboration among the different emergency departments, in particular their directors. Over a six-year period, these directors continued to meet to discuss new quality improvements.

Their overall efforts were also reflected in malpractice claims. As Table 17.1 indicates, malpractice claims diminished, with the years 1994 to 1997 averaging just under 18 claims per year, and 1998 to 2001 averaging 12 claims per year. For the specific diagnostic areas included in the Harvard Emergency Department Quality Study, the number of claims dropped from 6 per year to 4 per year.

Project 2: Ambulatory Care

In light of the success of the emergency department study, a second, similar study was undertaken in the area of ambulatory care. This study, known as the Ambulatory Medical Quality Improvement Project (AMQIP), took place in 1996 to 1998. The same format was followed as the Harvard Emergency Department Quality Study. An effort was made to design specific instruments to capture the quality of care in different areas of ambulatory care, feed information back to create interventions, and finally remeasure to understand whether improvement had occurred. This study was undertaken with the same methodological rigor as the Harvard Emergency Department Quality Study. However, certain other factors failed to fall into place, in particular participation of the clinical care directors of the project. These factors are discussed in the next section.

Project 3: Breast Care

Another major effort by RMF, again collaborating with health services researchers, was to address the rising number of claims involved in failure to diagnose breast cancer. In this particular circumstance, RMF did not feel as though it could countenance a long-term study of breast cancer claims. Indeed, a large amount of information had been gathered in the AMQIP study about abnormal mammograms and breast complaints (Haas et al. 2000). Therefore, RMF engaged quality improvement experts to develop a breast cancer algorithm, relying on expert involvement. Initially completed in 1995, the researchers pulled together another project

TABLE 17.1
Emergency
Department
Claims by
Loss Year

Year	No. of Claims
1990	13
1991	16
1992	9
1993	16
1994	16
1995	22
1996	15
1997	18
1998	13
1999	17
2000	7
2001	13
2002	3
2003	0
Total	**178**

committee in 2000 consisting of mammographers, breast surgeons, and primary care doctors. They reviewed the data from the AMQIP as well as the existing literature on quality of breast care. In addition, the committee engaged other experts to join a working group to oversee the development of an algorithm. Finally, a series of experts, including chairs of departments and leading oncologists, acted as reviewers of the algorithm.

The 2000 algorithm itself is comprehensive, and it is intended to be available to radiologists, primary care doctors, and surgeons.[1] It consists of five parts: risk assessment, a screening guideline, an abnormal nipple discharge portion, a breast pain section, and a palpable mass portion. The algorithm takes the physician through the various steps important in determining whether further intervention is necessary. It also recommends endpoints such as referral to a surgeon or continued follow-up by a primary care physician. Biopsy is the recommendation of several endpoints of the algorithm.

The breast care algorithm was endorsed enthusiastically by primary care doctors within the Harvard system. It quickly became well known and widely used. As with all good algorithms, it must be consistently updated and improved. Indeed, a second working group has gathered to update the algorithm, keeping up with changes in technology and thoughts about appropriate prevention.

The breast care algorithm study could not be validated by quality data in the same way that the emergency department care or ambulatory medical care studies could be. Instead, RMF had to rely on changes in malpractice claims. Over the course of the eight years since the algorithm was put into place, malpractice claims regarding failure to diagnose breast cancer diminished significantly, as Table 17.2 demonstrates. As with Table 17.1, one should note there is an average 12- to 18-month delay before claims are brought, so years 2002 and 2003 are likely to see more claims.

Keys to Success and Understanding Failure

Overall, the interventions based on these studies were quite successful. The successes are somewhat different in character, however. In the first case, the Harvard Emergency Department Quality Study, the approach was a large-scale PDCA cycle with gathering of thorough quality measurements, followed by enlightened interventions and another large-scale gathering of data. This was a relatively expensive study, probably absorbing more than $800,000 over several years. However, the data were of publishable quality, and the study was thought necessary to convince physicians to modify their behavior.

It appears that the entire undertaking was cost effective, especially when we look at the malpractice claims. As noted above, the keys for success in the emergency department study were the cohesiveness and excellent working relationship among the emergency department directors. They essentially became collaborators, rather than competitors; as a result, they were able to define interventions that would work. Moreover, they continued to perfect their interventions over time, bouncing ideas off one another. Therefore, the critical success factors of the Harvard Emergency Department Quality Study were strong guidance from malpractice claims experience, long-term commitment from leadership, crisp data on quality of care, and persistence of the teams at the various emergency departments as they waited for the data from the initial quality measurement and on the efficacy of their interventions. The collaborative nature cannot be overemphasized.

The same is not necessarily true with the AMQIP. The interest of the clinical leadership from the primary care practices proved much more

TABLE 17.2
Breast Cancer
Claims by
Loss Year

Year	No. of Claims
1987	1
1988	2
1989	4
1990	4
1991	5
1992	10
1993	4
1994	8
1995	5
1996	3
1997	4
1998	3
1999	1
2000	2
2001	0
2002	0
2003	0
Total	**56**

difficult to sustain. As with the Harvard Emergency Department Quality Study, gathering of large-scale epidemiological information on quality of care from 12 to 15 sites, while exciting for researchers, tended to cause the primary care leadership to lose attention. By the time relatively thorough information was available in each of the various problem areas, the ambulatory medicine directors had begun to lose interest and were drifting off to other projects.

As a result, it was never possible to identify specific improvement projects and then test to determine whether they had really improved the care. In some manner, the emergency department directors took the entire study more seriously, whereas many of the ambulatory medical directors saw it as an unnecessary burden in their already time-starved environment.

This was probably the fault of the quality improvement/researcher team. They did not sufficiently pique interest and keep it focused. The team did try to do so and even had consultation with colleagues at the Institute for Healthcare Improvement in an effort to invigorate the quality improvement effort. Unfortunately, nothing seemed to work, and the study team began to fall apart before significant interventions could be undertaken.

They did, however, learn from this experience. First, the valuable information on care of breast lumps and breast complaints was not lost completely. This information provided the basis for thinking about the breast care algorithm. Moreover, the team recognized that it would be impossible to always develop quality data on a publishable level. This process is long and exacting and tries the patience of busy clinicians who are participating in the project.

Therefore, instead of gathering new information on care of breast complaints, information from AMQIP was used when the breast care algorithm committee was called together. The team moved this committee quickly through analysis of the data and development of the algorithm. This was thought important because busy clinicians clearly wanted a tangible outcome, which the algorithm provided. Moreover, we did not set forth to validate the algorithm by looking at the rare outcome of when a breast complaint is mishandled. Hopefully, the quality of the algorithm team as well the comprehensiveness of the guideline itself are good selling points.

RMF has been very enthusiastic about the results of the breast care algorithm. Breast cancer claims are decreasing significantly. Moreover, we feel much more confident that we can bring about successful quality improvement efforts in the future without the broad efforts underlying the Harvard Emergency Department Quality Study or the AMQIP.

Study Questions

Like all good research, the studies discussed in this chapter raise more questions than they provide answers. However, some sufficient answers to identify the next set of questions exist. It is these the authors believe students of quality improvement should be studying.

1. What types of data from malpractice claims could one use for quality improvement? What types of systems issues would you hypothesize that the data would show?
2. If you were asked to make a presentation to providers on how different domains of quality may correlate with malpractice, what would you say?

3. If you were at the state level and in the position to make changes to the cyclical malpractice crisis, what would you consider, and why?
4. Will insurer-mediated safety efforts replace traditional risk management?

Note

1. For more information, see RMF's web site at www.rmf.harvard .edu/bca.

REFERENCES

Berwick, D. M. 1994. "Eleven Working Aims for Clinical Leadership of Health System Reform." *Journal of the American Medical Association* 2782: 797–802.

Brennan, T. A., and D. M. Berwick. 1996. *New Rules: Regulation, Markets and the Quality of American Health Care.* San Francisco: Jossey-Bass Publishers.

Burstin, H. R., A. Conn, G. Setnik, D. W. Rucker, P. D. Cleary, A. C. O'Neil, E. J. Oray, C. M. Sox, and T. A. Brennan. 1999. "Benchmarking and Quality Improvement: The Harvard Emergency Department Quality Study." *American Journal of Medicine* 107 (5): 437–49.

Cleary, P. D., S. Edgman-Levitan, M. Roberts, T. W. Moloney, W. McMullen, J. D. Walker, and T. L. Delbanco. 1991. "Patients Evaluate Their Hospital Care: A National Survey." *Health Affairs (Millwood)* 10 (4): 254–67.

Haas, J. S., E. F. Cook, A. L. Puopolo, H. R. Burstin, and T. A. Brennan. 2000. "Differences in the Quality of Care for Women with an Abnormal Mammogram or Breast Complaint." *Journal of General Internal Medicine* 15 (5): 321–28.

Institute of Medicine. 1999. *To Err Is Human: Building a Safer Health System.* Washington, DC: National Academy Press.

Mello, M. M., and T. A. Brennan. 2002. "Deterrence of Medical Errors: Theory and Evidence for Malpractice Reform." *Texas Law Review* 80 (7): 1595–1637.

Weiler, P. C., H. H. Hiatt, J. P. Newhouse, W. G. Johnson, T. A. Brennan, and L. L. Leape. 1993. *A Measure of Malpractice: Medical Injury, Malpractice Litigation, and Patient Compensation.* Boston: Harvard University Press.

ACCREDITATION: ITS ROLE IN DRIVING ACCOUNTABILITY IN HEALTHCARE

Greg Pawlson and Paul Schyve

There is a large, growing body of evidence that the current level of quality in healthcare is substantially lower than what is possible with currently available treatments and technology. This evidence was summarized in the Institute of Medicine (IOM 2001) report *Crossing the Quality Chasm*. Recognition of this gap and growing purchaser and consumer demand for information about healthcare quality have given rise to a call for more accountability in the healthcare system. This chapter examines the role of accreditation in both its past and prospective future roles in driving accountability in the healthcare system.

Background and Terminology

Accountability has been defined as "the procedure and process by which one party provides a justification and is held responsible for its actions by another party who has an interest in the action" (Emanuel and Emanuel 1996; Emanuel 1996). Accountability in healthcare has been characterized as being driven by three major forces: the marketplace, regulation, and professionalism. In healthcare, the parties that may seek accountability include those directly affected by health services (patients) and those who directly or indirectly pay for the services (insurers, employers, employees, or taxpayers). This chapter refers collectively to this group of interested parties as *the public*.

Accountability can be achieved by informal, subjective means or through the exchange of information using a formal set of metrics. One mechanism that has been used to create accountability is accreditation. *Accreditation* can be defined as a process in which an entity external to the organization providing goods or services evaluates that organization against a set of predetermined requirements or desirable attributes and publicly attests to the results.

The term *certification* is often used to denote a similar process, except that certification is more often used either in reference to the determination of an individual's (rather than an organization's) competency or in reference to the government's determination of eligibility of an organization to participate in a government program. While organizational accreditation or certification—as contrasted with licensure—is usually thought of as voluntary, the decision to seek accreditation can range from one that is truly optional to one that is linked to participation in an insurance program[1] or required for licensure by government at the federal or state level.[2] Throughout the world, organizational accreditation and certification can be provided through either private sector bodies or government agencies; in the United States, organizational accreditation is provided through private sector bodies, whereas certification can be provided through either private sector or government agencies. By contrast, *licensure* is always the domain of government, is nearly always mandatory, and requires meeting certain legally defined requirements to practice or exercise some activity.

Regulation and Accreditation

The bodies that provide accreditation have nearly always been originally created and governed by trade associations or professional societies within the field being evaluated. Thus, a major genesis of accreditation or private sector certification is often the desire of professionals to define adherence to professional norms and standards in the delivery of services at both the individual and organizational levels. However, both regulatory and market forces also have a strong influence on the presence of accreditation. Regulatory forces, including licensing and federal or state regulations or mandates, and the justice system, including malpractice litigation, are forces that often encourage professional groups to offer accreditation—both to encourage adherence to standards of performance beyond those required by licensure and as an alternative to additional regulatory control. The implicit delegation of some portion of accountability to accreditation is seen by some as a manifestation of the self-monitoring that society has historically granted—and expected—through implicit and explicit contracts it establishes with professionals. Market forces play a role in some forms of accreditation, as, for example, in the case of health maintenance organization (HMO) accreditation in which some private purchasers either encourage or require HMO accreditation as a prerequisite to inclusion in the insurance programs they offer to employees. Thus, in most situations, accreditation exists where there are both a professional drive to set and maintain standards and either regulatory or market pressures that support accreditation.

While a full discussion of the relative merits of accreditation versus government regulation in ensuring accountability is beyond the scope of this chapter, a few of the relative advantages of accreditation follow:

- Standards can be created, changed, and updated frequently based on science and professional norms, rather than relying on the political process required for amending laws or government regulations.
- The bar for passing can be set higher than the minimum needed for practice without constraining entry into the field.
- The feedback provided to the entity or individual being evaluated is usually richer than the pass-fail of licensure decisions and can include substantial information that can be used in quality improvement activities.

Relative disadvantages of accreditation include the following:

- If the accrediting body is perceived to be controlled by the industry being evaluated, concerns can arise that the standards and evaluation process are not rigorous enough to serve the public's interest.
- Where multiple accrediting bodies provide accreditation for the same type of healthcare entity, the competition—which in most circumstances can be expected to drive continuous improvement in products and services—creates the potential for each body to set more easily achievable standards to gain market share.

The Process and Content of Accreditation

Accreditation is based on the premise that it is possible both to define attributes that are critical (either required or highly desirable) to the quality and safety of a healthcare product or service and to create a method to measure whether some preset threshold of performance has been achieved. Critical attributes can be defined for both administrative and clinical activities, and they can be based on expert opinion, consensus (of providers or multiple stakeholders), or research studies (qualitative or quantitative studies). Measurement can involve onsite observation, review of policies, review or abstraction of data from administrative or clinical records, surveys, and interviews with provider staff or patients (see Figure 18.1). While many accreditation programs still rely only on onsite observation and review of reports and policies, this does not have to be the case when other types of measurement are feasible.

Following the measurement phase—the data collection by the accrediting body—the accreditor analyzes the data to transform them

Observation
Direct observation of structures or processes used by an entity

Interviews
Structured and unstructured interviews with patients and staff

Audits
Verification of the integrity and accuracy of data, including data collection and reporting processes

Review of written documentation (reports, policies, medical records)
Review, either onsite or remotely, and abstraction of data that have been recorded for either administrative or clinical purposes

Surveys
Collection and analysis of data from surveys of those using services (e.g., consumers, patients, physicians in HMOs) or supplying services (e.g., nurses, doctors, pharmacists in hospitals)

Derived information (claims, clinical reports)
Collection and analysis of data contained in either paper or electronic form and used in claims (e.g., office visit, laboratory, pharmacy, other services) or in reports on clinical processes (e.g., laboratory, pathology results)

into information about the evaluated entity's performance. An accreditation decision usually includes an overall assessment of the entity (organization or service) as a whole, and it may also include assessment of specific components, functions, or services that comprise the larger entity.

To complete the process, the accrediting body shares some level of information concerning the results of the evaluation to both the evaluated entity and those parties (e.g., consumers, patients, purchasers, insurers, government agencies) who desire accountability from the evaluated entity. The level and quantity of information shared with either those evaluated or outside groups are highly variable. The information can range from a simple list of those that passed (with no indication of which organizations did not apply or applied but failed to be accredited) to relatively detailed information on comparative performance, including performance on specific subsets of the requirements. The level of detail provided is often greater to those who undergo evaluation; where it is timely and sufficiently detailed, this information can be useful in quality improvement activities. Most accreditation bodies expect that the accredited organization will use this feedback to improve.

Scope and Use of Accreditation in Healthcare: Successes and Failures

Hospitals

Accountability for hospital quality in the United States has relied primarily on regulation and accreditation, both of which are highly influenced by professionalism and professionals. Like licensure for physicians, hospital licensure is codified in laws at the state level and usually overseen by state-appointed medical or hospital boards consisting largely of physicians. However, the federal government, in its role as the single largest purchaser of hospital care in the United States (through the Medicare program), has played the most prominent government role in defining hospital accountability. The 1964 legislation that created Medicare required that hospitals, to participate in the program, undergo a federal regulatory review and certification by the organization now called the Centers for Medicare & Medicaid Services (CMS). As an alternative to federal review, the legislation allowed hospitals to participate in Medicare through *deemed status* based on accreditation by a private accrediting body, the Joint Commission on Accreditation of Healthcare Organizations (Joint Commission). Thus, the accreditation of hospitals is tightly linked to the creation and evolution of the Joint Commission.[3]

Because Medicare pays for nearly 40 percent of all hospital bed days, the viability of most hospitals depends on their being able to participate in the Medicare program. Given both their distrust of direct government oversight and the need to participate in Medicare, it is not surprising that most U.S. hospitals seek Joint Commission accreditation (Greenberg 1998). In addition, 47 states also license hospitals based in whole or in part on attainment of Joint Commission accreditation.

Accreditation by the Joint Commission is based on receiving a passing score on a set of standards it promulgates. These standards encompass the requirements set out by CMS (called Conditions of Participation) that are required for the Medicare program. In addition to meeting basic standards, the Joint Commission requires hospitals to conduct quality improvement activities, including activities based on the collection and use of nationally standardized (core) performance measures from the Joint Commission's ORYX measurement sets. These measurement sets span a large number of clinical conditions related to hospital admission (e.g., heart failure, pneumonia, childbirth). Each hospital selects a subset of ORYX measures to report to the Joint Commission on a quarterly basis; these measurements are used to focus the Joint Commission's onsite survey of the hospital and examine the hospital's use of the measurement results to improve the quality and safety of care.

Until 2004, hospitals did not report on the same measures, so comparable data on all hospitals have not been available nor have the actual performance levels on the measures been used in the accreditation decision itself. However, as described below, all hospitals are now required to report comparable data on selected sets of ORYX measures. Since July 2004, comparative performance information based on these ORYX data is reported on the Joint Commission's public web site, along with the hospital's accreditation status.

For accreditation reviews beginning in January 2004, the Joint Commission has made significant changes in its approach that are designed to make accreditation a more continuous process for maintaining and improving a healthcare organization's performance and provide more useful information about healthcare organizations to the public. First, standards were rewritten and reorganized to make them as clear as possible, and those that are not strongly linked to patient safety and the quality of care were eliminated. The standards were also reformatted to explicitly itemize the elements of performance for which an organization is responsible to comply with each standard. Second, a requirement was introduced for organizations to conduct a performance evaluation against all the standards at the midpoint of the accreditation cycle, which is normally three years. This self-assessment at 18 months, accompanied by a corrective action plan to address any standard(s) not in compliance and with objective measures to be used in demonstrating successful correction, will be submitted to the Joint Commission for review, consultation, and approval. These findings and plans, if approved, will not affect the organization's accreditation status, to encourage a rigorous self-assessment and full disclosure to the Joint Commission. Third, information from multiple sources, including MedPar and ORYX data, will be fed into a priority focus tool, an algorithm that will identify critical areas on which to focus during the announced triennial onsite survey.

The fourth change made to the Joint Commission's approach is that, during the onsite survey, surveyors will examine these priority focus areas by using a tracer methodology, that is, by following individual patients' care throughout their hospitalization and observing care, interviewing patients and staff, and examining documents. Fifth, the Joint Commission surveyors will use their findings to conduct system analyses to identify, and consult on, strengths and weaknesses in the hospital's clinical and organizational systems. Sixth, because organizations will have undertaken a performance review at midcycle and implemented a Joint Commission–approved corrective action plan, they are expected to be in compliance with all the standards during the onsite survey. If an organization is out of compliance with only a few standards, it will have 45 days to provide evidence of compliance to the Joint Commission (90 days during the initial transition year, 2004). If the evidence is accepted, the organization will be labeled accredited. If it fails to provide sufficient evidence, the organization will be placed in provisional accreditation. If it either has too many standards out of compliance during the onsite survey or does not emerge from provisional accreditation in a timely manner, the organization will be conditionally accredited, and, with continued poor performance, not accredited. Thus, "accredited" will mean that the organization was found to be in compliance with all the standards. Seventh, the reports of organizations' performance placed on the Joint Commission public web site will include not only their accreditation status but also absolute and comparative performance with respect to discrete national patient safety goals and quality goals based on ORYX data (i.e., initially for acute myocardial infarction, heart failure, community-acquired pneumonia, pregnancy and related conditions, and, as they are developed, national standardized core measures for other diseases and conditions). In addition, this quality report will indicate whether the hospital has earned special certification for disease-specific services such as diabetes, asthma, or heart disease.

Beyond these changes, the Joint Commission board of commissioners has announced that all onsite accreditation surveys will be unannounced beginning in 2006, with organizations that volunteer receiving unannounced surveys in 2004 and 2005. Finally, beyond hospitals, the Joint Commission now accredits an array of other healthcare organizations including nursing homes, ambulatory surgery centers, ambulatory office practices, and integrated delivery systems.

Insurers

Prior to the emergence of HMOs, insurers were regulated primarily though state insurance laws. Through the 1980s, accountability for HMOs, which emerged in the late 1970s and early 1980s and combine insurance with varying degrees of oversight of clinical delivery functions, remained largely within an insurance regulatory framework. Accountability for care in HMOs that employed physicians or ran hospitals was subject to the same licensing and accreditation standards as for other hospitals and physicians. Initially, there was little or no oversight for the HMO functions related to utilization or quality management or contractually imposed controls on physicians or other providers.

In the face of these limited regulatory requirements, HMO accountability grew largely out of market forces, specifically pressures from the purchasers of healthcare for more detailed information on the quality of services provided by HMOs. One manifestation of this pressure was the creation of a voluntary accreditation process by the National Committee for Quality Assurance (NCQA). While other organizations accredit HMOs (including the Joint Commission, URAC, and the Accrediting Association for Ambulatory Health Care [AAAHC]), the majority of accredited HMOs are accredited by NCQA.

While some large employers (about half of the Fortune 100) and the Federal Office of Personnel Management require accreditation, relatively few other employers do so. Largely because voluntary accreditation by NCQA and others developed before the move by states to increase regulation of HMOs, about 25 states recognize private accreditation as fulfilling all or part of state HMO licensure requirements. In addition, in 2000, CMS issued rules that will allow HMOs to substitute deemed status for most CMS requirements related to HMO participation in the Medicare+ Choice program. However, because Medicare is a much smaller, and declining, proportion of HMO enrollment, Medicare requirements for HMOs— or deemed status for these requirements—are unlikely to have a significant effect on accountability. Thus, in contrast to the nearly universal hospital accreditation, only slightly more than half of all HMOs (although nearly all the largest plans) are accredited by a private accrediting group. Finally, for non-HMO forms of managed care, such as the rapidly growing preferred provider organization (PPO) market, virtually no accountability for quality exists beyond the market and basic state insurance regulations. Although NCQA and other accreditors offer voluntary accreditation programs for PPOs, fewer than 10 percent of PPOs are accredited.

Like most other accrediting bodies, NCQA began as part (actually, as its name implies, as a committee) of a trade organization related to health plans—the Group Health Association of America, the predecessor of the current Association of American Health Plans (AAHP). However, in addition to the interest from health plans themselves, NCQA's early development was strongly influenced by private purchasers' demands for accountability. As a result, NCQA became independent of AAHP in 1990 and has evolved independently such that its current board of directors includes a broad array of representatives from consumer, purchaser, provider, and other healthcare sectors. Only one of the 18 board members is affiliated with an HMO or other organization now accredited by NCQA—a board composition that is unusual among accrediting organizations.

Another factor that marked the early development of NCQA was the development and implementation of a set of clinical performance measures called the Health Plan Employer Data and Information Set (HEDIS). This data set was started by a small group of HMO leaders, with input from clinicians and purchasers. The goal was to create a reliable, valid, and standard set of measures of clinical performance that would provide useful information on quality for purchasers and at the same time limit the uncoordinated and disparate demands by large purchasers for clinical information from HMOs.

Beginning in 1999, NCQA accreditation has changed in important ways. First, the HEDIS measurement set has been substantially expanded, with the addition of measures related to management of major chronic illnesses. In addition, HEDIS now includes a version of the Consumer Assessment of Health Plans Survey (CAHPS 2.0H) developed by a research team coordinated and funded by the Agency for Healthcare Research and Quality. More than 80 percent of HMOs, including plans that do not opt for NCQA accreditation, now report most or all of the HEDIS measures annually to NCQA (Dybkare 1994). While not all measures are reported by all plans (e.g., some plans do not have enough members or lack critical data), the population base of the plans that do report a given measure usually exceeds 50 million people.

Beginning in 1999, NCQA began to incorporate performance on selected HEDIS measures as an integral and substantial portion (25 percent in 2001) of the overall accreditation score. This represents a major change in accreditation practice. As noted previously, nearly all accreditation and certification have relied exclusively on adherence to standards or on cognitive testing, rather than on an analysis of quantitative measures of performance. A major criticism of accreditation is that little empirical evidence links compliance with accreditation standards to outcomes of the service or care delivered. The inclusion in the accreditation process of reliable measures of clinical processes and outcomes of care increases the likelihood that accreditation status is a valid indication of the quality of care delivered.

NCQA accreditation decisions are now reported on a public web site as excellent, commendable, accredited, provisional, or denied (Romano 1993). The web site also includes plan-specific information about performance on accreditation standards and HEDIS measures grouped in five categories understandable to consumers (access and service, qualified providers, staying healthy, getting better, and living with illness). The NCQA report card is also linked to major commercial web sites, such as Medscape, America Online, and Compuserve. This level of reporting begins to provide the amount and type of detail that purchasers or consumer can use to select health plans based on differential quality. NCQA has also created a web-based reporting and self-assessment system for many of its accreditation processes, minimizing the need for onsite review of materials and programs. Finally, like the Joint Commission, NCQA has expanded its scope of accreditation programs to include managed behavioral health, disease management, and physician group practices. The Joint Commission and NCQA also have a joint venture for accreditation of human subject research protection programs.

In summary, for HMOs, the market—driven primarily by private purchasers and voluntary accreditation—has played a stronger role in the evolution of accountability than in the physician or hospital sectors. Regulation by state and federal governments is clearly moving beyond insurance regulation but is still not widespread or consistent, and, beyond HMOs, little accountability of insurers exists.

Nursing Homes

Accreditation has had limited penetration into nursing homes, largely because of the dominance of state Medicaid programs (Medicare accounts for less than 10 percent of nursing home expenditures) and self (private) pay as the means of financing nursing home care. CMS (Medicare and Medicaid) and the states (Medicaid) have developed both an extensive set of regulatory standards and a government survey and certification program to enforce nursing home regulations. Given the less-than-adequate quality and, in some instances, outright abuse of patients in nursing homes in the past, most public advocacy groups have been strongly opposed to allowing deemed status out of fear that the largely for-profit nursing home industry would try to lower current regulatory standards. Thus, no legislation authorizes CMS or states to allow deemed status in Medicare or Medicaid for private accrediting bodies to substitute for governmental survey and certification of nursing homes.

This is in contrast to hospitals, where there was a tradition of not-for-profit entities with strong professional involvement, and HMOs, for which private purchasers played a major role in requiring or encouraging accreditation. While the Joint Commission and others offer accreditation to nursing homes, only limited numbers apply because the deemed status and market benefits are not present. Nevertheless, those nursing homes that achieve accreditation have been shown to have significantly fewer serious deficiencies when surveyed by the government than do unaccredited nursing homes.

Ambulatory Care

While accreditation of ambulatory care practice (e.g., in sites where ambulatory surgery is performed) is growing, it remains far less developed than in the hospital or HMO sector. One exception is in renal dialysis, where the dominance of Medicare as a payer, and the creation by CMS of deemed status for some parts of the program, has created close to universal accreditation of programs. However, most insurers, including Medicare, have few, if any, requirements other than licensure for ambulatory care sites (e.g., physician groups, individual offices) to participate in their programs. Moreover, the traditional reliance on professionalism for assurance of high quality is arguably stronger in ambulatory care, which has been dominated by small, physician-owned practices. (The median size of a physician office practice is still under four physicians.)

The emergence of large regional or national for-profit entities providing imaging (MRI, mammography), renal dialysis, cancer treatment, or other services, combined with the growing recognition of purchasers, insurers, and the public of the wide variation in the quality and cost of ambulatory care services, is giving rise to an increasing number of programs and entities offering accreditation of ambulatory care programs. Some examples include accreditation of office-based surgery (e.g., by AAAHC, Joint Commission) and imaging centers (e.g., by the American College of Radiology, Joint Commission), but none of these activities has achieved close to universal acceptance, even when deemed by CMS (e.g., office-based surgery accreditation), with the exception of the deemed accreditation of mammography centers by the American College of Radiology. A notable unsuccessful attempt in ambulatory care accreditation was the American Medical Accreditation Program, created by the AMA to offer accreditation to physician office practices. A lack of any regulatory or market incentives from either the public or private sector and the concern of some specialty boards that a physician's office accreditation would be redundant to board certification of the individual physician appear to be the major factors that doomed the program.

The Future of Accreditation: Challenges and Changes

If accreditation is to remain an important part of ensuring accountability, it will need to evolve in response to market forces and the further evolution of the healthcare system. One of the most important challenges to accreditation is the proliferation of new services and products and of the types of organizations that provide them. For example, most of the growth in hospital revenues since the mid-1990s has been in ambulatory and ancillary services, such that some hospitals now receive the majority of their income from services other than inpatient care. This movement has also given rise to myriad outpatient facilities, such as urgent care centers, ambulatory surgery centers, and office-based surgery sites, that provide some component of inpatient services. Clearly, an accreditation process for hospitals that focused largely on inpatient standards would not address this new reality. In addition, services like disease management, mental health benefits management, and pharmacy benefits management, which were included in the services of a staff- or group-model HMO, are now provided by contract with separate entities—entities for which no system of accountability for quality and safety currently exists. Accreditation focused on hospitals or HMOs, even if it addresses delegated functions, does not fully capture these new activities and sites. Accreditation will need to evolve quickly toward a more flexible, multientity, performance-based process to serve both the public interest and that of these new activities. Accreditation will also need to address issues related to coordination and sharing of data between the increasingly fragmented entities involved in healthcare.

Another factor likely to grow stronger in the future is the public demand for information that would facilitate comparison of individual clinicians, clinical groups, and hospitals, as well as health plans. Sole reliance on structural and process standards to provide a limited range of accreditation decisions for a single entity provides only a limited amount of meaningful information to consumers or purchasers relevant to their decision making. That is, while this information helps to differentiate between accredited and unaccredited organizations, it provides less help in differentiating among accredited organizations with respect to specific services or programs. This is especially true in the hospital sector, where virtually all hospitals are accredited. And creating comparative information at the physician group or individual level will be even more costly and difficult than creating similar information with respect to HMOs or hospitals. Given the costs of gathering information and the lower fiscal margins in virtually all sectors of healthcare, accreditors and others will need to find ways to reduce the number of redundant standards and measures and the cost of data collection. Without these developments, efforts to enhance accountability at the provider level are likely to end in redundant and dysfunctional evaluations—and unnecessary costs—and raise the resistance of those being evaluated even further.

As noted, NCQA now includes performance measures as part of HMO accreditation and reports information on accreditation of HMOs and PPOs at multiple levels of accreditation performance. Likewise, as noted, the Joint Commission will, beginning in 2004, report comparative data on its web site that will be more useful to the public and purchasers in selecting healthcare provider organizations. At present, however, because of sampling size restrictions, information on clinical performance measures, although already collected at the individual physician level for some measures, cannot be reliably reported at the physician level. In addition, an individual physician's patient outcomes can be influenced by the system in which he or she provides care. Pennsylvania's release of surgeon-specific mortality data demonstrated that some surgeons who operated in multiple hospitals had better than (statewide) average results in one hospital, and worse than (statewide) average results in another hospital. Thus, obtaining the depth and quantity of information necessary to prepare reports that are reliable and valid at the physician group or individual physician levels will pose a formidable challenge. Nevertheless, accreditation cannot hope to play a central role in accountability in the future unless it can provide the public (purchasers, insurers, consumers, and patients) with reliable and valid comparative information on quality and safety.

A number of other groups not directly tied to accreditation have created report cards of varying types. Most rely on consumer surveys of varying reliability or validity. Few use random samples or have large enough sample sizes to allow valid comparisons between entities. Some larger HMOs rate providers, and even more furnish some basic demographic information about physicians in their clinical networks. A more sophisticated set of measures can be found in the ratings of HMOs and providers created by the Pacific Business Group on Health, which include physician group-practice information for larger physician groups in the California market. While some large purchasers are able to use current information on at least HMO quality as part of their purchasing decisions, most consumers feel overwhelmed by the number of sites and are distrustful of conflicting report cards or ratings. The result is that consumers still rely largely on word-of-mouth information from friends, relatives, coworkers, or their physicians in making healthcare choices.

Finally, the long-term hope for more effective accreditation and information about quality depends on enhancement of information technology use in healthcare. The wide availability of broad-band, web-enabled data collection may eventually allow accreditation to be based on real-time measurement of a rich array of clinical structure, process, and outcome performance measures that can also be used for quality monitoring, rather than on retrospective measures or survey-assessed compliance with standards alone.

Accreditation Sets the Bar Too Low

Issue

Accreditation, especially where it is a prerequisite for participating in large insurance programs like Medicare, must be constructed to set a basic level of acceptable quality that at least encompasses the minimal level required by law and regulation. If the threshold is set too far above this minimal level, many or most providers would not be able to achieve accreditation, thereby reducing the information about them that enables consumer choice and potentially adversely affecting access for many consumers. Perhaps most important, the fewer the organizations enrolled in the accreditation process, the less influence accreditation has in lifting the quality and safety of care. On the other hand, if the threshold is set too close to the regulatory minimum, providers with serious quality defects will gain access to the insurance program and patients will have less protection from being harmed. This dilemma is similar to that seen in licensing. This has led some to see accreditation as a basic floor of requirements that everyone doing business in the given area should achieve. Thus, if regulatory requirements are generally considered the minimum level of performance that must be achieved to remain in business, accreditation might be described as a basic level of quality and safety that should be achieved.

Where accreditation is truly optional, those who do not even attempt to achieve accreditation avoid both the cost of accreditation and any risk of not passing. With no pressure to participate, a high threshold could discourage providers from seeking accreditation because the risk of failing accreditation is far worse than not being evaluated at all. Even more challenging is the situation in which multiple accrediting bodies compete. It is not clear that many purchasers or consumers will distinguish one accrediting body's accreditation from that of another. In this instance, a move by one accrediting body to raise standards may be seen as an opportunity for its competitor(s) to gain market share by retaining a lower standard. If neither strong pressure from state regulation nor incentives (e.g., differential payment or selection) from private purchasers exists to encourage accreditation and push standards to high levels, there is a tendency among provider organizations to either move to the easiest accreditation program or drop accreditation altogether.

Finally, concerns have been raised about the governance of many accrediting organizations. As noted earlier in this chapter, accreditation has traditionally been a bridge between professionalism and regulation. In many instances, accrediting bodies have been created by professionals with the goal of both trying to drive quality assessment and improvement and reducing the need for direct government regulation. Many accrediting organizations have emanated from within professional groups themselves. While involvement of those within the profession is important in setting credible standards, if not balanced by the interests of other stakeholders, particularly consumers, there can also be pressure to keep from setting standards that could potentially put at a disadvantage some members of the professional organization that controls, or strongly influences, the accrediting organization. It should be noted that accrediting bodies given deemed status by the federal government must be not-for-profit, and, therefore, regardless of the composition of their governing boards, are to act in the interest of the public.

Analysis and Response

A decision on where to set the threshold for acceptable performance can often be challenging given these disparate forces. Such a decision is even more problematic to the degree that accrediting bodies are strongly influenced or controlled by either the providers they accredit or by consumer advocates who want higher quality but are often not willing to pay more for it. One approach to addressing this challenge is to seek broad input from both those being accredited and those desiring accountability though formal groups such as multi- and single-stakeholder advisory councils. Structuring the accrediting body's board of directors or oversight committees that have decision-making authority so that they are representative of all the relevant stakeholder groups is also likely to be helpful in addressing this challenge.

An important factor in the usefulness of accreditation is how carefully the importance and evidence base for a given standard are determined. Good standards must be based on a carefully structured determination of what evidence can be found and documented to support a conclusion that the standard in question is really critical to good quality and safety. The standards also must be closely linked to agreed-on definitions of quality. The definition most widely used is that published by IOM (2001): "The degree to which healthcare services for individuals or populations increase the likelihood of desired outcomes and are consistent with current professional knowledge."

In the case of endpoint outcomes, it could be argued that any endpoint seen by those with an interest in the action as being important and desirable should be a *standard*. However, a more formal, consensus process is valuable in determining the scope and definition of critical outcomes. While outcomes are often seen as the most desirable type of requirement or standard, numerous instances exist in which outcomes either are not measurable or are so infrequent (e.g., death from wrong-site surgery) or remote in time (e.g., myocardial infarction from untreated hypertension), that it is desirable to turn to a process or structural standard as a proxy. Any standard, and its corresponding metric, based on a structure, process, or intermediate outcome must be shown to be linked to some desired end outcome (Meyer and Massagil 2001). Structural or process standards can relate to either administrative or clinical systems. In the administrative realm, there are usually few, if any, experimental studies to suggest the linkages to health outcomes, and most linkages rely on face validity (including laws) and expert opinion. To avoid meaningless and burdensome administrative standards, careful dialog and review by experts *external to* the staff of the accrediting body itself are critical. In clinical services, evidence should come from experimental studies (e.g., studies on safe practices and infection-control procedures such as handwashing), and when possible, from randomized controlled trials (e.g., the standard that HbA1c levels in diabetics should be lower than 9.5).

To transform standards into information about an organization's performance, accreditation must include some metric or verification process to ensure that the standards and criteria have been met. Relatively few means of gathering data exist (see Figure 18.1). Most accreditation in the past has included only structural or process standards measured by reviews of documentation, interviews with patients or staff of the entity, or observation of some processes. Given the often subjective nature of this type of review, the level of expertise, experience, and survey training of the reviewers are crucial to valid measurement.

Since 1999, NCQA accreditation has included adherence to standards related to intermediate or physiological outcomes based on medical chart abstraction or electronic data and of surveys of patient perceptions of care. Since 2001, similar measures of intermediate and physiological outcomes have been included in Joint Commission accreditation. Clinical performance measures, especially when used for public accountability, are, in most cases, based on a much higher level of scientific evidence that links them directly to final outcomes (e.g., survival, quality of life) than are onsite reviews of structures or processes. Thus, performance measures provide a view of quality unavailable in structure and process review alone. In addition, if these performance measures are collected and reported in a timely manner and with a sufficient sampling frame, they can be used by those being evaluated as internal quality improvement measures. Thus, the potential exists for performance measures to serve as an effective and efficient means for both external reporting and internal quality improvement purposes. In fact, if a measure is not useful for internal quality improvement because it measures a process or outcome that is not under the control of the measured entity, the measure is probably not relevant as an accountability measure either. Accountability is based on the ability to control—at least in part—that for which one is held accountable.

While external measurement of outcomes may be the ultimate goal in most instances, in some areas, such as safety, risk-reducing measures are necessary even if the undesirable outcome never occurs. In such cases, verification of structural or process elements critical to quality and safety is part of accreditation. In addition, because of the lack of robust electronic information systems, coding and reporting problems, or insufficient sample sizes, there are many aspects of quality for which reliable or valid performance measures are currently either impossible or prohibitively expensive to collect. Thus, metrics other than performance measures still play a central and critical role in providing accountability for quality.

Accreditation Fails to Provide Critical Information Needed for Either Consumer Choice or Quality Improvement
Issue

In the past, most accreditation has been reported as pass-fail or, in many instances, a list of those who received accreditation, with no reporting of those who attempted and failed or those who did not even attempt accreditation. While this pass-fail level of information can be considered as meeting the basic intent of accreditation (to ensure that a basic floor—beyond the minimum—has been met), most accreditation processes now include a rich set of information that could be used for comparison or choice. Moreover, the scoring or determination of achieving a set threshold is not an exact science. Reasonable individuals can disagree on what requirements are most critical or should contribute most to the scoring. Finally, the level of data publicly reported may reflect the relative influence of those who want to limit external reporting and those who want more public accountability.

Analysis and Response

In most traditional forms of accreditation, the only information provided to those outside the entity being accredited was whether the entity received accreditation. In some cases, this information did not even include whether a group had been evaluated but was denied accreditation. While in some instances, such as airline safety, it may be enough for the public and businesses to know that a given airline, airplane, and pilot are certified, where personal services are involved, a reasonable argument that more detailed information is needed can be made. Given the growth of consumer and payer demand for more in-depth information about quality in healthcare (Pawlson and O'Kane 2002), information limited to simply being accredited or not is no longer sufficient. Given the strength of evidence of substantial variation in the quantity and quality of services provided by accredited healthcare providers (Fisher et al. 2003; Fisher and Wennberg 2003; Wennberg 1999; IOM 2001), purchasers and patients would benefit from basing their choices of healthcare providers on more information than just whether the entity is accredited, although accreditation itself is an important differentiation from nonaccredited status.

By using the information gathered in accreditation in a more robust manner, accreditation can play a much larger role than setting the basic floor in providing the public with much of the information critical to making choices about quality. As noted, some accreditation programs have expanded the set of metrics beyond inspection and verification. In addition, NCQA and the Joint Commission have moved beyond simple reporting of "accredited or not." In the case of NCQA, accreditation status is reported both as ranked categories based on accreditation scores (excellent, commendable, accredited, provisional) and ranking on specific areas of accreditation (from one to four stars in access and service, providers [credentials], staying healthy, getting better, and living with chronic illness). The Joint Commission provides similar levels of accreditation and, as described above, provides disease-specific information. In addition, NCQA provides data from its HEDIS measurement set for public purchasers through the Quality Compass, and the Joint Commission reports core performance data on its public web site. Other accrediting bodies (e.g., URAC, AAAHC) disclose only whether the organization has achieved accredited or certified status.

The Cost of Accreditation Is Not Worth the Benefit

Issue

The cost-benefit concern is most frequently raised by those undergoing (and directly paying for) accreditation. However, those who benefit from (as well as indirectly pay for) accreditation (i.e., purchasers and consumers) should see a net benefit. Indeed, the costs of accreditation, both indirect (e.g., preparation, data collection, reports) and direct (e.g., the fee paid to be reviewed), can be considerable. This is especially true of accreditation that relies exclusively or heavily on paper documentation of large quantities of data or on extensive onsite inspections. To the degree that accreditation is not required, or not used by purchasers or consumers, providers may feel that accreditation does not provide a cost-effective use of their constrained resources. Even where accreditation is required, concerns can exist about whether the standards reflect critical components of quality and safety and whether the evaluation methods used are the most efficient means for determining compliance to those standards. While any quality improvement or regulatory process has associated costs, it is clear that, given the high and rising costs of healthcare, investment in any form of accreditation that does not bring real value either to providers, through quality improvement, or to those using the services, through assurance of quality or choice, should be questioned.

Analysis and Response

In its traditional form, accreditation is a mechanism to enhance improvement in the quality and safety of healthcare *and* provide accountability of the accredited entity to other stakeholders (e.g., patients, consumers, purchasers, insurers, regulators). With respect to accountability, whether the benefits of accreditation exceed its costs is ultimately answerable by those who pay for the healthcare services and ask for accountability for those services. While a healthcare organization might choose to *undergo* accreditation by an outside entity as a benchmark for its overall internal quality improvement processes, this benefit may not be sufficient—in the absence of use of the results by purchasers and consumers—for the organization to *maintain* its accreditation. While some public purchasers (CMS and a few Medicaid programs), some regulators (26 states), and some private purchasers (mostly Fortune 100 companies) require accreditation of health plans as a precursor to contracting with them, the majority do not. Likewise, while most states and CMS accept (deem) hospital accreditation in lieu of government survey and certification, they do not *require* accreditation of hospitals—a (free) state survey for licensure and Medicare certification is always available. Surveys of consumers and private purchasers (specifically those selecting health plans) indicate a minimal understanding of the value or use of accreditation in decision making. This presents a mixed picture of how, in actual practice, the costs and benefits of accreditation are weighed. However, given the ongoing concerns about healthcare insurers and about the quality and safety of care in hospitals, some form of accountability seems needed. The most commonly stated alternatives to accreditation—reliance on professionalism and voluntary quality improvement, government regulation, or contractually defined performance measures—are far from proven as to their value in ensuring accountability.

Some feel that government regulation may be more desirable than, or a replacement for, voluntary (or deemed) accreditation. However, regulation is fraught with political problems and frequently lags behind changes in healthcare (Brennan 1998). The history of healthcare licensure, state mandates, and other regulatory processes provides ample evidence of the limitations of regulation as a means to accountability. Regulation is also often an adversarial process where political power, rather than evidence-based analysis, ends up determining the outcome. By contrast, accreditation can create a process by which there is an active dialog between those being held accountable and those desiring the accountability. In addition, because action by a legislature is not required, accrediting bodies can more quickly adjust to changes in the scope, modes, and technologies of services delivered. Finally, the voluntary nature of accreditation means that the evaluated healthcare provider entity has a desire to take ownership of and responsibility for its performance, rather than simply meeting an outside party's requirements. And, ultimately, the quality and safety of care for the public is controlled by those provider entities, not by either a government agency or accrediting body.

Conclusion

This chapter traces the development of accreditation as one approach to addressing accountability in healthcare. Accreditation in its traditional form has, in some areas of healthcare, provided a relatively successful approach to measuring and reporting accountability in the past. Enhanced accountability is clearly needed in healthcare. This demand encompasses not only a much more robust set of metrics but also accountability at multiple levels of the healthcare system. The challenge is whether accreditation can evolve to meet the expanded demand for accountability. It appears that an expanded scope of accreditation has a major role in meeting the expanding demand for accountability. However, major barriers must be overcome if accreditation is to achieve its potential in meeting this demand.

Study Questions

1. Compare and contrast the use of licensure and accreditation in terms of accountability and quality improvement.
2. What role can/should accreditation play in the future, given the prospect of a huge amount of information from electronic clinical and administrative data sources?
3. What role do the market, regulation, and professionalism play in defining and promoting the use of accreditation as a means of accountability? How would a much more prominent market for medical services affect the usefulness of accreditation? Or the implementation of a single-payer, government-financed system (e.g., if Medicare coverage were extended to everyone living in the United States)?
4. If the ultimate goal is better health outcomes for individuals and populations, can measurement of health outcomes alone substitute for structure and process measures? Why or why not?

Notes

1. For example, hospital accreditation by the Joint Commission on Accreditation of Healthcare Organizations (Joint Commission) or certification by the Centers for Medicare & Medicaid Services (CMS) is a prerequisite for hospitals to participate in the Medicare program. In this situation, accreditation by the Joint Commission is "deemed" (accepted as a substitute) for most elements of the CMS review and certification process.
2. About 25 states require HMOs to be accredited to sell insurance within the state or offer insurance to state employees. Currently, 47 states use Joint Commission accreditation to make hospital licensure decisions.
3. Originally called the Joint Commission on Accreditation of Hospitals (JCAH), the Joint Commission was founded in 1951 as an outgrowth of the American College of Surgeons (ACS) Hospital Standardization Program, itself established in 1918 to improve the quality of care in U.S. hospitals, which at that time were largely

unlicensed and unregulated. The JCAH board of commissioners was appointed by ACS, the American College of Physicians (ACP), American Hospital Association (AHA), and American Medical Association (AMA). (The Canadian Medical Association was also a founding member, but later withdrew, to be replaced in 1969 by the American Dental Association [ADA].) In the past two decades, six public members and a nurse at large have been added to the board, and 21 of the board's remaining 23 members are still appointed by ACP, ACS, ADA, AMA, and AHA.

REFERENCES

Dybkare, R. 1994. "Quality Assurance, Accreditation, and Certification: Needs and Possibilities." *Clinical Chemistry* 40 (7 Pt. 2): 1416–20.

Emanuel, E. J., and L. L. Emanuel. 1996. "What is Accountability in Health Care?" *Annals of Internal Medicine* 124 (2): 229–39.

Emanuel, L. L. 1996. "A Professional Response to Demands for Accountability: Practical Recommendations Regarding Ethical Aspects of Patient Care." Working Group on Accountability. *Annals of Internal Medicine* 124 (2): 240–49.

Fisher, E. S., D. E. Wennberg, T. A. Stukel, D. J. Gottlieb, F. L. Lucas, and E. L. Pinder. 2003. "The Implications of Regional Variations in Medicare Spending. Part 1: The Content, Quality, and Accessibility of Care." *Annals of Internal Medicine* 138 (4): 273–87.

Fisher, E. S., and J. E. Wennberg. 2003. "Health Care Quality, Geographic Variations, and the Challenge of Supply Sensitive Care." *Perspectives in Biology and Medicine* 46: 69–79.

Greenberg, E. L. 1998. "How Accreditation Could Strengthen Local Public Health: An Examination of Models from Managed Care and Insurance Regulators." *Journal of Public Health Management and Practice* 4 (4): 33–37.

Institute of Medicine. 2001. *Crossing the Quality Chasm: A New Health System for the 21st Century.* Washington, DC: National Academy Press.

Meyer, G. S., and M. P. Massagil. 2001. "The Forgotten Component of the Quality Triad: Can We Still Learn Something from 'Structure'?" *Joint Commission Journal on Quality Improvement* 27: 484–93.

Pawlson, L. G., and M. O'Kane. 2002. "Professionalism, Regulation, and the Market: Impact on Accountability for Quality of Care." *Health Affairs (Millwood)* 21 (3): 200–14.

Romano, P. M. 1993. "Managed Care Accreditation: The Process and Early Findings." *Journal of Healthcare Quality* 15 (6): 12–16.

Wennberg, J. E. 1999. "Understanding Geographic Variations in Health Care Delivery." *New England Journal of Medicine* 340 (1): 52–53.

Suggested Reading

Bell, D., and E. N. Brandt, Jr. 1999. "Accreditation by the National Committee on Quality Assurance (NCQA): A Description." *Journal of the Oklahoma State Medical Association* 92 (5): 234–37.

Braun, B. I., R. G. Koss, and J. M. Loeb. 1999. "Integrating Performance Measure Data into the Joint Commission Accreditation Process." *Evaluation & the Health Professions* 22 (3): 283–97.

Carlson, D. A. 1996. "Point of Care Testing: Regulation and Accreditation." *Clinical Laboratory Science* 9 (5): 298–302.

Flanagan, A. 1997. "Ensuring Health Care Quality: JCAHO's Perspective. Joint Commission on Accreditation of Healthcare Organizations." *Clinical Therapeutics* 19 (6): 1540–44.

Gonen, J. S., and S. L. Probyn. 1996. "The Evolution of Accreditation." *HMO* 37 (1): 52–57.

Halverson, P. K., R. M. Nicola, and E. L. Baker. 1998. "Performance Measurement and Accreditation of Public Health Organizations: A Call to Action." *Journal of Public Health Management and Practice* 4 (4): 5–7.

Irvine, D. 1997. "The Performance of Doctors: I: Professionalism and Self Regulation in a Changing World." *British Medical Journal* 314 (7093): 1540–42.

Joint Commission on Accreditation of Healthcare Organizations. 2000. *Benchmarking in Health Care: Finding and Implementing Best Practices.* Oakbrook Terrace, IL: Joint Commission.

Kassebaum, D. G., R. H. Eaglen, and E. R. Cutler. 1997. "The Meaning and Application of Medical Accreditation Standards." *Academic Medicine* 72 (9): 808–18.

Lansky, D., and S. Purdy. 1995. "Public Accountability for Health: New Standards for Health System Performance." *Managed Care Quarterly* 3 (3): 17–24.

Markson, L. E., and D. B. Nash. 1995. *Accountability and Quality in Health Care: The New Responsibility.* Oakbrook Terrace, IL: Joint Commission on Accreditation of Healthcare Organizations.

O'Leary, D. S., and P. M. Schyve. 1994. "The Role of Accreditation in Quality Oversight and Improvement Under Healthcare Reform." *Quality Letter for Healthcare Leaders* 5 (10): 11–14.

O'Leary, M. R. 1996. *Clinical Performance Data: A Guide to Interpretation.* Oakbrook Terrace, IL: Joint Commission on Accreditation of Healthcare Organizations.

O'Malley, C. 1997. "Quality Measurement for Health Systems: Accreditation and Report Cards." *American Journal of Health-System Pharmacy* 54 (13): 1528–35.

Scanlon, D. P., and T. J. Hendrix. 1998. "Health Plan Accreditation: NCQA, JCAHO, or Both?" *Managed Care Quarterly* 6 (4): 52–61.

Schyve, P. M. 1998. "Joint Commission Perspectives on Accreditation of Public Health Practice." *Journal of Public Health Management and Practice* 4 (4): 28–33.

Scrivens, E. 1998. "Widening the Scope of Accreditation—Issues and Challenges in Community and Primary Care." *International Journal for Quality in Health Care* 10 (3): 191–97.

Shaw, C. D. 2000. "External Quality Mechanisms for Health Care: Summary of the ExPeRT Project on Accreditation, EFQM and ISO Assessment in European Union Countries. External Peer Review Techniques. European Foundation for Quality Management. International Organization for Standardization." *International Journal for Quality in Health Care* 12 (3): 169–75.

Viswanathan, H. N. 2000. "Accrediting Organizations and Quality Improvement." *American Journal of Managed Care* 6 (10): 1117–30.

Walshe, K. 2000. *Accreditation in Primary Care: Towards Clinical Governance.* Abingdon, UK: Radcliffe.

HOW PURCHASERS SELECT AND PAY FOR QUALITY

Francois de Brantes

Healthcare cost trends continue to outpace inflation, and a study by RAND confirms others showing that quality of care is highly deficient (McGlynn et al. 2003; Schuster, McGlynn, and Brook 1998; Wennberg 1999). Faced with the decreasing value (costs increasing while quality stagnates) of resources committed to healthcare, purchasers have developed new strategies to select and pay for quality in the delivery of healthcare services.

In healthcare, the concept of *value-based purchasing* (VBP) was imported and applied based on the premise that plans would compete for employer/employee premium dollars by demonstrating greater effectiveness in caring for covered members and greater efficiency in paying for care services. The latter would be (and was) achieved by consolidating the purchasing power of payers and health plan sponsors and obtaining services from physicians, hospitals, and ancillary care providers at discounted rates. The former would be achieved by standardizing measures of quality across plans and creating a common way of assessing plan quality. The efforts by the National Committee for Quality Assurance (NCQA) described in Chapter 18 helped create the methodology to assess plan performance on effectiveness of care in a standard way.

Yet, even before VBP at the plan level lost its ability to improve quality and control costs for the majority of Americans covered by health insurance, purchasers had started to understand that providers did not change their behaviors for one plan alone. They changed their behaviors for all plans. As a result, little difference in the quality of care existed between managed care networks and nonmanaged networks (McGlynn et al. 2003; Schuster, McGlynn, and Brook 1998; Wennberg 1999). This became increasingly true as purchasers demanded that plans increase the size of their networks. And with the expansion of networks came the reduction in relative purchasing power. Purchaser focus has, as a result, shifted from individual plan performance to individual provider performance, as evidenced by the creation of the Leapfrog Group (Birkmeyer et al. 2000).[1] With the release of the Institute of Medicine's (IOM 2001) *Crossing the Quality Chasm* report, purchasers also realized that some very serious gaps continued to exist in the quality of care in the United States and that variations in quality at the individual provider level were significant as well. Reducing the variation in quality and increasing the overall level of quality has become a purchasing imperative, especially in light of renewed and rampant cost increases.

While Joint Commission on Accreditation of Healthcare Organizations (Joint Commission) accreditation of hospitals provides the beginning of an answer in measuring individual provider performance, it is insufficient to meet the needs of purchasers and consumers in the new definition of VBP because accreditation itself hides significant variations in quality performance. However, the individual measures of performance collected by the Joint Commission provide a robust answer to the extent they are made public.

What purchasers describe as VBP today is the ability to create competition at the provider level around effectiveness and efficiency of care. At equal quality, purchasers want to reward the most efficient provider. At different degrees of quality, purchasers want to reward providers who can demonstrate a higher level of quality. In addition, consumers have shown little or no interest in plan performance (in fact, consumers have continued to select their plans based on premium differences, not quality differences), but are increasingly interested in and motivated by provider performance (Hibbard and Jewett 1997; Marshall et al. 2000). Use of financial incentives such as different coinsurance or copayment levels, or use of tiering to differentiate providers, are causing consumers to demand comparative provider performance data.

This chapter describes the efforts undertaken by General Electric (GE) and other large purchasers, in cooperation with some health plans, leading provider organizations, and NCQA, to create a sustainable framework for VBP at the provider level. The effort is called Bridges to Excellence[2] because its objective is to create a bridge to cross the quality chasm; the primary components of that bridge are performance measures. Without performance measures, there is no way to understand the gaps in quality, nor any way to distinguish the level of performance from one provider to another with respect to the effectiveness of the care delivered. Because cost of care is an imperfect way to measure overall provider performance, initial efforts by purchasers have to be focused on defining measures of effectiveness and creating a business case for providers to compete on the basis of quality (Galvin 2001).

Background and Terminology

These concepts and initiatives have the potential for far-reaching consequences in healthcare organizations. A few are summarized here.

- *Managed care organizations.* Managed care organizations have touted their provider quality initiatives as a competitive advantage to increase their market share by winning new customers. However, many of these initiatives have failed to demonstrate robust returns on investment. In addition, they create dissonance at the provider level because of the disparity of initiatives between managed care organizations and the differences in the performance measures used. Starting with the Leapfrog Group (Birkmeyer et al. 2000), purchasers have increasingly urged plans and providers to focus on standardizing measures of effectiveness of care and creating a level playing field for comparing physicians and hospitals. This is especially important to purchasers/employers who offer multiple plans in a single geographical location. How can they explain to employees that each plan has identified a different set of top-quality providers? As a result, plans will increasingly have to stop variations in provider measurement and agree to focus on standards (e.g., Leapfrog, National Quality Forum, Bridges to Excellence/NCQA). However, they will continue to compete on the efficiency of care scores that they can maximize through innovative contracting mechanisms and benefit designs.

- *Provider organizations* (e.g., integrated delivery networks or large group practices). Having a standardized means of assessing internal performance and a business case for improving effectiveness of care will help organized provider groups to compete for patients because they have more resources to deploy in information technology and other support programs to help their physicians meet quality goals. In addition, the redesign of payment systems that encourage physicians to adopt better processes will put the decision making about using new technologies back into their hands. If they are judged and rewarded based on the effectiveness and efficiency of the care they provide, physicians and hospitals will have a vested interest to use technologies that are proven to be effective and efficient.

- *Accreditation organizations* (NCQA, Joint Commission). To meet purchaser and consumer needs, accreditation organizations will have to adapt their performance measures to make them more transparent and more detailed. As mentioned previously, it will be increasingly important for the Joint Commission to disclose the full hospital report card, not simply an overall accreditation score, which can mask significant variations in quality within an institution. Similarly, NCQA will have to continue its move toward individual physician measurement as opposed to planwide accreditation and use standardized measures that have been preferably reached through a consensus process.

- *Disease management and care management/coordination vendors.* Over time, vendors that currently provide a purchaser-based service to manage individual cases or populations with a specific condition should shift their sales and marketing strategy to the provider. If providers are measured on and rewarded for effectiveness of care, they will need to reengineer internal care processes and use the services of these vendors. Purchasers, on the other hand, should no longer need to buy the services of these vendors because they will be paying for them at the point of care.

- *Technology vendors.* In a real VBP model, the bundling of payments around episodes of care creates a mechanism for providers to reap the benefits of adopting technologies that are proven to be effective and efficient in managing patients and delivering better outcomes. As such, technology vendors will have to focus their products and services on these factors. At the same time, technology vendors will no longer have to rely on the approval of various managed care organizations to deploy their products because physicians will be free to adopt them directly.

This chapter also looks at other like experiments in the market and draws some early lessons and implications.

Bridges to Excellence

The report *Crossing the Quality Chasm* (IOM 2001) documented the quality shortfalls in the U.S. healthcare system and provided a road map for change. Subsequent publications have substantiated the quality issues, including a report that indicated that 20 percent of physicians and 25 percent of the public have had personal experiences of serious harm caused by avoidable errors (Blendon et al. 2002). A key point made by IOM is that the current reimbursement system does not encourage, and frequently discourages, quality improvement. Healthcare purchasers, concerned about the rising costs of healthcare, believe that improving quality will mitigate unnecessary cost increases and, through the Leapfrog Group, a voluntary organization of 130 healthcare purchasers, established rewarding quality as a fundamental principle of purchasing healthcare services. Leading providers and provider organizations also recognize the instability of the status quo.

Although several studies have demonstrated that quality can reduce overall costs, no consensus that this is true exists. Part of the problem in establishing a business case is that results vary by type of quality improvement (i.e., reduction in overuse, misuse, or underuse), reimbursement system (i.e., fee-for-service or prepaid), and recipient of the reward (i.e., payers or providers). A fundamental premise in the Bridges to Excellence initiative is that both payers and providers must experience a positive return on investment for the project to be sustainable.

In sectors outside healthcare, an underlying belief is that higher quality lowers cost; within healthcare, a growing consensus is that better quality should be rewarded (see Table 19.1 for details on various pay-for-quality initiatives). GE, through its adoption of a quality improvement methodology called Six Sigma (Harry and Schroeder 1999), has demonstrated billions of dollars in savings since 1995. Working with a group of organizations and individuals representing different stakeholders of the healthcare system (provider, payer, plan, measurement experts), GE applied the same Six Sigma methodology (called Design for Six Sigma [DFSS]) to develop Bridges to Excellence that it uses to design all new products, from jet engines to long-term care insurance products. The program defined a clear mission: to create an adaptable healthcare model that rewards quality performance, in particular, but not exclusively, for chronic care, simultaneously for both providers or provider organizations and purchasers. The rewards are based on objective measures of processes of care that (1) prevent defects (misuse, overuse, underuse) and (2) are valued, actionable, and auditable by providers, consumers/patients, and purchasers.

Such a framework is the building block of VBP in that agreed-on measures of quality and rewards linked to them are required to encourage providers to participate. While Bridges to Excellence focused on a design that gives bonuses to those who meet standard performance measures, an extension would be to redesign the overall payments to providers, making bonuses an integral part of the design.

Design for Six Sigma

The DFSS process, summarized in Figure 19.1, lays out a series of steps, grouped in tollgates, and statistical tools that guide the development of a new product or service. Unique concepts in Six Sigma are *CTQs*—program attributes that are critical to quality and define what the customer needs—and *CTPs*—design attributes of the product or service that are critical to process and will ensure that CTQs are met. The application of these concepts increases the likelihood of success of new products or services.

Defining the CTQs

This step in the DFSS process is the most important because it requires all stakeholders to agree on a core set of important principles (customer and stakeholder needs) that will define the program's design. Given the nature

TABLE 19.1
Pay-for-
Quality
Initiatives

Inpatient	Outpatient
Anthem Cardiac Surgery Recognition Program: Anthem's program is one of the largest in the United States and rewards hospitals that meet certain performance measures for cardiac surgery, in addition to giving hospitals a benchmark to compare their relative performance against	CMS—Physician Group Practice Demonstration: In this demonstration project, CMS will bundle payments for Medicare Parts A and B and tie them to specific performance measures including selected HEDIS measures (e.g., HbA1c for diabetes, ECG for congestive heart failure); the goal is to create an incentive for physicians to better manage their patients and be rewarded by decreasing hospitalizations
BlueShield of California Hospital Tiering Program: BlueShield of California, like many plans across the United States, has started to tier its hospitals based on how well they perform with respect to both cost and quality; the quality measures used are a combination of Leapfrog measures and other statewide hospital performance data	The Integrated Healthcare Association (IHA): This organization includes the largest plans in California; together, they have agreed to measure physician performance in a common way, although each plan will independently determine the rewards; measures used include HEDIS indicators, measures of use of information technology to decrease errors, and a patient experience of care survey
Hannaford Brothers Hospital Copay Program: Employers as diverse as Hannaford Brothers and Boeing are using benefit design changes to vary the copayments between hospitals according to certain quality measures, driving more patients to higher-quality facilities	Plans—Aetna, CIGNA, Highmark, Anthem, BlueCross BlueShield Illinois, BlueCross California, Indiana Health Many plans across the United States reward physicians for meeting certain performance measures (primarily HEDIS indicators), although, for the most part, this performance is never made public
Empire BlueCross and BlueShield's Leapfrog Program: Empire was the first plan to launch a reward program for hospitals that meet the Leapfrog measures; rewards are bonuses that represent a certain percentage of existing fees (up to 4%)	Anthem of Maine's Systems of Care Initiative: Anthem of Maine has launched a program that will reward physicians for adopting information technology tools in their practices to help them better manage their patients

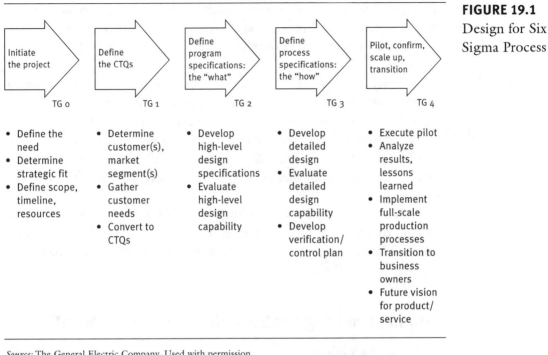

Source: The General Electric Company. Used with permission.

FIGURE 19.1
Design for Six
Sigma Process

of the Bridges to Excellence program—a performance-based incentive program with performance measures to be made public—both physicians and consumers/patients are considered customers; all other parties, including purchasers, are stakeholders. This distinction is critical because the customers' needs drive most of the product's design.

Identifying, sorting, and ranking customer needs, or CTQs, was accomplished through a combination of interviews, focus groups, and literature searches. In prior work (de Brantes and Galvin 2001), GE had defined key attributes consumers/patients require of healthcare-related information and of their interaction with consumers. Physician needs were collected through focus groups and later validated by work done on incentive programs (Bailit and Dyer 2002). A consensus view is that rewards and incentives have to be (1) meaningful enough to more than compensate for the added cost associated with data collection and measurement of processes; (2) perceived to be fair and equitable; (3) attainable; (4) periodically reviewed; and (5) incremental, with small-step increments, as opposed to a "cliff." The incentives should be based on measures that are standard and well accepted by experts, and they should only measure what is actionable by the physician or provider being measured. Finally, if performance measures are linked to outcomes, patient incentives should be deployed to align patient behavior with the performance measures. These provider CTQs are summarized in Table 19.2.

Other key attributes of successful physician-based incentive programs include simplicity and standardization of processes; no added burden on staff or office; low intensity of data requirements; increased income while giving high-quality care; ability to educate and motivate patients to seek out high-quality providers; ability to educate staff and enable them to be better teachers; and avoidance of putting the physician at odds with the patient.

As the design of the program evolved from high-level to detailed design, providers were regularly interviewed and consulted to make sure that the incentives and rewards would meet their needs and stimulate their desire to achieve the performance measures.

Defining the Program Specifications—The "What"

Performance Measures

The performance measures had to meet specific requirements. They had to help achieve the six aims for better care identified in IOM's report: safe, timely, effective, efficient, equitable, and patient centered. The measures also had to be clearly measurable, actionable, and under the control of the provider being measured.

With these critical attributes defined, the cross-functional team identified a series of processes that could affect these attributes to varying degrees. The Six Sigma tool used in this phase of the design is called a Quality Functional Deployment (see Figure 19.2).

It took the team several weeks and then a full day working together to agree on how to rank each of the key processes of care with respect to how they affected the critical attributes. The consensus on how each process would affect a customer need (high, medium, low) and the importance of that need relative to others yielded a ranking of 16 processes. The highest was "information and resources for both clinicians and patients in managing specific, high-intensity conditions—typically, but not always, after an acute episode or hospitalization." The balance grouped in three tiers, with the top two tiers including 11 processes that fit in three distinct categories (see Figure 19.3): clinical information systems with evidence-based decision support, patient education and support, and care management. These three categories of processes are consistent with the areas of focus identified by IOM in its

Incentives and Rewards	Performance Measures	TABLE 19.2
• Ensure incentive is meaningful to providers • Establish clear expectations for performance • Reward in a timely manner • Evaluate the incentive program regularly; modify as needed • Focus incentives on a limited number of measures • Collaborate and consult with providers to obtain and retain buy-in • Develop an incentive approach that is easy to understand and administer • Predictable costs and benefits of program • Incentives that occur regularly for actions over which providers have control • Insurers and purchasers work collaboratively to overcome small market share • Meaningful enough to more than compensate for the added cost associated with data collection and measurement of process • Perceived to be fair and equitable • Incremental, with small-step increments as opposed to a cliff • Nonpunitive—a carrot, not a stick	• Select performance measures that are well defined and within the provider's control • Select thresholds that are a stretch, but attainable over time • Accurate and comprehensive data • Timely data to provide feedback to the provider and staff on what to improve • Absolute benchmarks of performance • Utilize an independent entity for measuring performance • Address noncompliance by creating patient incentives • Minimize burden on staff and duplication of effort	Provider Critical-to-Quality (CTQ) Factors

Crossing the Quality Chasm report (IOM 2001), have also been highlighted in a number of studies, and are the focus of like initiatives.

Turning these three categories of care processes into meaningful measures led to a canvassing of existing performance measures to determine whether any set would map back to the three groups of processes. One program emerged as a good candidate: The American Diabetes Association–NCQA Diabetes Physician Recognition Program (DPRP). This program is a self-report (with audit) by individual physicians of their practices' performance on a set of measures of the care of diabetic patients. The DPRP has shown that recognized physicians systematically improve their performance upon resubmission. While the criteria used to score physicians are primarily outcomes based, achieving these outcomes requires a certain reengineering of a practice.

FIGURE 19.2
Quality Functional Deployment

Customer Expectation	Importance	Data capture and management for patient tracking	Data capture and management of patient compliance with standards of care	Data capture and management of provider compliance with standards of care	Evidence-based clinical treatment decision support focused on error prevention	Evidence-based clinical treatment decision support focused on guidelines for care	Value-based decision support focused on an integrated radiology program	Value-based decision support focused on an integrated PBM program	Information and resources enabling the patient to make fully informed decisions for treatment of condition	Information and resources enabling the patient to make fully informed decisions for managing health	Proactive management of patient care—Disease management programs	Proactive management of patient care—Coordination of multispecialty teams	Proactive management of patient care—Effective systems of communication across providers	Proactive management of patient care—Effective systems of communication between patients and providers	Proactive management of patient care—Risk factor screenings	Proactive management of patient care—Support systems for patient lifestyle changes	Information and resources for both clinicians and patients in managing specific, high-intensity conditions—typically, but not always, after an acute episode or hospitalization	Total
Safe—care for, not harm the patient	5	L	H	M	H	M	H	H	M	L	M	H	H	M	L	L	H	370
Effective—care is evidence based and designed to help the patient get better as soon as appropriate	5	M	H	H	M	H	L	H	H	M	H	H	M	M	H	M	M	480
Patient centered—focused on the patient's values, physiology, respecting the patient's needs for information and support	5	L	M	L	L	M	L	M	H	H	H	H	H	H	H	H	H	470
Timely—care is given when needed, with minimum delays, efficient flow, as appropriate	4	L	M	M	M	M	M	M	M	L	M	H	H	H	M	L	H	256
Efficient—care given represents the best use of resources to get the best value for money spent	5	M	H	H	M	M	H	M	M	M	M	M	H	M	M	L	H	440
Equitable—appropriate standards of care are applied to all irrespective of gender, color, creed, socioeconomic background, culture, etc.	4	H	H	H	H	H	L	M	M	L	H	M	M	L	H	L	H	368
Measurable—processes used are measurable	4	H	H	M	M	H	H	M	L	L	M	L	L	M	H	M	M	328
Portable—processes defined are adaptable from one care system/setting to another	3	H	H	H	L	H	L	M	H	H	L	L	M	H	H	H	H	288
Actionable—processes defined are implemented by providers or provider organizations	5	H	H	H	H	H	H	H	H	H	M	M	H	H	H	H	H	690
Impactful—processes defined favorably affect the largest amount of patients possible	2	H	H	M	M	H	M	H	M	M	M	M	H	H	H	M	L	176
Customer-centric—convenient to the patient and delivered with a high level of customer service	3	L	M	L	L	L	H	H	H	H	M	H	H	H	M	H	H	258
Total		209	309	257	189	273	211	333	253	205	249	253	301	259	293	195	335	

Source: The General Electric Company. Used with permission.

FIGURE 19.3
Process
Groupings

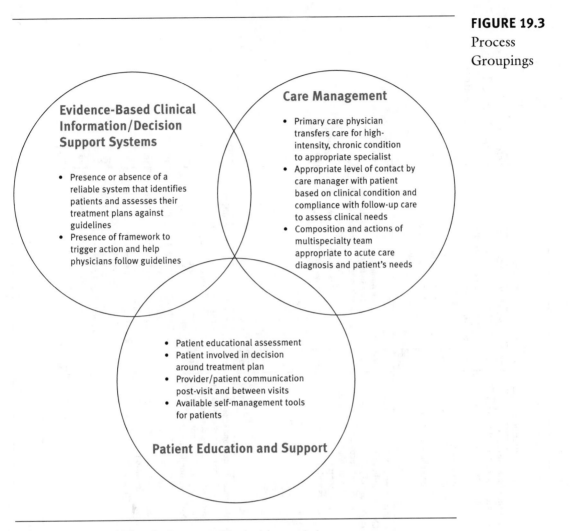

Evidence-Based Clinical Information/Decision Support Systems

- Presence or absence of a reliable system that identifies patients and assesses their treatment plans against guidelines
- Presence of framework to trigger action and help physicians follow guidelines

Care Management

- Primary care physician transfers care for high-intensity, chronic condition to appropriate specialist
- Appropriate level of contact by care manager with patient based on clinical condition and compliance with follow-up care to assess clinical needs
- Composition and actions of multispecialty team appropriate to acute care diagnosis and patient's needs

- Patient educational assessment
- Patient involved in decision around treatment plan
- Provider/patient communication post-visit and between visits
- Available self-management tools for patients

Patient Education and Support

Source: The General Electric Company. Used with permission.

Given that at most only 6 percent of consumers under age 65 are diabetic, measuring provider performance only on this dimension cannot achieve the broad impact specified in the original mission statement. As such, the Bridges to Excellence program decided to bifurcate its effort by (1) adopting the DPRP and turning it into an incentive program (Diabetes Care Link) and (2) refining the three groups of core measures into measurable performance indicators (Physician Office Link) using existing surveys that had been developed in similar efforts in other parts of the country as a guide (see Figure 19.4). Some elements in the survey are explored in more detail in Chapter 12.

FIGURE 19.4
Summary of Physician Office Link Measures

Clinical Information Systems/Evidence-based Medicine

Basic Registries and Follow-up	Pts
1. Type of registry used for chronic conditions	10
2. Percentage of patients in registry	10
3. Use of registry to identify patient populations	40
4. Use of paper or electronic system to track and follow upon referrals and test results	40
	100

Electronic Registries, Prescription and Test Ordering	Pts
1. Types of patient information in registry	10
2. Capabilities of an electronic system for prescriptions and tests	20
3. Use of electronic system for ordering prescriptions and checking for safety and efficiency	40
4. Use of electronic system to order and retrieve tests	10
5. Use of electronic system to track missing test results, distinguish abnormal results, and prompt follow-up on test results	20
	100

Electronic Medical Records	Pts
1. Types of patient information in an EMR	10
2. Percentage of patients who have information in the EMR	20
3. EMR's capability to report across practice on multiple fields	30
4. EMR's capability to use decision support to prompt physician interventions	30
5. EMR's capability to capture services ordered, delivered, or paid	5
6. Use of EMR to track referrals and test results	5
	100

Patient Education and Support

Educational Resources	Pts
1. Assessment of patient language preferences and risk factors	30
2. Identification of preferred languages in patient population	35
3. Provision of educational resources in preferred languages for risk factors and chronic conditions	35
	100

Referrals for Risk Factors and Chronic Conditions	Pts
1. Percent of patients who have specific risk factors	50
2. Provision of referrals for education and support to patients with risk factors and chronic conditions	50
	100

Quality Measurement and Improvement	Pts
1. Identification of opportunities for improving outcomes or processes	20
2. Setting goals for performance for identified opportunities of improvement	20
3. Measurement of performance and identification of goals not met	20
4. Implementation of improvement activities	40
	100

Care Management

Care of Chronic Conditions	Pts
1. Identification of the practice's top three chronic conditions	10
2. Structured process for disease management for patients with the top three conditions	45
3. Use of resources to assist with medication compliance, appointments, and barriers to care	45
	100

Preventable Admissions	Pts
1. Using data to identify patients who are at risk for emergency admissions	20
2. Identification of the reasons for and prevalence of emergency admissions	20
3. Structured system to prevent emergency admissions	60
	100

Care of High-Risk Medical Conditions	Pts
1. Resources for managing patients with high-risk conditions	5
2. Number and percentage of patients who receive high-risk care management	5
3. Contents of the high-risk care management program	30
4. Qualifications of the high-risk care manager	10
5. Types of information in database of patients with high-risk conditions	15
6. Frequency of communication between physician and care manager	5
7. Frequency of communication between care manager and patient	30
	100

Source: The General Electric Company. Used with permission.

Incentives and Rewards

In focus groups, physicians defined three broad categories and types of incentives, as well as their importance: direct financial incentives (most important), indirect financial incentives, and nonfinancial incentives (least important).

The existing data on cost savings accrued because improvements in treating diabetics or managing information flow in a physician office are not definitive. However, purchasers, with their bias toward action, believe sufficient evidence exists to move forward. Actuarial models indicate that potential short- and long-term savings of about 7 percent of total costs can be achieved by improving outcomes for diabetic patients. In addition, potential short-term savings of 4 percent of total cost of care (or overall premiums) can be achieved by a more thorough reengineering of physician practices (e.g., adoption of the processes in the Physician Office Link).

Since purchasers will require a return on any additional monies paid to physicians, it is reasonable for them to keep 50 percent of the expected savings and share the other 50 percent, setting those funds aside as the incentive pool available to those who meet the performance measures. This analysis and parsing of the savings pool led to having a bonus of $100 per diabetic patient per year for physicians meeting the DPRP performance measures and $55 per patient per year for physicians meeting the Physician Office Link performance measures.

The DPRP performance bonus is a cliff in that physicians either get it or they do not; physicians indicate that this is not their preferred method of receiving bonuses (see incentive CTQs in Table 19.2). However, the Physician Office Link bonus is structured to be gradual and provide the physician with seed money to invest in better systems of care. Figure 19.4 shows nine modules of measures, each independent from the other. The physician bonuses are structured to encourage physicians to meet an increasing number of modules over three years. In the first year, they can qualify for the full bonus ($55) by meeting any one of the modules in each column, for a total of three modules. In the second year, physicians have to meet two of three in each column, for a total of six modules, and in the third year, they must meet all nine modules. If a physician does not improve his or her performance from one year to another, they still qualify for a bonus, albeit a lower one than in the prior year. This system of providing a graduated increase in performance while still providing an opportunity to qualify for the maximum bonus seems to resonate with physicians more than the cliff-type bonuses.

While nonfinancial rewards—in particular, public recognition programs via some form of rating system—are not of uniform importance to providers (in fact, some providers have expressed strong antipathy for public data dissemination), purchasers and consumers have demonstrated a need and a strong demand for comparative provider performance data. Until 2003/2004, however, these data sets have not been widely adopted, and research has shown that most provider report cards are not understandable to consumers (Hibbard and Jewett 1997). To better meet the needs of consumers/patients in this domain, a research project was launched to gather critical input from consumers, enabling the design of an enhanced provider directory that could incorporate all of the data elements important for consumers to make informed decisions. An initial series of focus groups was conducted during which consumers delineated all the data elements they wanted and categorized those data into intuitive groupings. Subsequent focus groups used a pencil-and-paper exercise during which the groups of measures and associated labels were tested. The result is a prototype, shown in Figure 19.5, that needs further validation and testing to determine its effectiveness in helping consumers select physicians and hospitals.

Consumer-Based Elements

Consumers/patients are engaged in the program through the provision of information on physicians that they heretofore had not had, as illustrated above. In addition, consumers/patients with diabetes are engaged to better understand their condition and are encouraged to improve or stabilize it. Work by Bodenheimer, Wagner, and Grumbach (2002) has demonstrated that obtaining the full yield from a chronic care management model is impossible without robust patient involvement. That view was strongly echoed by physicians who reviewed Bridges to Excellence. They were adamant that if part of their performance measurement was based on patient outcomes, patients should have similar incentives to improve outcomes.

The result is a novel program called Diabetes Care Rewards, which includes tools for patients with diabetes to monitor their self-care activities and provides them with points for lowering their HbA1c levels and following care guidelines. Patients can accumulate points to qualify for rewards offered by the participating employers/purchasers. In some cases, those rewards are vouchers for lower copayments on physician office visits or on prescriptions. In other cases, they are coupons that can be redeemed at sites that offer patients with diabetes products not routinely covered by health benefits (e.g., sugar-free candies).

In focus groups, consumers/patients indicated that having a monetary or quasimonetary reward was very important to them and would keep them focused on achieving better outcomes. However, these rewards did not have to be large, but rather simply achievable (thus echoing what physicians said was important for their own incentives).

FIGURE 19.5
Physician
Report Card
Prototype

Doctor Information	Address & Hours	Staffing	Credentials	Hospital Affiliation
Dr. Robert Smith FAMILY PRACTICE ID NO. 0004668883 03 My Philosophy of Care 518.472.4584 518.472.4620 fax dr.smith@aol.com	997 Glen Cove Avenue Glen Head, NY 11545 Monday - Thursday 10-5 Friday, Saturday 11-4	• 2 Nurses • 3 Technicians • 1 on-call doctor	NY Medical College, M.D., 1989 St. Lukes–Roosevelt, 1992 AM Board of Internal Medicine, 1994	Mt. Sinai Medical Center Westchester Medical Center Columbia Presbyterian Medical Center

Performance Report:

Effectiveness of Care

	Overall	Diabetes Care	Cardiac Care
Overall			

◑ Doctor:
◑ Average Score:

Patient Experience of Care

	Overall

◑ Doctor:
◑ Average Score:

Clinical Information Systems And Evidence-based Medicine		Patient Education and Support		Care Management	
Basic Registries and Follow-up	✓100%	Educational Resources	✓100%	Care of Chronic Conditions	✓100%
Electronic Registries, Prescription and Test Ordering		Referrals for Risk Factors & Chronic Conditions		Preventable Admissions	
Electronic Medical Records		Quality Measurement and Improvement		Care of High-Risk Medical Conditions	

Key
✓ | Provider has fulfilled the requirements for the measures

Key
| | Your Provider |
| | Average Provider |

Doctor-Patient Interactions
- Communication
- Interpersonal Treatment
- Knowledge of Patient
- Health Practices
- Integration
- Patient Trust
- Relationship Duration

Access and Office Systems
- Organizational Access
- Visit-based Continuity
- Clinical Team

Source: The General Electric Company. Used with permission.

Designing the Program Implementation—The "How"

Three CTQs drove the majority of the operational design for Bridges to Excellence: (1) make the rewards as meaningful as possible by consolidating the bonuses in a single payment; (2) make the program administratively simple for purchasers, plans, and providers; and (3) do not cause plans to open up their provider contracts or do anything that would disrupt current network arrangements.

These CTQs forced elimination of many options (e.g., having each plan administer and pay the bonuses) that would have been easy for purchasers to implement but counter to what the customers and other stakeholders wanted. One of the core principles in designing a new program using the Six Sigma methodology is not to retrofit a solution into an existing infrastructure; the existing infrastructure may not meet the needs of your customers.

As a result, the operational framework chosen by Bridges to Excellence was to hire an independent third party as the general contractor, Medstat, a subsidiary of the Thomson Company. Medstat's role is to aggregate data files from plans, creating a master patient/physician/purchaser grid that defines the number of patients per physician for whom a bonus could be paid and enables the participating purchaser to quickly gauge its maximum exposure if all physicians met the performance measures. In addition, Medstat invoices each purchaser on a quarterly basis, reflecting all the bonuses that have to be paid to physicians who meet the performance measures, and then pays the physician a lump-sum bonus across all participating purchasers.

This structure ends up being administratively simple because it is not dependent on a specific health plan or network arrangement and does not require a plan to modify its existing contractual arrangements with network physicians. In fact, the health plan's role is limited to sending the data file to Medstat, although the plan can also become involved in helping physicians in their networks meet the performance measures and in engaging patients with diabetes to enroll in the self-care tools. For employers, the program does require signing a few agreements so that the data can flow between their plan and Medstat, and they are bound by the terms of the program to pay the bonuses and engage their employees in better self-care.

Conclusion

Designing any new product or service in a system as fragmented as healthcare—and with stakeholders that can have, at times, highly divergent needs—is far from easy. However, the framework provided by the DFSS process enabled all stakeholders to make trade-offs between their needs and those of other stakeholders and ensured that the design would, overall, have wide appeal to purchasers, providers, plans, and patients.

Key principles of a successful design include making sure that

- Incentives will meet provider CTQs, in particular, are attainable and meaningful;
- Measures meet provider and purchaser CTQs, create a return on investment for purchasers, are achievable yet not easy, and are standard as opposed to custom; and
- Operational structure meets purchaser and plan CTQs, is simple and easy for purchasers to implement, and keeps the administrative burden for plans to an absolute minimum.

Study Questions

1. Why are purchasers increasingly interested in a new model for value-based purchasing?
2. Once purchasers and plans have created enough rewards to attract physicians to meet high performance measures, and enough physicians do so, what is the next phase in creating a robust value-based purchasing model?
3. How would a value-based purchasing model look compared to the existing plan-based delivery system?

Notes

1. For more information, see www.leapfroggroup.org.
2. For more information, see www.bridgestoexcellence.org.

REFERENCES

Bailit, M., and M. B. Dyer. 2002. *Provider Incentive Models for Improving Quality of Care*. Washington, DC: National Health Care Purchasing Institute.

Birkmeyer, J. D., C. M. Birkmeyer, D. E. Wennberg, and M. Young. 2000. *Leapfrog Patient Safety Standards: The Potential Benefits of Universal Adoption*. Washington, DC: The Leapfrog Group.

Blendon, R. J., C. M. DesRoches, M. Brodie, J. M. Benson, A. B. Rosen, E. Schneider, D. E. Altman, K. Zapert, M. J. Herrmann, and A. E. Steffenson. 2002. "Views of Practicing Physicians and the Public on Medical Errors." *New England Journal of Medicine* 347 (24): 1933–40.

Bodenheimer, T., E. H. Wagner, and K. Grumbach. 2002. "Improving Primary Care for Patients with Chronic Illness." *Journal of the American Medical Association* 288: 1775–79, 1909–14.

de Brantes, F., and R. S. Galvin. 2001. "Creating, Connecting and Supporting Active Consumers." *International Journal of Medical Marketing* 2 (1): 73–80.

Galvin, R. S. 2001. "The Business Case for Quality." *Health Affairs (Millwood)* 20 (6): 57–58.

Harry, M., and R. Schroeder. 1999. *Six Sigma: The Breakthrough Management Strategy Revolutionizing the World's Top Corporations*. New York: Doubleday.

Hibbard, J. H., and J. J. Jewett. 1997. "Will Quality Report Cards Help Consumers?" *Health Affairs (Millwood)* 75: 395–414.

Institute of Medicine. 2001. *Crossing the Quality Chasm: A New Health System for the 21st Century*. Washington, DC: National Academy Press.

Marshall, M. N., P. G. Shekelle, S. Leatherman, and R. H. Brook. 2000. "The Public Release of Performance Data: What Do We Expect to Gain? A Review of the Evidence." *Journal of the American Medical Association* 283: 1866–74.

McGlynn, E. A., S. M. Asch, J. Adams, J. Keesey, J. Hicks, A. DeCristofaro, and E. A. Kerr. 2003. "The Quality of Health Care Delivered to Adults in the United States." *New England Journal of Medicine* 348: 2635–45.

Schuster, M. A., E. A. McGlynn, and R. Brook. 1998. "How Good Is the Quality of Healthcare in the United States?" *Milbank Quarterly* 76 (4): 517–63.

Wennberg, J. A. 1999. "Understanding Geographic Variations in Health Care Delivery." *New England Journal of Medicine* 340: 52–53.

APPENDIX 1.
CONTROL CHART FORMULAS

Attributes Data: Proportion Measures (p-Chart)

Proportion measures are analyzed using the p-chart. The following data elements (organization level) are used to construct a p-chart.

Data Element	Notation*
Number of denominator cases for a month	n_i
Number of numerator cases for a month	x_i
Observed rate for a month	p_i

* The subscript (i) represents individual months.

Statistical formulas for calculating the centerline and control limits are given below. Note that the control limits are calculated for individual months, and the limits vary by month unless the number of denominator cases from each month is the same for all months.

Centerline of the chart

$$\bar{p} = \frac{\sum x_i}{\sum n_i} = \frac{x_1 + x_2 + \ldots + x_m}{n_1 + n_2 + \ldots + n_m},$$

where *m* is the number of months (or data points).

Upper and lower control limits for each month

$$\bar{p} \pm 3 * \sqrt{\frac{\bar{p}*(1-\bar{p})}{n_i}}$$

Small sample size adjustments

When the sample sizes are very small, a standard p-chart cannot be used because the statistical assumption needed to create a p-chart (i.e., normal approximation to the binomial distribution) is not valid. Specifically, the small sample sizes are defined as follows:

$$\bar{n} * \bar{p} < 4 \ or \ \bar{n} * (1 - \bar{p}) < 4,$$

where n-bar is the average number of denominator cases and the p-bar is the centerline (i.e., weighted average of individual month = s observed rates).

In this situation, an adjusted p-chart using an exact binomial probability (i.e., probability limit method) is used. To calculate the upper and lower control limits using the probability limit method, the smallest x_U and the largest x_L satisfying the following two binomial probability distribution functions should be calculated first:

$$\sum_{x=x_U}^{n} \binom{n}{x} p^x (1 - p)^{n-x} \leq 0.00135 \ \ and \ \ \sum_{x=0}^{x_L} \binom{n}{x} p^x (1 - P)^{n-x} \leq 0.00135.$$

Then the upper and the lower control limits for the observed rate are obtained by dividing x_U and x_L by the number of denominator cases n for the month. Alternatively, instead of the binomial probability distribution, an incomplete beta distribution may be used to calculate the probability limits (SAS 1995).

Attributes Data: Ratio Measures (u-Chart)

Ratio measures are analyzed using the u-chart. A u-chart is created using the following data elements (HCO level).

Data Element	Notation*
Number of denominator cases for a month	n_i
Number of numerator cases for a month	x_i
Observed rate for a month	u_i

* The subscript (I) represents individual months.

Centerline of a u-chart

$$\bar{u} = \frac{\sum x_i}{\sum n_i} = \frac{x_1 + x_2 + \ldots + x_m}{n_1 + n_2 + \ldots + n_m},$$

where m is the number of months (or data points).

Control limits for each month

$$\bar{u} \pm 3 * \sqrt{\frac{\bar{u}}{n_i}}$$

* If the ratio is to be calculated based on a prespecified denominator basis (or a scaling factor), the control chart must be appropriately scaled using that information. For example, the denominator basis for a ratio measure number of falls per 100 resident days is 100. In this case, all values in the control chart, including the centerline and control limits, and observed ratio must be multiplied by 100.

Small sample size adjustments

Like p-charts, a standard u-chart should not be used when the sample size is very small. This is because the statistical assumption for u-chart (normal approximation to the Poisson distribution) fails if the sample size is very small. Small sample size for ratio measures is defined as:

$$\bar{n} * \bar{u} < 4,$$

where n-bar is the average number of denominator cases and u-bar is the centerline of the u-chart.

In this situation, an adjusted u-chart based on Poisson probability is used. The upper and lower control limits are obtained by first calculating x_U and x_L and then dividing each value by the number of denominator cases n for the month. To obtain x_U and x_L, following two Poisson probability distribution functions should be solved in such a way that the smallest x_U and the largest x_L satisfying these conditions are obtained:

$$\sum_{x=x_U}^{\infty} \frac{e^{-u} u^x}{x!} \leq 0.00135 \quad and \quad \sum_{x=0}^{x_L} \frac{e^{-u} u^x}{x!} \leq 0.00135.$$

Alternatively, a chi-square distribution may be used instead of the Poisson probability distribution to calculate the probability limits (SAS 1995).

Variables Data (X-bar and S Chart)

Variables data or continuous-variable measures are analyzed using the X-bar and S chart. To construct an X-bar and S chart, the following data elements (HCO level) are needed.

Data Element	Notation*
Number of cases for a month	n_i
Mean of observed values for a month	x_i
Standard deviation of observed values for a month	s_i

* The subscript (i) represents individual months.

The center line and control limits for an X-bar and S chart are calculated using the formulas below. Note that the control limits vary by months depending on the denominator cases for individual months.

Centerline

1) X-bar chart

$$\bar{x} = \frac{\sum n_i * x_i}{\sum n_i}$$

2) S chart
(a) Minimum variance linear unbiased estimate (SAS 1995)

$$\bar{s_i} = c_4 * \frac{\sum h_i * \frac{s_i}{c_4}}{\sum h_i}, \quad \text{where } h_i = \frac{c_4^2}{1 - c_4^2}$$

(b) Pooled standard deviation (Montgomery 1996)

$$\bar{s} = \sqrt{\frac{\sum (n_i - 1) * s_i^2}{\sum n_i - m}}$$

* These two methods result in slightly different values, but the differences are generally negligible.

* c_4 is a constant that depends on the sample size. As the sample size increases, c_4 approaches to 1. The exact formula for c_4 is:

$$c_4 = \sqrt{\frac{2}{n_i - 1}} * \frac{\Gamma(\frac{n_i}{2})}{\Gamma(\frac{n_i - 1}{2})}$$

Control limits

1) X-bar chart

$$\bar{x} \pm 3 * \frac{\bar{s}}{c_4\sqrt{n_i}}$$

2) S chart

$$\bar{s} * (1 \pm \frac{3}{c_4} * \sqrt{1 - c_4^2})$$

Small Sample Size Adjustments

If the sample size is 1 for all data points, an XmR chart is used instead of an X-bar and S chart, assuming the observed mean value as a single observation for the month (Lee and McGreevey 2000).

Source:
The content of Appendix 1 is largely based on Lee and McGreevey (2000).

References:
Lee, K. Y., and C. McGreevey. 2000. *Mining ORYX Data 2000—A Guide for Performance Measurement Systems.* Oakbrook Terrace, IL: Joint Commission on Accreditation of Healthcare Organizations.

Montgomery, D. C. 1996. *Introduction to Statistical Quality Control.* New York: John Wiley & Sons.

The SAS Institute. 1995. SAS/QC Software: Usage and Reference, Version 6, 1st ed., vol. 2. Cary, NC: The SAS Institute.

APPENDIX 2.
COMPARISON CHART FORMULAS

Comparison Analysis: Proportion Measures

Three data elements listed below are used in the comparison chart analysis for proportion measures. The expected rate is either risk-adjusted rate (if risk adjusted) or overall observed rate for the comparison group (if not risk adjusted or risk-adjusted data are not available).

Data Element Name	Notation
Number of denominator cases for a month	n
Observed rate for a month	p_o
Expected rate for a month	
A) Risk-adjusted rate, or	p_e
B) Overall observed rate	p_e

1) Analysis is based on the score test (Agresti and Coull 1998). This test is based on the difference between the observed and the expected rates divided by the standard error of the expected rate as below.

$$Z = \frac{P_o - P_e}{\sqrt{\frac{P_e * (1 - P_e)}{n}}}$$

This value (or Z-statistic) follows a normal distribution when the sample size is not very small. Any value less than -2.576 or greater than 2.576 signals statistically significant difference between the two rates at 1% significance level.

2) The confidence interval for observed rate is obtained by expanding the above formula with respect to the expected rate (Agresti and Coull 1998; Bickel and Doksum 1977). Its upper limit (U_o) and lower limit (L_o) for a month are calculated as follows.

$$U_o = \frac{\left(p_o + \dfrac{Z^2_{1-\frac{\alpha}{2}}}{2*n}\right) + Z_{1-\frac{\alpha}{2}} * \sqrt{\dfrac{Z^2_{1-\frac{\alpha}{2}}}{4*n^2} + \dfrac{p_o*(1-p_o)}{n}}}{1 + \dfrac{Z^2_{1-\frac{\alpha}{2}}}{n}} \quad , \quad \text{where } Z_{1-\frac{\alpha}{2}} = 2.576$$

$$L_o = \frac{\left(p_o + \dfrac{Z^2_{1-\frac{\alpha}{2}}}{2*n}\right) + Z_{1-\frac{\alpha}{2}} * \sqrt{\dfrac{Z^2_{1-\frac{\alpha}{2}}}{4*n^2} + \dfrac{p_o*(1-p_o)}{n}}}{1 + \dfrac{Z^2_{1-\frac{\alpha}{2}}}{n}} \quad , \quad \text{where } Z_{1-\frac{\alpha}{2}} = 2.576$$

Statistical significance can also be determined by comparing the expected rate (p_e) with the confidence interval (L_o, U_o). If p_e is within the interval, the observed rate is not different from the expected rates, hence it is not an outlier. If p_e is outside the interval, it is an outlier.

This information is depicted on the comparison chart by converting the confidence interval around the observed rate into the expected range (or acceptance interval) around the expected rate (Holubkov et al. 1998). The upper limit (U_e) and lower limit (L_e) of the expected range is calculated as below.

$U_e = p_e + (p_o - L_o)$ [if $U_e > 1$ then $U_e = 1$]

$L_e = p_e + (p_o - U_o)$ [if $L_e < 0$ then $L_e = 0$]

The interpretation of comparison chart now involves the relative location of observed rate with respect to the expected range. If the observed rate (p_o) is within the expected range (L_e, U_e), it is not a statistical outlier (i.e., not statically significantly different) at 1% significance level. If the observed rate is outside the expected range, the observed rate is a statistical outlier.

Comparison Analysis: Ratio Measures

Three data elements are used in the comparison chart analysis for ratio measures. The expected rate is either risk-adjusted rate (if risk adjusted) or overall observed rate for the comparison group (if not risk adjusted or risk-adjusted data are not available).

Data Element Name	Notation
Number of denominator cases for a month	n
Observed rate (ratio) for a month	u_o
Expected rate (ratio) for a month	
A) Risk-adjusted rate, or	u_e
B) Overall observed rate	u_e

1) Similar to proportion measures, analysis for ratio measures is based on the score test (Joint Commission 2000). This test is based on the difference between the observed and the expected number of numerator cases divided by the standard error of the expected number of events.

$$Z = \frac{n * u_o - n * u_e}{\sqrt{n * u_e}}$$

This value (or Z-statistic) is assumed to follow a normal distribution when the sample size is not very small. Any value less than -2.576 or greater than 2.576 signals statistically significant difference between the two rates at 1% significance level.

2) The confidence interval is derived from the above test statistic (Agresti and Coull 1998; Bickel and Doksum 1977).

    The upper limit and the low limit of the confidence interval are given as follows.

$$U_o = \frac{\left(n * u_o + \frac{Z_{1-\frac{\alpha}{2}}^2}{2}\right) + \frac{Z_{1-\frac{\alpha}{2}}}{2} * \sqrt{Z_{1-\frac{\alpha}{2}}^2 + 4 * n * u_o}}{n}, \quad where\ Z_{1-\frac{\alpha}{2}} = 2.576$$

$$L_o = \frac{\left(n * u_o + \frac{Z_{1-\frac{\alpha}{2}}^2}{2}\right) + \frac{Z_{1-\frac{\alpha}{2}}}{2} * \sqrt{Z_{1-\frac{\alpha}{2}}^2 + 4 * n * u_o}}{n}, \quad where\ Z_{1-\frac{\alpha}{2}} = 2.576$$

The upper limit (U_e) and lower limit (L_e) of the expected range is calculated as below (Holubkov et al. 1998).

$$U_e = u_e + (u_o - L_o)$$

$$L_e = u_e + (u_o - U_o), \quad [\text{if } L_e < 0 \text{ then } L_e = 0]$$

Using the comparison chart, one can determine statistical significance by comparing the observed rate (u_o) with the expected range (L_e, $U_{=e}$). If the observed ratio (u_o) is within the expected range (L_e, U_e), it is not a statistical outlier at 1% significance level. If the observed ratio is outside the expected range, the observed rate is a statistical outlier.

Continuous Variable Measures

Four data elements listed below are used in the comparison chart analysis for continuous variable measures. The expected value is either risk-adjusted value (if risk adjusted) or overall mean observed value for the comparison group (if not risk adjusted or risk-adjusted data are not available).

Data Element Name	Notation
Number of cases for a month	n
Mean of observed values for a month	X_o
Standard deviation of observed values	S_o
Mean of expected values for a month	
A) Mean risk-adjusted value, or	X_e
B) Overall mean observed value	X_e

1) The statistical test is based on normal distribution. Specifically, the following formulas are used depending on the sample size.

$$Z = \frac{X_o - X_e}{S_o / \sqrt{n}}$$

(a) $n >= 25$

This value (or Z-statistic) is assumed to follow a normal distribution when the sample size is not very small. Any value less than -2.576 or greater than 2.576 signals statistically significant difference between the two rates at 1% significance level.

(b) $n < 25$

$$t = \frac{X_o - X_e}{S_o / \sqrt{n}}$$

This value (or t-statistic) is assumed to follow a t distribution. Unlike a normal distribution, the t distribution depends on the sample size. For example, if the sample size is 15, any value less than -2.977 or greater than 2.977 signals statistically significant difference between the two rates at 1% significance level.

2) Based on the test statistic, an expected range is calculated using the following formula.

Expected upper limit: $U_e = x_e + (x_o - L_o)$
Expected lower limit: $L_e = x_e + (x_o - U_o)$,

where

$$U_o = x_o + Z_{1-\frac{\alpha}{2}} * \frac{S_o}{\sqrt{n}} \text{ and } L_o = x_o - Z_{1-\frac{\alpha}{2}} * \frac{S_o}{\sqrt{n}} \text{ if } n \geq 25$$

or

$$U_o = x_o + t_{1-\frac{\alpha}{2}, n-1} * \frac{S_o}{\sqrt{n}} \text{ and } L_o = x_o - 1 - \frac{\alpha}{2}, n-1 * \frac{S_o}{\sqrt{n}} \text{ if } n < 25$$

If the observed value (x_o) is within the expected range (L_e, U_e), it is not a statistical outlier (i.e., not statically significantly different) at 1% significance level. If the observed value is outside the expected range, the observed rate is a statistical outlier (Lee and McGreevey 2004).

Source:
The content of Appendix 2 is largely based on Lee and McGreevey (2000).

References:
Agresti, A., and B. A. Coull. 1998. "Approximate Is Better than Exact for Interval Estimation of Binomial Proportions." *The American Statistician* 52 (2).

Bickel, P. J., and K. A. Doksum. 1977. *Mathematical Statistics*. San Francisco: Holden-Day, Inc.

Holubkov, R., V. L. Holt, F. A. Connell, and J. P. LoGerfo. 1998. "Analysis, Assessment, and Presentation of Risk-Adjusted Statewide Obstetrical Care Data: The StORQS II Study in Washington State." *Health Services Research* 33 (3, Pt. I).

Joint Commission on Accreditation of Healthcare Organizations. 2000. *A Guide to Performance Measurement for Hospitals.* Oakbrook Terrace, IL: Joint Commission on Accreditation of Healthcare Organizations.

Lee, K. Y., and C. McGreevey. 2000. *Mining ORYX Data 2000—A Guide for Performance Measurement Systems.* Oakbrook Terrace, IL: Joint Commission on Accreditation of Healthcare Organizations.

APPENDIX 3.
CASE STUDIES

Case 1. C-Section Rate—Proportion Measure

A healthcare organization (HCO) started to collect data for a proportion measure C-section rate on July 1, 1998. As of November 1, 1999, this organization has collected 12 months of observed C-section rates (p_o). Since this measure is risk adjusted, the organization calculated predicted rate (p_e) for individual months as below.

	7/98	8/98	9/98	10/98	11/98	12/98
n	81	75	88	89	66	67
x	13	14	18	8	9	7
p_o	0.1605	0.1867	0.2046	0.0899	0.1364	0.1045
p_e	0.1546	0.2046	0.1846	0.1046	0.1116	0.1126

	1/99	2/99	3/99	4/99	5/99	6/99
n	68	79	84	81	75	85
x	11	10	11	13	14	11
p_o	0.1618	0.1266	0.1310	0.1605	0.1867	0.1294
p_e	0.1326	0.1326	0.1426	0.1526	0.1626	0.1526

Control Chart (p-Chart)

A standard p-chart can be created for this HCO because (1) at least 12 months passed since the data collection start date, (2) more than two non-missing data points are available, and (3) the sample sizes are not small.

$$\overline{p} = \frac{13+14+18+8+9+7+11+10+11+13+14+11}{81+75+88+89+66+67+68+79+84+81+75+85} = 0.1482$$

Centerline

Control limits

(a) Upper control limit (UCL) for July 1998

$$UCL = 0.1482 + 3 * \sqrt{\frac{0.1482*(1-0.1482)}{81}} = 0.2666$$

$$LCL = 0.1482 + 3 * \sqrt{\frac{0.1482*(1-0.1482)}{81}} = 0.0298$$

(b) Lower control limit (LCL) for July 1998

$$UCL = 0.1482 + 3 * \sqrt{\frac{0.1482*(1-0.1482)}{85}} = 0.2638$$

(c) Upper control limit (UCL) for June 1999

$$LCL = 0.1482 + 3 * \sqrt{\frac{0.1482*(1-0.1482)}{85}} = 0.0326$$

(d)   Lower control limit (LCL) for June 1999
* The calculations above were done with a rounding to four decimal points for illustration. A p-chart using the above data is shown below. (Centerline is rounded to two decimal points.)

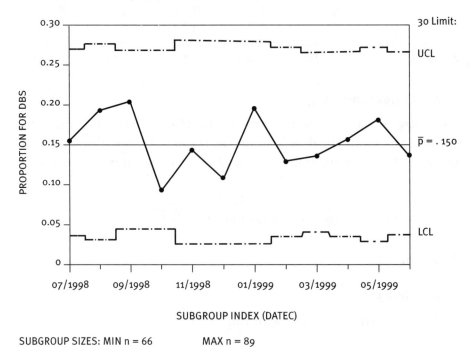

PMS ID = 1   HCO ID = 1   MEAS ID = 1

SUBGROUP SIZES: MIN n = 66   MAX n = 89

Comparison Chart

For the month of July 1998:

$$U_o = \frac{0.1605 + \frac{2.576^2}{2*81} + 2.576 * \sqrt{\frac{2.576^2}{4*81^2} + \frac{0.1605*(1-0.1605)}{81}}}{1 + \frac{2.576^2}{81}} = 0.2904$$

$$L_o = \frac{0.1605 + \frac{2.576^2}{2*81} + 2.576 * \sqrt{\frac{2.576^2}{4*81^2} + \frac{0.1605*(1-0.1605)}{81}}}{1 + \frac{2.576^2}{81}} = 0.0820$$

The expected range is:

$U_e = 0.1605 + 0.1546 - 0.0820 = 0.2331$

$L_e = 0.1605 + 0.1546 - 0.2904 = 0.0247$

Since $|Z| = 0.147 < 2.576$, the C-section rate for July 1998 is not a statistical outlier at 1% significance level. The same conclusion can be drawn about the July 1998 performance using the expected range approach because the observed rate 0.1605 is within the expected range (0.0247, 0.2331).

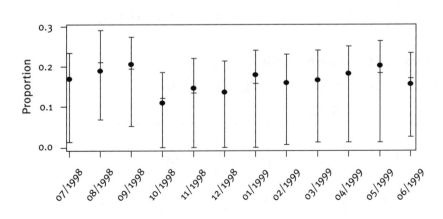

PMS ID = 1   HCO ID = 1   MEAS ID = 1

Case 2. Number of Adverse Drug Reactions per 100 Patient Days—Ratio Measure

Suppose an HCO collected data for a ratio measure number of adverse drug reactions per 100 patient days for the period from July 1, 1998, to June 30, 1999. U_o and U_e represent actual rate and comparison group rate, respectively.

	7/98	8/98	9/98	10/98	11/98	12/98
n	164	170	145	179	185	155
x	8	11	4	5	7	6
U_o	0.0488	0.0647	0.0276	0.0279	0.0378	0.0387
U_e	0.0315	0.0415	0.0415	0.0315	0.0425	0.0435

	1/99	2/99	3/99	4/99	5/99	6/99
n	165	189	175	166	156	176
x	9	4	7	5	6	9
U_o	0.0545	0.0212	0.0400	0.0301	0.0385	0.0511
U_e	0.0415	0.0315	0.0435	0.0415	0.0465	0.0485

Control Chart (u-Chart)

A standard u-chart can be created for this HCO because (1) at least 12 months passed since the data collection start date, (2) more than two non-missing data points are available, and (3) the sample sizes are not small.

Centerline

$$\bar{u} = \frac{8+4+\ldots+9}{164+189+\ldots+176} = 0.04\,(4\ ADRs\ per\ 100\ patient\ days)$$

Control limits for each month

a)   Upper control limit (UCL) for July 1998

$$UCL = 0.04 + 3*\sqrt{\frac{0.04}{164}} = 0.0869\,(8.69\ ADRs\ per\ 100\ patient\ days)$$

b)   Lower control limit (LCL) for July 1998

$$LCL = 0.04 + 3*\sqrt{\frac{0.04}{164}} = -0.0069\,(0)$$

c)   Upper control limit (UCL) for June 1999

$$UCL = 0.04 + 3*\sqrt{\frac{0.04}{176}} = 0.0852\,(8.52\ ADRs\ per\ 100\ patient\ days)$$

d)   Lower control limit (LCL) for June 1999

$$UCL = 0.04 + 3 * \sqrt{\frac{0.04}{176}} = -0.0052\ (0)$$

* Note that the lower control limit calculations for July 1998 and June 1999 resulted in negative values and were replaced by 0 because u-chart must include only nonnegative values. Below is a u-chart created using these data.

PMS ID = 1   HCO ID = 1   MEAS ID = 2

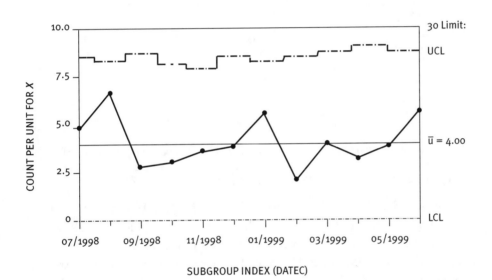

SUBGROUP INDEX (DATEC)

Comparison Analysis

For July 1998:

$$Z = \frac{164 * 0.0488 - 164 * 0.0315}{\sqrt{164 * 0.0315}} = 1.248$$

$$U_o = \frac{(164 * 0.0488 + \frac{2.576^2}{2}) + \frac{2.576}{2} * \sqrt{2.576^2 + 4 * 164 * 0.0488}}{164} = 0.1179$$

and

$$L_o = \frac{(164 * 0.0488 + \frac{2.576^2}{2}) + \frac{2.576}{2} * \sqrt{2.576^2 + 4 * 164 * 0.0488}}{164} = 0.0202$$

PMS ID = 1   HCO ID = 1   MEAS ID = 2

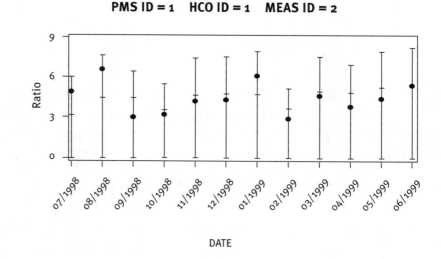

DATE

The expected range is:

U_e = 0.0488 + 0.0315 – 0.0202 = 0.0601 (6.01 ADRs per 100 patient days)

L_e =0.0488 + 0.0315 – 0.1179 = –0.0376 (0)

Since $|Z|$ = 1.248 < 2.576, the observed ratio for July 1998 is not a statistical outlier at 1% significance level. The same conclusion for July 1998 performance can be drawn using the expected range approach because the observed ratio 0.0488 (4.88 ADRs per 100 patient days) is within the expected range (0, 0.0601). The comparison chart using these data is shown below.

Case 3. CABG Length of Stay—Continuous Variable Measure

Suppose an HCO has collected data for a continuous-variable measure CABG length of stay during the 12 month period from July 1, 1998, to June 30, 1999 (see below).

	7/98	8/98	9/98	10/98	11/98	12/98
n	35	36	45	32	36	45
x_o	6.53	8.61	7.93	6.53	7.61	7.93
s_o	3.11	4.04	3.77	4.11	3.04	4.35
x_e	6.76	7.16	7.06	7.00	7.76	7.76

	1/99	2/99	3/99	4/99	5/99	6/99
n	32	36	45	32	36	45
x_o	6.53	8.61	7.93	6.53	7.61	7.93
s_o	3.11	3.04	3.71	3.11	3.04	3.57
x_e	7.16	7.96	7.56	7.46	7.76	7.76

Control Chart (X-bar and S chart)

An X-bar and S chart can be created for this HCO because (1) at least 12 months passed since the data collection start date, (2) more than two non-missing data points are available, and (3) the sample sizes are not small.

Centerline

1) X-bar chart

$$\bar{x} = \frac{35*6.53 + 36*8.61 + ... + 45*7.93}{35 + 36 + ... + 45} = 7.58$$

2) S-chart (June 1999)

$$\bar{s}_{12} = 0.9943 * \sqrt{\frac{\frac{0.9927^2}{1-0.9927^2} * \frac{3.11}{0.9927} + ... + \frac{0.9943^2}{1-0.9943^2} * \frac{3.57}{0.9943}}{\frac{0.9927^2}{1-0.9927^2} + ... + \frac{0.9943^2}{1-0.9943^2}}} = 3.53$$

* c_4 is 0.9927 for $n = 35$ and 0.9943 for $n = 45$.

Control limits

1) X-bar chart

$$LCL(\bar{x}) = 7.58 - 3 * \frac{3.53}{0.9943\sqrt{45}} = 5.99$$

$$UCL(\bar{x}) = 7.58 + 3 * \frac{3.53}{0.9943\sqrt{45}} = 9.17$$

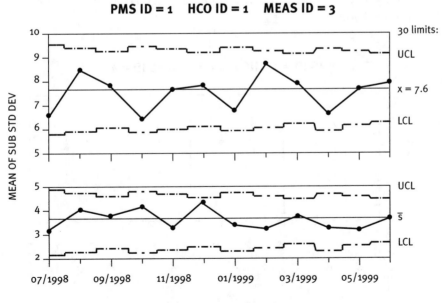

PMS ID = 1   HCO ID = 1   MEAS ID = 3

SUBGROUP INDEX (DATEC)

2) S Chart

$$UCL(\bar{s}) = 3.53 * (1 + \frac{3}{0.9943}\sqrt{1 - 0.9943^2}) = 4.67$$

$$LCL(\bar{s}) = 3.53 * (1 - \frac{3}{0.9943}\sqrt{1 - 0.9943^2})\ \ 2.39$$

Comparison Analysis

For June 1999:

$$Z = \frac{7.93 - 7.76}{3.57 / \sqrt{45}} = 0.319$$

$$U_o = 7.93 + 2.576 * \frac{3.57}{\sqrt{45}} = 9.30$$

$$L_o = 7.93 - 2.576 * \frac{3.57}{\sqrt{45}} = 6.56$$

Then, the expected range is:

$$U_e = 7.76 + 7.93 - 6.56 = 9.13$$

$$L_e = 7.76 + 7.93 - 9.30 = 6.39$$

Since $|Z| = 0.319 < 2.576$, the observed value for June 1999 is not a statistical outlier at 1% significance level. The same conclusion for June 1999 performance can be drawn using the expected range approach because the observed value 7.93 is within the expected rage (6.39, 9.13) (Lee and McGreevey 2000).

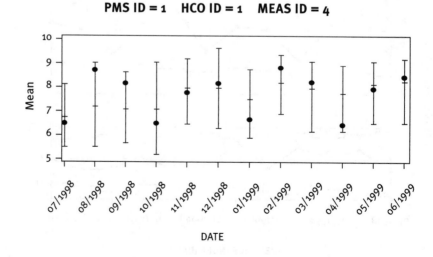

PMS ID = 1   HCO ID = 1   MEAS ID = 4

DATE

Source:

The content of Appendix 3, including all figures, is largely based on Lee and McGreevey (2000). © Joint Commission Resources: *Mining ORYX™ Data 2000: A Guide for Performance Measurement Systems.* Oakbrook Terrace, IL: Joint Commission on Accreditation of Healthcare Organizations, 2000. Reprinted with permission.

Reference:

Lee, K. Y., and C. McGreevey. 2000. *Mining ORYX Data 2000—A Guide for Performance Measurement Systems.* Oakbrook Terrace, IL: Joint Commission on Accreditation of Healthcare Organizations.

INDEX

ABOUT THE AUTHORS

About the Editors

Scott B. Ransom, D.O., FACHE, is director of the program for health-care improvement and leadership development and associate professor of obstetrics, gynecology, health management, and policy at the University of Michigan in Ann Arbor. He continues clinical practice in obstetrics and gynecology at the University of Michigan Health System and the VA Ann Arbor Healthcare System. He serves as scientific director of the Griffith Leadership Center and as research scientist at the Center for Practice Management and Outcomes Research of the VA. Dr. Ransom conducts research in areas related to improving the healthcare delivery system, leadership development, and women's health policy. He is past president of the American College of Physician Executives, the president of the Certifying Commission in Medical Management, and a member of the House of Delegates of the American Medical Association. He is a fellow in many professional organizations, including the American College of Obstetrics and Gynecology, American College of Surgeons, American College of Physician Executives, and American College of Healthcare Executives. Dr. Ransom received his master of public health degree from Harvard University in Boston; his master of business administration degree from the University of Michigan in Ann Arbor; his doctor of osteopathy degree from the University of Health Sciences in Kansas City, Missouri; and his bachelor of arts degree from Pacific Lutheran University in Tacoma, Washington. He is also a graduate of United States Marine Corps Officer Candidate School in Quantico, Virginia.

Maulik S. Joshi, Dr.P.H., is president and chief executive officer of the Delmarva Foundation. A not-for-profit national quality improvement organization of 250 employees, Delmarva's mission is to improve health in the communities that it serves in more than 15 states. Delmarva provides an essential link between government agencies, healthcare providers, and consumers to ensure the highest quality care. Prior to his work at Delmarva,

Dr. Joshi was vice president at the Institute for Healthcare Improvement in Boston, cofounder and executive vice president of DoctorQuality, senior director of quality at the University of Pennsylvania Health System in Philadelphia, and executive vice president of The HMO Group. He received his doctor of public health degree and master of health services administration degree from the University of Michigan in Ann Arbor and his bachelor of science degree in mathematics from Lafayette College in Easton, Pennsylvania. Dr. Joshi was selected by the American Society for Quality as one of the "21 Voices for Quality for the 21st Century" by the *Philadelphia Business Journal*, as one of the "40 Under 40 Outstanding Leaders" for contribution to the Philadelphia community, and as one of the "Up and Comers" by *Modern Healthcare*/Witt Kieffer. Dr. Joshi is adjunct faculty at the Harvard School of Public Health's Department of Health Policy and Management and is on the board of the Quality Health Foundation.

David B. Nash, M.D., is the Dr. Raymond C. and Doris N. Grandon Professor and chair of the department of health policy at Jefferson Medical College of Thomas Jefferson University in Philadelphia, Pennsylvania. Dr. Nash, a board-certified internist, founded the original Office of Health Policy in 1990. From 1996 to 2003, he served as the first associate dean for health policy at Jefferson Medical College. In 2004, he was named codirector of the masters program in public health at Jefferson. He has published more than 60 articles in major journals and in a dozen edited books, including *A Systems Approach to Disease Management* and *Connecting with the New Healthcare Consumer*. Named by *Modern Healthcare* as one of the top 100 most powerful persons in healthcare in , his national activities include an appointment to the Joint Commission on Accreditation of Healthcare Organizations Advisory Committee on Performance Measurement and to the Foundation for Accountability board and membership on the board of directors of the Disease Management Association of America-three key national groups focusing on quality measurement and improvement. Dr. Nash received his bachelor of arts degree in economics (graduating Phi Beta Kappa) from Vassar College in Poughkeepsie, New York; his doctor of medicine degree from the University of Rochester School of Medicine and Dentistry in Rochester, New York; and his master of business administration degree in health administration (graduating with honors) from the Wharton School at the University of Pennsylvania in Philadelphia. While at Penn, he was a Robert Wood Johnson Foundation clinical scholar and medical director of a nine physician faculty group practice in general internal medicine.

About the Contributors

A. Al-Assaf, M.D., CQA, is Presbyterian Health Foundation Presidential Professor and professor and director of the master of public health degree and certificate programs in the Department of Health Administration and Policy of the College of Public Health at the University of Oklahoma Health Sciences Center in Oklahoma City.

David J. Ballard, M.D., Ph.D., is senior vice president and chief quality officer of Baylor Health Care System (BHCS) and executive director and BHCS Endowed Chair at the Institute for Health Care Research and Improvement in Dallas, Texas.

Donald Berwick, M.D., is chief executive officer of the Institute for Healthcare Improvement and adjunct professor of health management and policy at Harvard University in Boston.

Troyen A. Brennan, M.D., J.D., is professor of law and public health in the Department of Health Policy and Management at the Harvard School of Public Health in Boston; professor of medicine at the Harvard Medical School; and president and chief executive officer of Brigham and Women's Physician Organization in Boston.

John Bulger, D.O., is director of inpatient medical services in the Department of General Internal Medicine at Geisinger Health System in Danville, Pennsylvania.

John J. Byrnes, M.D., is senior vice president for system quality at Spectrum Health in Grand Rapids, Michigan.

Francois de Brantes is program leader of healthcare initiatives for eHealth Initiative at General Electric Corporation in Fairfield, Connecticut.

Susan Edgman-Levitan, PA, is executive director of the John D. Stoeckle Center for Primary Care Innovation at Massachusetts General Hospital in Boston and a fellow of the Institute for Healthcare Improvement in Boston.

Adam Evans, M.D., is with the Department of Health Policy at Jefferson Medical College in Philadelphia, Pennsylvania.

Frances A. Griffin, RRT, is director of patient safety at the Institute for Healthcare Improvement in Boston.

Linds S. Hanold is director of the Department of Performance Measurement and Health Informatics at the Joint Commission on Accreditation of Healthcare Organizations in Oakbrook Terrace, Illinois.

Robert Hanscom, J.D., is director of loss prevention and patient safety at the Risk Management Foundation in Cambridge, Massachusetts.

Carol Haraden, Ph.D., is vice president of the Institute for Healthcare Improvement in Boston.

Robert S. Hopkins III, Ph.D., is director of strategic development for the Institute for Health Care Research and Improvement at the Baylor Health Care System in Dallas, Texas.

Michael L. Jones is with the Medical College of Wisconsin in Milwaukee.

Narendra Kini, M.D., is senior vice president and chief medical officer of Trinity Health System in Novi, Michigan.

Richard G. Koss is director of the Department of Health Policy Research at the Joint Commission on Accreditation of Healthcare Organizations in Oakbrook Terrace, Illlinois.

Kwan Y. Lee, Ph.D., is former project director of biostatistics and data analysis at the Joint Commission on Accreditation of Healthcare Organizations in Oakbrook Terrace, Illinois.

Robert C. Lloyd, Ph.D., is director of performance at the Institute for Healthcare Improvement in Boston.

Jerod M. Loeb, Ph.D., is executive vice president for research at the Joint Commission on Accreditation of Healthcare Organizations in Oakbrook Terrace, Illinois.

John L. McCarthy is president of the Risk Management Foundation in Cambridge, Massachusetts.

David Nicewander is with the Institute for Health Care Research and Improvement at Baylor Health Care System in Dallas, Texas.

L. Gregory Pawlson, M.D., is executive vice president of the National Committee for Quality Assurance in Washington, DC.

Michael D. Pugh is principal at Pugh Ettinger McCarthy Associates, LLC, in Pueblo, Colorado; faculty for the Institute for Healthcare Improvement in Boston; and adjunct faculty of the health administration program at the University of Colorado in Denver.

Ann Louise Puopolo, R.N., is with the Department of Medicine at Brigham and Women's Hospital in Boston.

Elizabeth R. Ransom, M.D., is vice chair of the board of governors of Henry Ford Medical Group in Detroit, Michigan, and residency director of the Department of Otolaryngology, Head and Neck Surgery at Henry Ford Health System in Detroit.

James L. Reinertsen, M.D., is senior fellow at the Institute for Healthcare Improvement in Boston and president of the Reinertsen Group in Alta, Wyoming.

Luke Sato, M.D., is chief medical officer at the Risk Management Foundation in Cambridge, Massachusetts.

Paul Schyve, M.D., is senior vice president of the Joint Commission on Accreditation of Healthcare Organizations in Oakbrook Terrace, Illinois.

Mike Stoecklein is senior operations consultant at Catholic Health Initiatives.

Richard E. Ward, M.D., is chief executive officer at Reward Health Sciences Inc. in Windsor, Ontario, and chief medical informatics officer at Anceta, LLC.

Valerie Weber, M.D., is director of the Department of General Internal Medicine at Geisinger Health System in Danville, Pennsylvania.

Leon Wyszewianski, Ph.D., is associate professor of the Department of Health Management and Policy in the School of Public Health at the University of Michigan in Ann Arbor.